Download Your Included Ebook Today!

Your print purchase of *Virtual Simulation in Nursing Education* **includes an ebook download** to the device of your choice—increasing accessibility, portability, and searchability!

Download your ebook today at:
http://spubonline.com/virtualsim
and enter the access code below:

17VPEKBA3

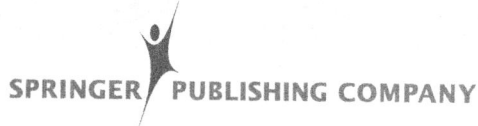

springerpub.com

Randy M. Gordon, DNP, FNP-BC, is an assistant professor in the MSN family nurse practitioner (FNP) specialty track at Chamberlain University in the College of Nursing. He brings more than 20 years of experience in clinical nursing and academia to the position. Dr. Gordon holds BSN and MS degrees from the University of South Florida and a DNP degree from the University of South Alabama. His clinical career includes work in emergency departments as an RN and in family practice and dermatology as an FNP. Dr. Gordon continues his clinical practice as an advocate and regular FNP volunteer for the Remote Area Medical organization, a nonprofit, airborne medical relief corps that provides free healthcare, dental care, and eye care, as well as technical and educational assistance, to people in remote areas of the United States and around the world.

Dr. Gordon began his academic career as a clinical preceptor for the University of South Florida and Lake Erie College of Osteopathic Medicine, Erie, Pennsylvania. Prior to joining Chamberlain, Dr. Gordon was a graduate faculty instructor in the Community and Mental Health department at the University of South Alabama College of Nursing and adjunct faculty/clinical instructor for the FNP program at Walden University. He has served as manuscript reviewer for the *JDNA Journal of the Dermatology Nurses' Association* for over 10 years. Dr. Gordon has authored articles in *Clinical Simulation in Nursing, Seminars in Oncology Nursing, Advances in Skin & Wound Care, The Nurse Practitioner,* and *Advance for Nurse Practitioners.* He has professionally reviewed and written numerous chapters in textbooks, including *The Complete Guide to Geriatric Rehabilitation* (3rd ed.), *The NP Guide: Essential Knowledge for Nurse Practitioner Practice* (2nd ed.), *Synergy for Clinical Excellence: The AACN Synergy Model for Patient Care* (2nd ed.), *Primary Care: A Collaborative Practice* (5th ed.), and *Clinical Guidelines in Primary Care* (2nd ed.) on clinical topics such as skin disorders, skin cancer, and skin cancer screening, as well as virtual simulation and debriefing. The impetus for this text, *Virtual Simulation in Nursing Education,* stemmed from several years of working to integrate innovative technology with the FNP curriculum. He was nominated for the Novice Faculty Excellence in Clinical Teaching Award 2015–2016 offered by the AACN and is a recipient of the Chamberlain College Faculty Honoree: Discovery Award (2015), which honors faculty who regularly engage in discovery and share that knowledge with others. In 2016, Dr. Gordon received the Ron Taylor Award from the DeVry Education Group for exemplary performance that truly exceeds performance expectations, going above and beyond normal job function.

Dee McGonigle, PhD, RN, CNE, FAAN, ANEF, directs the Virtual Learning Environments (VLE) and is a professor in the graduate program at Chamberlain University in the College of Nursing. She brings more than 40 years of experience in nursing and nursing informatics to this position. She co-founded the *Online Journal of Nursing Informatics* (OJNI), a professional, scholarly, peer-reviewed journal in 1996, for which she was the Editor in Chief for 17 years, through 2013. OJNI is currently published by the Healthcare Information and Management Systems Society (HIMSS). In 2014, Dr. McGonigle was the first one honored as a Platinum Award recipient from the *Online Journal of Nursing Informatics.* This text, *Virtual Simulation in Nursing Education,* is her fourth co-authored textbook. The nursing informatics text, *Nursing Informatics and the Foundation of Knowledge* took second place as AJN's 2014 Information Technology/Social Media Book of the Year in its third edition. The fourth edition was released in 2018. *The Informatics for Health Professionals* text was published in 2016. The text written for nurse educators to help them assimilate technology to enhance teaching and learning, *Integrating Technology into Nursing Education: Tools for the Knowledge Era,* was AJN's 2010 first place Technology Book of the Year.

Her continuous and enduring impact on nursing informatics and nursing education has been recognized; she is a Fellow in the American Academy of Nursing and a Fellow in the NLN Academy of Nursing Education. She was president of the Division of Learning and Performance Environments (DLPE) for the Association for Educational Communications and Technology (AECT). Currently, she is a member of the Serious Gaming & Virtual Environments Special Interest Group for the Society for Simulation in Healthcare and a member of International Nursing Association for Clinical Simulation and Learning (INACSL). As a member of the Nursing Informatics Research Team (NIRT), she led the development of an online self-assessment tool for level 3 and level 4 nursing informatics competencies, NICA L3/L4, which was cited in the American Nursing Informatics Association's (2014) *Nursing Informatics Today* and the American Nurses Association's (2015) *Nursing Informatics: Scope and Standards of Practice.* Dr. McGonigle was a research team member for the development of the online self-assessment tool, TIGER-based Assessment of Nursing Informatics Competencies (TANIC), for basic level 1 and level 2 nursing informatics competencies based on the Technology Informatics Guiding Education Reform (TIGER) initiatives. This team's current research proposal will compare nursing informatics students' perceived informatics competencies in a virtual world practicum (VWP) and a real-world practicum (RWP).

Virtual Simulation in Nursing Education

Randy M. Gordon, DNP, FNP-BC
Dee McGonigle, PhD, RN, CNE, FAAN, ANEF

Editors

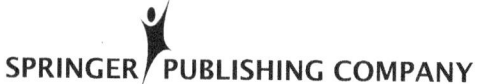

Copyright © 2018 Springer Publishing Company, LLC

All rights reserved.

No part of this publication may be reproduced, stored in a retrieval system, or transmitted in any form or by any means, electronic, mechanical, photocopying, recording, or otherwise, without the prior permission of Springer Publishing Company, LLC, or authorization through payment of the appropriate fees to the Copyright Clearance Center, Inc., 222 Rosewood Drive, Danvers, MA 01923, 978-750-8400, fax 978-646-8600, info@copyright.com or on the Web at www.copyright.com.

Springer Publishing Company, LLC
11 West 42nd Street
New York, NY 10036
www.springerpub.com

Acquisitions Editor: Joseph Morita
Associate Managing Editor: Kris Parrish
Compositor: Exeter Premedia Services Private Ltd.

ISBN: 978-0-8261-6963-1
ebook ISBN: 978-0-8261-6964-8

Instructor's Manual: 978-0-8261-3853-8
Instructor's PowerPoints: 978-0-8261-3847-7

Instructor's Materials: Qualified instructors may request supplements by emailing textbook@springerpub.com

18 19 20 21 22 / 5 4 3 2 1

The author and the publisher of this Work have made every effort to use sources believed to be reliable to provide information that is accurate and compatible with the standards generally accepted at the time of publication. Because medical science is continually advancing, our knowledge base continues to expand. Therefore, as new information becomes available, changes in procedures become necessary. We recommend that the reader always consult current research and specific institutional policies before performing any clinical procedure. The author and publisher shall not be liable for any special, consequential, or exemplary damages resulting, in whole or in part, from the readers' use of, or reliance on, the information contained in this book. The publisher has no responsibility for the persistence or accuracy of URLs for external or third-party Internet websites referred to in this publication and does not guarantee that any content on such websites is, or will remain, accurate or appropriate.

Library of Congress Cataloging-in-Publication Data

Names: Gordon, Randy M., editor. | McGonigle, Dee, editor.
Title: Virtual simulation in nursing education / Randy M. Gordon, Dee
   McGonigle, editors.
Description: New York, NY: Springer Publishing Company, LLC, [2018] |
   Includes bibliographical references and index.
Identifiers: LCCN 2017058487 | ISBN 9780826169631 | ISBN 9780826169648 (ebook)
   | ISBN 9780826138538 (instructors manual) | ISBN 9780826138477
   (instructors PowerPoints)
Subjects: | MESH: Education, Nursing—methods | Simulation Training—methods
Classification: LCC RT55 | NLM WY 18 | DDC 610.73076—dc23
LC record available at https://lccn.loc.gov/2017058487

> Contact us to receive discount rates on bulk purchases.
> We can also customize our books to meet your needs.
> For more information please contact: sales@springerpub.com

Printed in the United States of America.

CONTENTS

Contributors   vii
Preface   ix
Acknowledgments   xi
Authors' Note   xiii

SECTION I: THE EVOLVING VIRTUAL LEARNING LANDSCAPE

1. Assessing the Virtual Learning Landscape   3
   Dee McGonigle

2. Faculty Administrators Students Technology Strategic Integration Model©   25
   Randy M. Gordon

3. Application of the Faculty Administrators Students Technology Strategic Integration Model© as the Basis for Integrating Virtual Educational Technologies   31
   Randy M. Gordon

4. Technology's Impact on Society and Culture   43
   Michael H. Reitzel

SECTION II: FACULTY PERSPECTIVE—PEDAGOGICAL APPLICATIONS AND SPECIFIC INTEGRATION STRATEGIES

5. Opportunities and Advantages With Virtual Technology Integration   59
   Megan Keiser and Carman Turkelson

6. Challenges and Disadvantages With Virtual Technology Integration   71
   Rebecca A. Burhenne, Kristin A. Kerling, and Randy M. Gordon

7. Faculty Role in Integrating Virtual Simulations   87
   Dee McGonigle, Randy M. Gordon, and Diana Meeks

8. Preparing the Instructional Environment   97
   Julie McAfooes

9. Nexus of Game Development: Curricular Integration and Faculty Development   113
   Eric B. Bauman, Penny Ralston-Berg, and Gregory E. Gilbert

10. Design and Creation of Virtual Gaming Simulations in Nursing Education   127
    Jennifer L. Lapum, Margaret Anne Verkuyl, Michelle Hughes, Oona St-Amant, Daria Romaniuk, Lorraine Betts, and Paula Mastrilli

11. Virtual Gaming in Nursing Education   143
    Natália Del Angelo Aredes, Suzanne Hetzel Campbell, and Luciana Mara Monti Fonseca

12. **Nursing Student Simulation Scenarios Within a Virtual Learning Environment**   159
    Pamela L. Grant

13. **Enhancing the Rigor of Virtual Simulation**   175
    Simon JR Cooper and Fiona Bogossian

SECTION III: STUDENT PERSPECTIVE—WORKING WITH STUDENTS TO IMPLEMENT VIRTUAL LEARNING STRATEGIES: MAXIMIZE LEARNING AND SUPPORT TRANSITION TO PRACTICE

14. **A Student's Journey Encountering a Virtual Learning Environment: A Pathway From Novice to Expert**   195
    Karen West

15. **Mentor Role in Virtual Simulation–Mediated Learning**   211
    Rebecca J. Sisk

16. **Creating Interprofessional Simulation Scenarios in Virtual Learning Environments**   223
    Ellen Jakovich

17. **Advancing Nursing Informatics Knowledge and Skills Using a Virtual Learning Environment**   233
    Carolyn Sipes

SECTION IV: ADMINISTRATIVE PERSPECTIVE—NAVIGATING THE CHASM WHEN A PROFOUND DIFFERENCE EXISTS AMONG STAKEHOLDERS, VIEWPOINTS, AND FEELINGS REGARDING VIRTUAL SIMULATION

18. **Administrative Perspective**   247
    Suzanne Hetzel Campbell

19. **Administrator Role**   261
    Dee McGonigle and Randy M. Gordon

Epilogue: Faculty Administrators Students Technology Strategic Integration Model©: Analysis, Synthesis, and Application   269
Appendix A: Simulation Integration Strategies   273
Appendix B: Proposal Strategies   275
Abbreviations   281
Glossary   283
Index   297

CONTRIBUTORS

Natália Del Angelo Aredes, PhD, RN, Adjunct Professor, University of São Paulo, Brazil

Eric B. Bauman, PhD, FSSH, RN, Innovation Senior Leadership Team, Adtalem Global Education; Managing Member, Clinical Playground LLC, Madison, Wisconsin

Lorraine Betts, RN, MN, CHSE, Nursing Professor, George Brown College, Toronto, Ontario, Canada

Fiona Bogossian, PhD, MPH, RN, RM, DipAppSci(NEd), BAppSci (with distinction), FACM, Professor, University of Queensland, St Lucia, Queensland, Australia

Rebecca A. Burhenne, DNP, RN, Assistant Dean of Faculty, Chamberlain University, Downers Grove, Illinois

Suzanne Hetzel Campbell, PhD, RN, IBCLC, IBCLC Director, Associate Professor, University of British Columbia School of Nursing, Vancouver, British Columbia, Canada

Simon JR Cooper, PhD, MEd, RN, BA (Hons), FHEA, Professor, Federation University, Melbourne, Victoria, Australia

Luciana Mara Monti Fonseca, PhD, RN, Professora da EERP/USP, University of São Paolo, Brazil

Gregory E. Gilbert, EdD, MSPH, PStat®, Adjunct Assistant Professor, Ross University School of Medicine, Roseau, Commonwealth of Dominica, West Indies

Randy M. Gordon, DNP, FNP-BC, Assistant Professor, Chamberlain University in the College of Nursing, Downers Grove, Illinois

Pamela L. Grant, EdD, MSN, RN, Adjunct Faculty, Chamberlain University, St. Louis, Missouri

Michelle Hughes, MEd, BScN, RN, Professor, Centennial College, Toronto, Ontario, Canada

Ellen Jakovich, MSF, MAFM, CPA, Professor, Keller Graduate School of Management, DeVry University, Arlington, Virginia

Megan Keiser, DNP, RN, CNRN, SCRN, ACNS-BC, NP-C, Director of Undergraduate Nursing Affairs, Assistant Professor, University of Michigan–Flint, Michigan

Kristin A. Kerling, DNP, RN, Assistant Dean of Faculty, Chamberlain University, Downers Grove, Illinois

Jennifer L. Lapum, PhD, MN, BScN, RN, Associate Professor, Daphne Cockwell School of Nursing, Ryerson University, Toronto, Ontario, Canada

Paula Mastrilli, PhD, MScN, RN, Sally Horsfall-Eaton School of Nursing, George Brown College, Toronto, Ontario, Canada

Julie McAfooes, MS, RN-BC, CNE, ANEF, FAAN, Web Development Manager, Chamberlain College of Nursing, Downers Grove, Illinois

Dee McGonigle, PhD, RN, CNE, FAAN, ANEF, Director of Virtual Learning Environments, Chamberlain University College of Nursing, Dillon, South Carolina

Diana Meeks, PhD, RN, MSN, CS, FNP, CNE, NE-BC, Professor, Chamberlain University College of Nursing, Marietta, Georgia

Penny Ralston-Berg, MS, Senior Research Instructional Designer, Penn State, World Campus, University Park, Pennsylvania

Michael H. Reitzel, PhD, JD, Professor, DeVry University, Austin, Texas

Daria Romaniuk, PhD, RN, Associate Professor, Daphne Cockwell School of Nursing, Ryerson University, Toronto, Ontario, Canada

Carolyn Sipes, PhD, CNS, APN, PMP, RN-BC, Associate Professor, MSN Specialty Track, Chamberlain College, College of Nursing, Conifer, Colorado

Rebecca J. Sisk, PhD, RN, CNE, Professor, Chamberlain University, Downers Grove, Illinois

Oona St-Amant, PhD, RN, Acting Assistant Professor, Ryerson University, Toronto, Ontario, Canada

Carman Turkelson, DNP, RN, CCRN, CHSE, Assistant Professor, Associate Director of Nursing Simulation Lab, School of Nursing at the University of Michigan–Flint, Flint, Michigan

Margaret Anne Verkuyl, MN, NP-PHC, Professor, Nursing, Centennial College, Toronto, Ontario, Canada

Karen West, MSN, RN, Support Specialist for White Mouse Productions, Working with Chamberlain College of Nursing, Downers Grove, Illinois

PREFACE

The integration of technology with nursing curricula is a dynamic and increasingly necessary step in the evolution of nursing education. Numerous disciplines, including physics, medicine, psychology, public health, business, and emergency medical services (EMS), use virtual environments in academic settings. Schools of medicine have been using some form of virtual patient for over 40 years. Nursing institutions are following in a similar direction. For more than a decade, the National League for Nursing has endorsed simulation as a teaching methodology to prepare nurses for practice across the healthcare continuum. Administrators and faculty are encouraged to explore engaging learning experiences that leverage technology to reduce instructional costs, the cost of tuition, and student fees. Numerous textbooks promote the inclusion of simulation as a fundamental educational tool, but few books offer practical integration strategies or provide instances of how integration may occur. The impetus for this textbook and the overarching goals were to offer nursing educators and administrators thoughtful and well-planned simulation integration strategies, as well as to illustrate how students may use technologies to maximize learning and support practice. The editors of this textbook present, explore, reflect, and expand on a new model for technology integration with nursing curricula. The **Faculty Administrators Students Technology Simulation Integration Model**© (FAST SIM) provides a framework for guiding and evaluating the technology integration process and is the model that frames and underpins the content of this text. Throughout this textbook, faculty, researchers, and administrators from academic institutions around the world share expertise and exemplars of innovative virtual simulation integration with undergraduate and graduate curricula to showcase and inspire you on how to leverage resources and reform nursing education. This book is dedicated to students, teachers, and administrators who are pioneers and willing to blaze the trail. The goals of this text are to help the reader:

1. Appreciate the evolution of instructional technology tools.
2. Make sense of the various terms being used in relation to virtual reality, virtual simulation, and virtual learning environments.
3. Determine trends and issues with technology integration.
4. Explore a variety of expert's insights and applications related to technology integration from the perspectives of faculty, administrators, and/or students.
5. Implement technology tools prescriptively and purposefully by providing the FAST SIM© conceptual framework and numerous ideas and exemplars.

The definition of *technology* varies with the context in which it is used. Educational technology resources include, but are not limited to, computers and specialized software, network-based communication systems, electronic products, software, and devices, as well as infrastructure. *Integration* refers to combining or incorporating into one. The editors of this textbook broadly define *technology integration* as the use of technology to enhance and support the educational environment. Discordant definitions of *virtual reality*, *virtual simulation*, and *virtual learning environments* in higher education illuminate the fact that a shared understanding has not been developed of what constitutes these terms. To foster a mutual understanding, the following definitions serve to establish the context from which this text is written. A **virtual learning environment** is the integration of computer and Internet technologies into teaching and learning to improve learning. **Virtual reality** is the use of computerized applications to create interactive and immersive three-dimensional environments in which the user is given the impression of being physically present. **Virtual simulation** is a simulation that can occur in a virtual learning or virtual reality environment that replicates real-life situations. The user plays a central role by participating and interacting in the virtual environment by exercising motor-control, communication, and decision-making skills. A **virtual world** is a digital or computer-based online world or environment designed for interaction in which customized simulations can be developed. Users can interact with one another as avatars, as well as with objects in the environment based on the customized programming. *Virtual world* also refers to the use of a virtual learning environment such as Second Life® so that learners can enact their learning activities or real-life experiences in a virtual setting. Virtual simulation–mediated learning is active learning that is facilitated by a human mentor who helps engage the learner in the simulation to gain insights, reflect on the intent of the learning, and connect the dots to translate the learning to their practice. Throughout the book, the terms *faculty*, *teacher*, and *educator*, and *students* and *learners*, as well as *pilot test* and *trial* are used interchangeably by the authors.

Academic institutions of nursing are increasingly challenged to provide high-quality clinical experiences for students. Educators are turning toward simulation as a way to provide rich learning experiences that can replicate actual clinical experiences. Virtual simulation can standardize clinical experiences in this time of unpredictable and often unequal clinical learning opportunities. Furthermore, virtual simulation focused on interprofessional learning objectives provides the opportunity for nursing students to learn with, from, and about their peers in other healthcare disciplines. Regardless of the simulation modality, simulation helps learners in bridging the gap between knowledge and practice through deliberate application of skills and reflective debriefing. As the use of simulation in nursing education increases, more regulations, guidelines, and standards are being developed to assist nursing programs to obtain the best outcomes. The editors and authors of this textbook invite you to explore and apply this critically important and useful content. This book offers technology-enhanced simulation solutions from the perspectives of international authors and provides readers with ideas to integrate virtual simulation into existing curricula while exploring ways to develop and/or enhance current teaching strategies.

Randy M. Gordon
Dee McGonigle

ACKNOWLEDGMENTS

We are intensely appreciative of the contributors who provided this virtual simulation text with a wealth, range, and diversity of substantive information. Their contributions have added expertise and authentic practice exemplars to the text.

Randy wishes to acknowledge JC for his support, expressing his deepest gratitude, especially for the continued encouragement when times got rough. Randy also wishes to thank Dee for her unwavering inspiration and collaboration for which he is truly grateful. He would also like to express his gratitude to his friends and family who offered unending support and motivation.

Dee acknowledges the undying love, support, patience, and continued encouragement of her best friend and husband, Craig, and her son, Craig, who has made her so very proud. She sincerely thanks her dear friends for their support and encouragement, especially Renee, Rose, Kate, Kathy, and Deb.

SPECIAL ACKNOWLEDGMENTS

We want to express our sincere appreciation to the staff at Springer Publishing, especially Joe Morita, Rachel Landes, Ryan Famanila, and Jill Ferguson, for their assistance and support during the writing process and publication of our book.

AUTHORS' NOTE

This text provides an introduction, exploration, and validation of virtual simulation. The reader should focus on the relationship of virtual simulation to nursing education. Explore how learning outcomes are met through innovative virtual simulation strategies and reflect on ways that virtual simulation can be implemented within a learning episode, course, and/or curriculum. We want you to not only enjoy the text, but also be able to apply virtual simulation strategies and validate innovative educational practices!

THE EVOLVING VIRTUAL LEARNING LANDSCAPE

To integrate technologies into the educational arena, one must change his or her perceptual lens from focusing on what has been done to expand to what can be accomplished in an innovative and transforming learning landscape. It is imperative that we foresee and generate technology integration that will impact not only our facilities, teaching, learning, and nursing education, but also the nursing profession; it will ultimately improve patient outcomes. Administrators and teachers must discover opportunities to design educational solutions that are learner centered and authentic. This text was written to provide the reader with the information and knowledge needed to transform the practice of education.

Section I presents the evolving learning landscape, the Faculty Administrators Students Technology Strategic Integration Model© (FAST SIM; Figure I.1), and the ethical, cultural, and societal implications of technology. The four chapters in this section set the stage for the remainder of the text.

In Chapter 1, the reader will be introduced to the current trends and issues in technology integration, nursing and ethics, credentials and badging, and technological pedagogical content knowledge. The trends in technology integration, massive open online courses (MOOCs), serious games, augmented reality, terminology, and learning impact associated with virtual simulation is reviewed. Learner-centered events are underpinned with a constructivist approach that reflects on the data, information, knowledge, wisdom (DIKW) pathway. The ETHICAL Model for ethical decision making is reviewed and applied in relation to virtual simulation.

Chapters 2 and 3, as the basis for integrating virtual educational technologies, introduce, describe, and apply the FAST SIM©. Technology is a fundamental tool that can be used to transform nursing education. The FAST SIM© discusses how to integrate technology into the nursing curriculum because it is not intuitive. The FAST SIM© is a conceptual model intended to impart a richer understanding of the relationships between integration influences when contending with the process of developing thoughtful and well-planned educational strategies. The purpose of this model is to provide a framework to guide the process of integrating technology into the nursing curriculum because the literature lacks systematic strategies. Each administrative, faculty, and student influence drives virtual simulation development and must be considered equally when evaluating the success or failure of the simulation integration.

The FAST SIM© can be used to bridge pedagogical approaches to curriculum design and development with the tools educators have at their disposal. The model helps teachers articulate and organize concepts while providing a basis for further development of knowledge and educational episodes.

All three components, contributors, or influencers—teacher, administrator, and student—are discussed in relation to the importance of respecting and appreciating each of these influences and the way that it impacts the success of the technology integration. It is important to seamlessly integrate technology that effectively supports the learning outcomes dictated by the curriculum. However, it is important to consider that a goal of flawless integration is complicated by the dynamic synergies of the curriculum and technology because both are continually being redefined and evolving. The FAST SIM© is more than the sum of its parts because the components truly complement one another. Successful integration requires a coordinated and cooperative environment in which faculty, administrators, and students can interact in positive ways to enrich the technologically enhanced learning landscape.

Chapter 4, describes how a class on technology, culture, and society could be augmented by integrating the technology of a virtual world. This chapter illustrates how the virtual world of Second Life® could provide a rich learning experience for teamed students. The students are able to reflect on and apply their understanding of the impact of technology on culture and society in the concept of a capstone course with standard deliverables. It is interesting if the students are able to see that real-life concerns are mirrored in the virtual world. As technology is constructed by us, our technology constructs us and our lives.

The FAST SIM© captures the complex influences surrounding virtual simulation integration. Throughout the chapters in this section, *The Evolving Virtual Learning Landscape*, the readers should reflect on how the model can be applied to the integration of technology in their specific teaching and learning contexts.

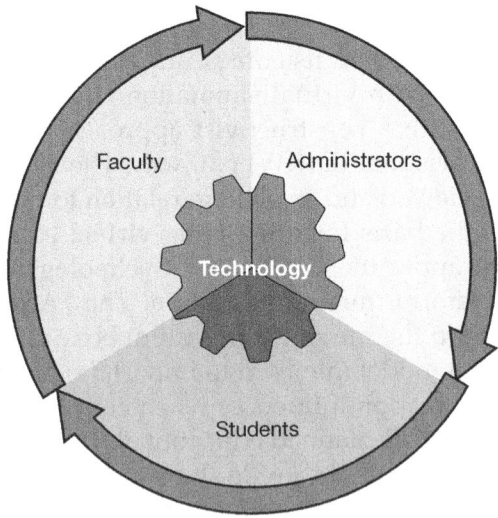

FIGURE I.1 Components of FAST SIM© (Faculty Administrators Students Technology Strategic Integration Model).

CHAPTER 1

Assessing the Virtual Learning Landscape

DEE McGONIGLE

LEARNING OBJECTIVES

Upon completion of this chapter, the reader will be able to:

- Appreciate the evolution of technological tools.
- Assess virtual simulation in nursing education.
- Determine trends and issues with technology integration.
- Describe nursing informatics (NI) and the data, information, knowledge, wisdom (DIKW) pathway in relation to nursing practice and virtual simulation in nursing education.
- Explore constructivism.
- Implement the ETHICAL Model in ethical decision making.

KEY TERMS

Asynchronous
Augmented reality (AR)
Badges
Constructivism
Credentials
Data
Data, information, knowledge, wisdom (DIKW) pathway
Edutainment
E-learning
Engage
Ethical
Gameplay
Game mechanics
Immersion
Information
Knowledge
Latex-based simulation
Learner centered
Micro-credentials
Nursing informatics (NI)
Serious game
Simulation
Simulation scenario
Synchronous
Technology integration
Virtual patient
Virtual reality (VR)
Virtual simulation
Virtual world
Wisdom

In the past decade, new technologies have changed our world in ways that we have yet to fully comprehend. The evolution of social media, communication tools, and virtual spaces, have impacted the way that we interact with one another in our personal lives and are reflected in new ethical challenges and transformed social behaviors. Even our patients are using apps and entering virtual worlds to improve their health and to connect to others with similar concerns or illnesses.

The social characteristics of teaching and learning are changing; innovative teachers and administrators have recognized the learning potential of the technological tools available and harnessed them to enhance learning. This is creating a paradigm shift, and many teachers and administrators are trying to make sense of this new learning landscape that is not tied to brick-and-mortar physical spaces or set times. The online practices of the past are being transformed into high-quality, immersive, and engaging virtual learning environments that foster interaction: teacher/student, student/student, teacher/mentor, and mentor/student. Teachers, administrators, and students need help in understanding the technological tools and their educational capabilities. We are still grappling with the ways in which the roles of teacher and student continue to change. We must prepare teachers to assume their new role and embrace this changing learning landscape. We do not want a lack of understanding or poor educational skills to limit the impact of virtual learning.

Administrators must grasp the potential of this new mode of delivery in securing funding, dealing with accreditation and other issues, and transforming their institution to support this new educational environment. Teachers must be willing to accept new roles as they explore and implement these instructional technologies. Students must be prepared for the educational impact of these new technologies. Even if they use them personally, they must now understandwhat the educational intent is and what is expected of them during each learning episode. The framework for this text is our Faculty Administrators Students Technology Strategic Integration Model© (FAST SIM). Refer to Chapter 2 for more details on this model.

The learning landscape continues to evolve as new technological tools enable teachers to deliver robust learning experiences. It is important to help teachers, administrators, and students know where to begin so that the transition to virtual learning is smooth, without educational loss. This chapter consists of two sections: (a) current trends and issues in **technology integration** and (b) technological pedagogical content knowledge. The first section briefly reviews the trends in instructional or educational technologies that are causing administrators, teachers, and students to reflect on and modify their thinking about learning and educational content delivery. As we know, issues arise with change because the new ideas, knowledge, and skills must be analyzed and synthesized into our own knowledge base. The second section explores constructivism, the scientific underpinnings of **nursing informatics (NI)**, and ethics. Nurse educators must also address the ethical challenges brought about by this evolving learning landscape. The ETHICAL Model for Ethical Decision Making addresses ethical challenges; it is reviewed and applied. After reading this chapter, you should understand current trends and issues, as well as the influence of NI and ways to approach new ethical dilemmas.

CURRENT TRENDS IN TECHNOLOGY INTEGRATION

As we explore what is looming on the horizon, it is important to note that we must be judicious adopters and users of instructional technologies. The best technology must be chosen to address students' learning needs, and that is not always the newest one.

For example, Second Life®, a three-dimensional virtual world, has been in existence since 2003. Many institutions, programs, and individual teachers believe it is still the most stable virtual world in existence and continues to evolve to meet their needs. As nurse educators, we must remember the educational intent when selecting technologies and be sure that the technology chosen enhances the learning process.

Kelly (2016) interviewed experts and concluded that nine educational technology trends are looming:

1. Makerspaces
2. Competency-based education
3. **Virtual reality (VR)**
4. Data analytics and machine learning
5. Accessibility
6. Mobile first
7. Wearables
8. Video
9. Wireless infrastructure

Makerspaces provide administrative and teaching changes that promote collaboration and provide test beds for new technology tools and innovations in practice.

Competency-based education (CBE) is an administrative change and a move from the current credit-hour paradigm. CBE breaks learning down into competencies instead of organized courses or subject matter. This allows for modular learning episodes that can be easily scaled into stackable **credentials** or programs. According to Horn (2016),

> Credentials can be more discreet and smaller than a traditional degree—so-called **micro-credentials** or **badges**. This in turn could allow you to create stackable credentials—credentials that fit together in well understood ways such that students could assemble them together to create a bigger representation of the expertise they have (para. 16).

The learner might not end up with a degree but could be credentialed or badged in a way that employers are seeking.

VR has been used in education since the early 1990s. VR continues to evolve, and products such as Oculus Rift and Google Cardboard have increased accessibility. VR is being used for digital storytelling and serious gaming. It is certainly a trend to watch in relation to virtual simulation.

Data analytics and machine learning combine algorithms and predictive analytics. The models we build are determined by the algorithms that work best for different problems. These same algorithms help establish the evaluative criteria that are used to assess the models we develop.

Accessibility reminds us that as we push the boundaries, remove current limitations, and transform education for faculty, administrators, and students, we want it to be inclusive rather than exclusive. Everyone should be in the loop, and no one should be left behind.

Mobile first refers to the ongoing, evolving impact that mobile devices have on teaching and learning. As we move forward, our educational technology tools must be accessible from mobile devices whenever and wherever our students, faculty, and administrators work.

Wearables bring technological advancements to the forefront. Once, a mainframe computer took up an entire floor of a building; now, this computing power fits into the palm of your hand and continues to shrink and cost while increasing in capability. Wearables break down computing and dispense it throughout our personal spaces, including our bodies. It is in the fabrics of our clothing, jewelry, watches, phones, and head-mounted devices such as Google Glass and Google Cardboard. Education is beginning to capitalize on the data-capturing features, collaborative ability, and access that these tools provide. Faculty must continue to explore and expand their pedagogical use throughout the curriculum.

Video has evolved with tools such as Vine, Periscope, and Snapchat. They are moving it from a one-way delivery to an interactive experience. YouTube has allowed its users to be producers and affords global distribution for its users' video products as people from all over the world can view their videos.

Wireless infrastructure is the conductor for the interactivity afforded by these evolving technology tools. It is not uncommon for one individual to own and operate multiple technological devices simultaneously. One 16-year-old that this author knows owns a laptop, a tablet, a phone, a watch, four drones, a digital camera, and Google Glass; she uses all of these technologies while engaged in the learning process, as well as in her personal life. She is the oldest of five children; the entire household of seven (two parents) are all technologically enabled and work wirelessly. As teachers, we must be able to **engage** these students and harness these technologies at the point of learning.

Dhuha International School (2016) discussed the nine education technology trends for 2016:

1. Artificial intelligence
2. VR
3. M-learning
4. Tablets and laptops
5. Social media
6. Smart boards
7. Cloud-based technology
8. Massive open online courses (MOOCs)
9. Video

Artificial intelligence can be used to achieve greater levels of individualized learning. VR enables educational interactivity within a 3D environment. M-learning refers to learning using mobile devices. Typically, it is done through phones and learning apps developed for the educational arena. Tablets and laptops, instead of books, are being used. Traditional teaching methods are outdated, and administrators and teachers must evolve and integrate the technology tools being used today.

Social media has become a crucial component of education, with teachers and learners connecting for group meetings. Smart boards create an interactive environment, with teachers and learners actively participating in the learning process. Cloud-based technology is used to create cloud-based classrooms, share files, and interact. Massive open online courses (MOOCs) refer to a web-based model for delivering free online courses to an unlimited number of participants. MOOCs are known for their scalability because they can accommodate large numbers of learners. Coursera and Udacity are among dozens of platforms offering hundreds of classes to millions of users. Administrators and faculty must assess their use within their curriculum. The new revival of videos has been discussed.

Other trends include *serious games* and **augmented reality (AR)**. Serious games are "computer-based games designed for training purposes. They are poised to expand their role in medical education" (Wang, Demaria, Goldberg, & Katz, 2016, p. 41). Games can provide learner-centered experiences. "Our goal is the contextualization and the individualization of the gaming experience and therefore learning experience for each learner according to his own needs" (Debabi & Bensebaa, 2016, p. 138). AR is an application of technologies to enhance a physical space or object, with relevant information presented in a digital medium. Learners can drive the development of the AR learning episode or experience. AR is diffusing into the educational arena slowly (Miller & Dousay, 2015). As mobile devices enter the learning space, AR should be increasingly integrated. Petrucco and Agostini (2016) state that "the relationship between augmented reality, mobile learning, gamification and non-formal education methods provide a great potential" (p. 115).

As you can see, virtual learning is expanding and is expected to continue to grow, becoming integrated into nursing curriculums across the country. It is up to faculty to work with administrators as they begin to explore these technologies. Faculty must identify and pilot technologies to facilitate learning so that they can assess them and provide solid rationales for their choices to their administrators. This text is designed to help teachers, administrators, and students throughout the process of exploration, piloting, adoption, and support of instructional technologies used in virtual simulation.

VIRTUAL SIMULATION IN NURSING EDUCATION

The newest frontier in nursing education is virtual simulation. Its learning impact is being recognized and discussed at venues that have been dominated by latex-based simulation. Teachers, administrators, and students must all learn how to support learning in this new educational delivery modality. Virtual simulation immerses the learner in the experience. **Immersion** refers to fully involving the learner in the experience or learning episode. Throughout this text, you will learn about technology integration and virtual simulation.

Issues in Integrating Virtual Simulation in Nursing Education

As more institutions try to address the issues of the nurse educator shortage while competing for finite clinical settings, they must expand their horizons to include other mechanisms for achieving the learning results they desire. As administrators and faculty begin to explore alternative venues, such as virtual simulation, another issue that arises is confusing terminology. We will review some of the common terms and see what they actually mean.

E-learning, or online learning, occurs outside of a traditional classroom and uses electronic educational technologies to provide the content, pedagogical methodology, and assimilation of digital tools and resources that support teaching and learning. This delivery modality is typically **asynchronous** in nature. Asynchronous means that the learners and teachers can access the content, assignments, and discussion forums, for example, at any time from anywhere.

Simulation is a replication of a real-life event or situation. In nursing education, simulation refers to a practice setting scenario developed to provide an opportunity for learners to perform in an artificial situation in a safe environment. Simulation can consist of role play, scenarios, and assumption of nursing duties. When it occurs in a **virtual world**, it is considered **virtual simulation** versus a brick-and-mortar simulation laboratory with manikins, known as **latex-based simulation**. Virtual simulation can be asynchronous or **synchronous** in nature. Latex-based simulation is typically synchronous. Synchronous delivery means that the simulation is completed at a set time either individually or while working with others.

Simulation scenario is an episode, event or case developed in a simulation setting to imitate an authentic practice situation. A game is a structured activity initiated for enjoyment. A **serious game** is a game with an intent such as for learning and not just for entertainment (refer to Product Bytes 1.1). When we make learning fun, it is referred to as **edutainment**. Therefore, if our learner is having fun, we have edutained our learner. The rules, directions, and concepts that the learner interacts with while playing the game are referred to as **game mechanics**. As nurse educators, we must ensure that our game mechanics not only engage. but are also satisfying to, the learner. The interactions with the game or the playing of the game is known as **gameplay**. Game mechanics and gameplay are important to appreciate how the game works and how learners behave, play, and learn. Games are typically goal oriented, competitive, and fun but are not always socially interactive as users can play the game by themselves.

PRODUCT BYTES 1.1 Examples of Serious Games

Virtual Pain Manager
online serious nursing game simulating use of patient controlled analgesia machine—students are taught pain management theory in the classroom and then they can access the simulation platform. The student nurse must control and reduce the patient's pain within 48 game hours

VA Critical Thinking
serious game allowing nurses to practice assessment, treatment and prevention of patient health conditions related to skin integrity and pressure ulcers

(continued)

PRODUCT BYTES 1.1 Examples of Serious Games (*continued*)

Florence
multipurpose serious game for nurses focused on blood transfusion, fire safety, and infectious hazard

Virtual ECG
online serious game for accurate electrocardiographs

Code Orange
serious game based in a virtual hospital where players work with first aid staff of a hospital to save people injured by a weapon-of-mass-destruction

3DiTeams
serious game set in a virtual hospital that introduces the player to teamwork and communication skills that they must apply in a virtual scenario

Burn Center
serious game to practice triage and resuscitation

Zero Hour: America's Medic
serious game designed to train emergency medical services operators to respond to mass casualty incidents such as earthquakes and terrorism

Pulse!!
serious game to practice clinical skills to better respond to catastrophic incident injuries

Free Dive
serious game designed to entertain and distract children experiencing painful medical procedures

Time After Time
serious game and interactive decision aid for men diagnosed with localized prostate cancer

Source: Ricciardi, F., & De Paolis, L. (2014). A comprehensive review of serious games in health professions. *International Journal of Computer Games Technology, 2014,* 1–11. doi:10.1155/2014/787968

GAME2LEARN
asks the users various computer science questions in order to fight the bug.

Ware Aurora toolset
user is an apprentice wizard who must learn programming of statements and nested loops

(*continued*)

> **PRODUCT BYTES 1.1 Examples of Serious Games** (*continued*)
>
> Code Studio
> an introduction to computer science designed to demystify code
>
> Prog & Play
> is a real-time, multiplayer, strategy game
> students write programs to control units in a battlefield.
>
> CoLoBot: Colonize with Bots
> real time 3D game of strategy and an initiation to programming
>
> PlayLogo3D
> role playing game, especially designed for children aged 6-13 years
>
> M.U.P.P.E.T.S.: The Multi-User Programming Pedagogy for Enhancing Traditional Study
> web-based, collaborative three dimensional game that aims to teach the basic concepts of object-oriented programming
>
> *Source:* Debabi, W., & Bensebaa, T. (2016). Using serious game to enhance algorithmic learning and teaching. *Journal of e-Learning and Knowledge Society, 12*(2), 117–140. doi:10.20368/1971-8829/1125

Simulated nursing experiences must contain the prebrief, enactment, debrief, assessment (PEDA) elements to provide the information and opportunities for learners to think critically using judicious clinical decision making, as well to hone skills in a safe, controlled environment (McGonigle & Mastrian, 2018).

Prior to beginning any simulation experience, it is important to provide learners with a prebrief or overview of the activity, an orientation to the environment, and the ground rules. Students should receive pertinent information regarding the simulation activity, including goals, objectives, virtual learning outcomes, related course/program outcomes, and related competencies. Students must be provided with unambiguous, easy-to-understand instructions, including how to prepare for the activity and what is expected of them, and they should be provided with the background necessary to be able to fully enact their role in the activity and with the specifics about how their performance will be evaluated. Students must also be given the parameters within which the learning activities must be completed.

Virtual simulation is a simulation that can occur in a virtual learning or VR environment that replicates real-life situations. During enactment, the virtual simulation environment is prepared to facilitate the activity, and the student enacts the role assigned during the established timeframe. Learners play central roles by interacting in the virtual environment, exercising motor control and communication skills, and practicing decision making.

An essential component of the virtual learning experience is debriefing, which should be led by faculty and conducted one-on-one or with groups of students. Ideally, the number of students in a group should not exceed a predetermined student to faculty ratio, thereby maintaining intimacy, confidentiality, and trust between participants. The responsibilities and role of the faculty should guide the debriefing experience.

Students should be provided with a detailed explanation of how they will be assessed and evaluated in relation to the goal, educational outcomes, and if applicable, course/program outcomes. The assessment process must be shared during prebriefing. If the activity is not being graded, there should be a self-assessment provided for the students so that they know how to evaluate their own performance (Gordon, 2017).

A **virtual patient** or virtual standardized patient is a digital patient or computer-generated patient in an interactive simulation that allowing learners to assume their assigned nursing roles to develop and refine their patient-related clinical skills. Interacting with the virtual patient, learners make clinical decisions, explore diagnoses, and implement and evaluate care choices. Many applications permit interaction using text or voice, and learners make their own path through the simulation.

Games are typically competitive and fantastical. Simulations are more realistic and generally not competitive in nature. Virtual worlds are not fun or competitive unless they are designed that way, although they may include fantasy. Even though distinctions exist, there is a great deal of similarity and overlap among simulations, serious games, and virtual worlds. Simulations could have game mechanisms, and a serious game can be developed to be played in a virtual world. Virtual simulations can also be developed for virtual worlds. Nurse educators can control the simulated experiences of the learner within a virtual world.

By implementing the use of virtual patients and virtual simulation, learners can experience a broader range of learning opportunities than those provided in a real setting. As administrators, nurse educators, and learners become more skilled in the use of these technologies, the experiences can be customized to meet learners' needs. Teachers and learners can collaborate to enhance the learning process. Through shared experiences and collaborations such as this text, we will see widespread acceptance and integration of these tools in the coming decade.

Some of the other issues that come into play when deciding on virtual simulation tools are the system requirements for faculty and students, as well as the available support. These issues are addressed in more detail in upcoming chapters.

TECHNOLOGICAL PEDAGOGICAL CONTENT KNOWLEDGE

Constructivism

There are many learning theories, but the authors believe that all educational episodes must be **learner centered** and that **constructivism** is applicable to virtual learning experiences that are learner centered. The learner-centered paradigm shifts the instructional focus from the teacher to the learner. This is accomplished through engaging the learner in the learning process, teaching learners how to think critically, encouraging collaboration, and facilitating reflection. The authors believe that the most important aspect of learner-centered experiences is having learners reflect on what they are learning.

Constructivism focuses on thinking and understanding instead of rote memorization and refers to individuals constructing their own perception and knowledge of the world by experiencing the world through active and passive participation in activities with others and reflecting on their experiences. The learner can interact with other learners or the teacher, or the learner can interact with the environment. Therefore, it is important for the teacher to create learning activities that cause the learner to ponder and reflect on the content or substance of the lesson or activity and the actual process of learning. We all have our own perceptual screen that defines and organizes our world. As data, information, and knowledge are acquired, they are influenced by our past learning, experiences, knowledge, and skills. The internal synthesis with our own knowledge base results in our personal viewpoint or perspective that we present or exhibit externally through our perceptual screen.

Learning is an active, social process that is contextual and grounded in the authentic, real-world context. We must be motivated and involved to learn. Learners construct knowledge for themselves and are encouraged to question, analyze, interpret, and predict information, as well as to reflect on their learning. We learn from others, our environment, and ourselves. As one constructs meaning, one learns. One learns how to learn and how to construct systems of meaning, learning in relationship to what we know and believe. These constructed systems of meaning are transferable to other learning episodes. In a constructivist approach, assessment becomes part of the learning process.

Virtual learning technologies support asynchronous and synchronous learning experiences. The asynchronous learning episode allows learners to interact with the environment when their schedule permits, whereas the synchronous component requires learners to enter at a predetermined time to collaborate and interact with the teacher and/or other learners. Throughout this text, you are asked to reflect on the content in relation to the FAST SIM©.

Scientific Foundation of NI

NI is an evolving nursing specialty. It has been defined by McGonigle and Mastrian (2018) as:

> ... the synthesis of nursing science, information science, computer science, and cognitive science for the purpose of managing, disseminating and enhancing health care data, information, knowledge, and wisdom to improve collaboration and decision making, provide high quality patient care and advance the profession of nursing (p. 573).

NI helps all areas of nursing practice to improve patient care and evolve the profession.

NI is being integrated into nursing education; this integration is helping to advance nursing education. The technology tools that are available must be used carefully and selected by reflecting on and applying knowledge and wisdom to the learning process. The teacher must consider teaching and learning styles. Nurse educators are gaining competence in NI, and VR in education is becoming a reality in academia. Students in Generation Next and beyond continue to prompt nurse educators to experiment with VR to engage these technologically savvy learners.

Students, educators, and administrators are moving from the simple applications of email, presentation packages, word processing, or spreadsheets, to leverage NI competencies to provide simulations, VR, and game mechanics. Virtual worlds immerse students into the learning episode to practice complex skills in a safe environment while receiving feedback and engaging in self-reflection to assess their own learning. Using NI skills and educational prowess, nurse educators carefully select technology that enhances the learning episode. We must remember that technology can perform only to the level of the pedagogy that underpins and sustains it.

DATA, INFORMATION, KNOWLEDGE, WISDOM PATHWAY

To understand the impact of NI, it is imperative that you understand the **data, information, knowledge, wisdom (DIKW) pathway** and the way that we move from data to wisdom in our professional lives. **Data** are raw facts. **Information** is processed data or data that have been given meaning. **Knowledge** is related information, and **wisdom** is the correct application of knowledge to a specific situation. Refer to Practice Bytes 1.1 and 1.2.

PRACTICE BYTES 1.1 DIKW Pathway Example

If we state the number 99, how would you classify this number?
   99 is a raw fact or *data* and has no meaning by itself. It could stand for a radio station or an examination score.
Next, if you see this, how would you classify it?
   Mrs. Hendis   9 a.m.   99°
   This is now *information* that has meaning. You know that at 9 a.m., Mrs. Hendis' temperature was 99°.
Now, review and classify this:
   Mrs. Hendis
   9 a.m.   99°
   11 a.m.   100°
   1 p.m.   102°
   This is now *knowledge* because you have related information. Three temperature measurements indicate that Mrs. Hendis' temperature is rising.
You refer to your standing orders and then implement the medication protocol for a temperature greater than 101° and schedule vital signs to be taken hourly. Is this *wisdom*? Why or why not?

PRACTICE BYTES 1.2 DIKW Pathway Clinical Example

Renee has been an RN for 3 years and works in an ICU in a teaching hospital. She admits Mrs. Grovie to the unit. Mrs. Grovie is a 45-year-old who was in the hospital visiting another patient when she collapsed and is unresponsive.

(continued)

> **PRACTICE BYTES 1.2 DIKW Pathway Clinical Example (*continued*)**
>
> She has been in the emergency department (ED) for 4 hours in this state. While Renee is assessing the patient, Mrs. Grovie becomes alert and scared. She does not know where she is and wants to know what happened. Renee explains the situation and asks if this has ever happened before. Mrs. Grovie is now fully alert and oriented and has never had anything like this happen before. Renee asks her to describe her health history. She is the mother of 5, and those are the only times she was admitted to a hospital. Mrs. Grovie describes herself as a 5'4" woman who weighs approximately 130 pounds and is healthy and energetic. Renee assesses Mrs. Grovie's vital signs and heart monitor, noticing that she has a rapid pulse rate of 110. Renee determines that her pulse oximetry and everything else look fine. As she continues to converse with the patient, she sees that her pulse rate slows to 90. Renee continues to assess the patient because she does not appear to be in any immediate distress and determines that her vital signs, heart rhythm, and neurologic checks are all normal. All testing performed in the ED is within normal limits. Renee feels that she should observe Mrs. Grovie but that no other action is needed at this time. Mrs. Grovie's husband arrives with three of her older children at the same time as the attending physician. They are very concerned because she has always been healthy. The physician asks them to give her a minute while she assesses Mrs. Grovie and reviews her test results.
>
> How would you describe the DIKW pathway as it relates to this case?
> Renee relied on the *data* and *information* she was given to build *knowledge* about Mrs. Grovie's situational context and used her *wisdom* based on the data, information, and knowledge she obtained to determine that this patient was not in any immediate danger, that the patient should just be observed, and that she did not need to intervene at this time.

As we construct our simulations, we must keep the DIKW pathway in mind. How will students gather data? How much assistance will be provided in processing the data into information? How will they process knowledge and advance to wisdom? How will we assess each step of the DIKW pathway, especially the knowledge gained and the learner's resulting wisdom? It is important to remember that data, information, and knowledge are gleaned from our external interactions and that wisdom comes from within us as we synthesize new information and new knowledge with our experiences, knowledge base, and skills (see Appendix A).

Ethical Considerations Using the ETHICAL Model

The healthcare arena is constantly changing, and along with the changes arise numerous ethical challenges. Nursing education also experiences **ethical** dilemmas. As we assess the technologies that are emerging and their impact in education, we must always consider the ethical implications they bring with them. Technologies are evolving faster than ethical and social norms. Ethical issues and dilemmas abound. We must have a way to methodically explore the dilemmas we are facing. Ethics is a system of systematically investigating how we should interact or behave with others, as well as deal with differing views linked to the moral questions of right or wrong. While facing a moral question of right or wrong, one must have a method for studying the consequences of one's actions. The ETHICAL Model for Ethical Decision Making was designed to help you apply an ethical process or approach to instructional technology concerns (refer to Box 1.1).

> **BOX 1.1 ETHICAL Model for Ethical Decision Making**
>
> Examine the ethical dilemma (conflicting values exist).
> Thoroughly comprehend the possible alternatives available.
> Hypothesize ethical arguments.
> Investigate, compare, and evaluate the arguments for each alternative.
> Choose the alternative you would recommend.
> Act on your chosen alternative.
> Look at the ethical dilemma and examine the outcomes while reflecting on the ethical decision.
>
> **HOW TO APPLY THE ETHICAL MODEL**
>
> **Examine the ethical dilemma:**
>
> - Use your problem-solving, decision-making, and critical-thinking skills.
> - What is the dilemma you are analyzing? Collect as much information about the dilemma as you can, making sure to gather the relevant facts that clearly identify the dilemma. You should be able to describe the dilemma you are analyzing in detail.
> - Ascertain exactly what must be decided.
> - Who should be involved in the decision-making process for this specific case?
> - Who are the interested players or stakeholders?
> - Reflect on the viewpoints of these key players and their value systems.
> - What do you think each of these stakeholders would like you to decide as a plan of action for this dilemma?
> - How can you generate the greatest good?
>
> **Thoroughly comprehend the possible alternatives available:**
>
> - Use your problem-solving, decision-making, and critical-thinking skills.
> - Create a list of the possible alternatives. Be creative when developing your alternatives. Be open minded; there is more than one way to reach a goal. Compel yourself to discern at least three alternatives.
> - Clarify the alternatives available and predict the associated consequences—good and bad—of each potential alternative or intervention.

(continued)

> **BOX 1.1 ETHICAL Model for Ethical Decision Making (*continued*)**
>
> - For each alternative, ask the following questions:
>   - Do any of the principles or rules, such as legal, professional, or organizational, automatically nullify this alternative?
>   - If this alternative is chosen, what do you predict as the best-case and worst-case scenarios?
>   - Do the best-case outcomes outweigh the worst-case outcomes?
>   - Could you live with the worst-case scenario?
>   - Will anyone be harmed? If so, how will they be harmed?
>   - Does the benefit obtained from this alternative overcome the risk of potential harm that it could cause to anyone?
>
> **Hypothesize ethical arguments:**
>
> - Use your problem-solving, decision-making, and critical-thinking skills.
> - Determine which of the five approaches apply to this dilemma.
> - Identify the moral principles that can be brought into play to support a conclusion as to what ought to be done ethically in this case or similar cases.
> - Ascertain whether the approaches generate converging or diverging conclusions about what ought to be done.
>
> **Investigate, compare, and evaluate the arguments for each alternative:**
>
> - Use your problem-solving, decision-making, and critical-thinking skills.
> - Appraise the relevant facts and assumptions prudently.
>   - Is there ambiguous information that must be evaluated?
>   - Are there any unjustifiable factual or illogical assumptions or debatable conceptual issues that must be explored?
> - Rate the ethical reasoning and arguments for each alternative in terms of their relative significance.
>   - 4 = extreme significance
>   - 3 = major significance
>   - 2 = significant
>   - 1 = minor significance
> - Compare and contrast the alternatives available with the values of the key players involved.
> - Reflect on these alternatives.
>   - Does each alternative consider all of the key players?
>
> *(continued)*

BOX 1.1 ETHICAL Model for Ethical Decision Making (*continued*)

- ○ Does each alternative take into account and reflect an interest in the concerns and welfare of all of the key players?
- ○ Which alternative will produce the greatest good or the least amount of harm for the greatest number of people?
- Refer to your professional codes of ethical conduct. Do they support your reasoning?

Choose the alternative you would recommend:

- Use your problem-solving, decision-making, and critical-thinking skills.
- Make a decision about the best alternative available.
  - ○ Remember the Golden Rule: Does your decision treat others as you would want to be treated?
  - ○ Does your decision take into account and reflect an interest in the concerns and welfare of all of the key players?
  - ○ Does your decision maximize the benefit and minimize the risk for everyone involved?
- Become your own critic; challenge your decision as you think others might. Use the ethical arguments you predict they would use and defend your decision.
  - ○ Would you be secure enough in your ethical decision-making process to see it aired on national television or sent out globally over the Internet?
  - ○ Are you secure enough with this ethical decision that you could have allowed your loved ones to observe your decision-making process, your decision, and its outcomes?

Act on your chosen alternative:

- Use your problem-solving, decision-making, and critical-thinking skills.
- Formulate an implementation plan delineating the execution of the decision.
  - ○ This plan should be designed to maximize the benefits and minimize the risks.
  - ○ This plan must take into account all of the resources necessary for implementation, including personnel and money.
- Implement the plan.

Look at the ethical dilemma and examine the outcomes while reflecting on your ethical decision:

- Use your problem-solving, decision-making, and critical-thinking skills.

(*continued*)

> **BOX 1.1 ETHICAL Model for Ethical Decision Making (*continued*)**
>
> - Monitor the implementation plan and its outcomes. It is extremely important to reflect on specific case decisions and evaluate their outcomes to develop your ethical decision-making ability.
> - If new information becomes available, the plan must be reevaluated.
> - Monitor and revise the plan as necessary.
>
> *Source:* The ETHICAL model for ethical decision making, developed by Dr. Dee McGonigle, is the property of Educational Advancement Associates (EAA). Mr. Craig R. Goshow, Vice President, EAA, has granted permission for it to be included in this text.

It is paramount that ethical decisions be made as instructional technologies advance and are integrated into the learning process by administrators and faculty who are shaping the future of education. Administrators, nurse educators, and students are joining together to create learning episodes that are changing the learning landscape. The day-to-day reality produced by the adoption of virtual simulation technologies not only provides new learning opportunities, but also poses challenges as we navigate this unchartered frontier. These challenges must be addressed ethically (see Practice Byte 1.2). We must apply an ethical process or approach to address technological dilemmas; refer to Application Byte 1.1.

> **APPLICATION BYTE 1.1 Examine an Ethical Dilemma Using the ETHICAL Model for Ethical Decision Making**
>
> This Application Byte is intended to help you reflect on the ETHICAL Model and how it can be applied to dilemmas that arise as you implement virtual simulations in your institutions. The first step is to make sure you have reviewed the ETHICAL Model. Next, read through the dilemma that is presented, use the ETHICAL Model to address it, and determine the decision you would make before you review how we approached this dilemma using the model.
>
> ***Dilemma***
>
> An instructor developed a virtual simulation using the school's new virtual world. Her students are required to complete this activity prior to entering the clinical area to care for a real patient. She is the first instructor using this virtual simulation area and has provided students with the orientation and support information necessary to satisfactorily complete it.
>
> As the instructor conducts her preconference (prebrief), she quickly realizes that 5 of the 10 students in her clinical rotation have not completed the virtual simulation. She meets with the students and asks them why. They tell her that they
>
> *(continued)*

APPLICATION BYTE 1.1 Examine an Ethical Dilemma using the ETHICAL Model for Ethical Decision Making (*continued*)

feel she should help them learn, that they should not have to learn another software program, and that they need their clinical time. She tells the students that since they were not prepared, they must leave the unit and complete the simulation before they return for their next clinical day. This means that the students failed this clinical day. The students are not planning to comply and drive to the school to meet with the dean, whom they tell they do not feel that they should have to do the heavy lifting of their education but should be helped more by the faculty member. Now they are failing a day of clinical because they were dismissed from the clinical unit. Their instructor did not even try to help them...

Examine the Ethical Dilemma

The instructor issued a clear directive and assigned the students to complete the virtual simulation. The expectations were clear because 5 students completed the assigned virtual simulation and arrived at the clinical unit prepared to care for their patients. The instructor realized that 5 students were not prepared because they had not completed the required virtual simulation. The students were not ready to properly care for patients, so she solved the dilemma by dismissing them from the unit and failing them for the clinical day.

Thoroughly Comprehend the Possible Alternatives Available

The possible alternatives available include the following: (a) The instructor could have reviewed the information with the unprepared students and delayed working with the 5 prepared students, or (b) the instructor could have asked them to leave clinical, review the virtual simulation, and return to the clinical unit later so they would not fail the entire clinical practice day.

Hypothesize Ethical Arguments

The utilitarian approach can apply to this situation. An ethical action provides the greatest good for the greatest number; the underlying principle in this perspective is nonmaleficence, or do no harm. The rights to be considered are as follows: right of individuals to choose for themselves (autonomy), right not to be injured, and right to what has been promised (fidelity). The instructor is responsible for the care provided to the patients and ensuring their safety. The students each chose to come to the clinical unit unprepared because they did not want to complete the virtual simulation learning activity. The principles to consider are autonomy, right not to be injured, and fidelity.

As for fairness or justice, how fair or just is an action? Does the action treat everyone in the same way, or does it show favoritism or discriminate against anyone? Did the instructor discriminate against any of the students?

Virtue postulates that one should strive toward certain ideals; it is an attitude or character trait that facilitates an individual to be and act in ways that

(*continued*)

> **APPLICATION BYTE 1.1 Examine an Ethical Dilemma using the ETHICAL Model for Ethical Decision Making (*continued*)**
>
> develop their maximum potential. The virtuous person is ethical. The principles considered are fidelity, nonmaleficence, and justice. In this dilemma, the students were not prepared to care for the real patients because they chose not to comply with the educational requirement and did not complete the virtual simulation. The instructor is responsible for the safety of the patient and the quality of care the patient receives as well as the quality of education provided to the students. Does the patient care responsibility or obligation outweigh the obligation to the student's education and clinical practice? Yes, it should.
>
> Virtue ethics suggests that individuals use their power to bring about human benefit. One must consider the needs of others and the responsibility to meet those needs. The instructor must simultaneously provide quality patient care, prevent harm, provide quality educational experiences, and maintain professional relationships.
>
> The instructor may want to effect a long-term change in the educational institution's policy for the common good and be accountable to the patients being cared for, as well as to the students' learning. It is reasonable to assume that this will not be an isolated event and that the problem could recur. Is the instructor's decision supported by the institution, and can policies be amended to include virtual simulation in addition to other educational means required for providing safe clinical practice?
>
> The International Council of Nurses (2006) code of ethics stated that "the nurse uses judgment in relation to individual competence when accepting and delegating responsibilities" (p. 5). This statement applies to this dilemma. You must identify the moral principles that can be brought into play to support a conclusion as to what ought to be done ethically in this dilemma or other comparable or similar dilemmas.
>
> Ascertain whether the approaches generate converging or diverging conclusions about what ought to be done. From the analysis, it is clear that the best immediate solution was to require the students to be prepared; however, this is the first virtual simulation activity that has been developed and required.
>
> ***Investigate, Compare, and Evaluate the Arguments for Each Alternative***
>
> *Alternative 1:* The instructor could have reviewed the information with the unprepared students and delayed working with the prepared students.
>
> - Good consequences: Patient safety
> - Bad consequences: It is not the best use of the instructor's time, and the prepared students would be delayed because of the unprepared students.
> - Do any rules nullify? No

(continued)

> **APPLICATION BYTE 1.1 Examine an Ethical Dilemma using the ETHICAL Model for Ethical Decision Making** (*continued*)
>
> Expected outcome:
> Best
>
> - The unprepared students would be prepared to properly care for these patients.
>
> Worst
>
> - Some of the unprepared students would not be able to care for their patients and need additional help.
> - The prepared students would not be able to fully care for their patients due to reduced clinical practice time.
>
> Potential benefit: Patients are protected; patients' rights take precedence over students' needs.
>
> *Alternative 2:* The instructor could have asked the unprepared students to leave clinical, review the virtual simulation, and return to the clinical unit later so that they would not fail the entire clinical practice day.
>
> - Good consequences: The prepared students would be able to care for their patients, and the unprepared students would be held accountable for their learning.
> - Bad consequences: The unprepared students would not comply and try to return to the clinical unit, causing more disruption for the prepared students.
> - Do any rules nullify? No
>
> Expected outcome:
> Best
>
> - The unprepared students would be responsible and return prepared to care for their patients.
>
> Worse
>
> - The students do not comply, do not return to clinical, or cannot complete the virtual simulation in time to return and salvage a portion of their clinical practice day.
>
> Potential benefit: The students are held accountable and do not fail the entire clinical practice day.
>
> ***Choose the Alternative You Would Recommend***
>
> The best immediate solution is for the instructor to ask them to leave the clinical area, review the virtual simulation, and return to the clinical unit later so they would not fail the entire clinical practice day and she could assist the prepared students. The best long-term solution is to make sure the educational

(continued)

> **APPLICATION BYTE 1.1 Examine an Ethical Dilemma using the ETHICAL Model for Ethical Decision Making (*continued*)**
>
> institution supports the virtual simulation requirement and the faculty and students using this learning modality.
>
> ***Act on Your Chosen Alternative***
>
> The instructor should ask them to leave clinical, review the virtual simulation, and return to the clinical unit later so that they would not fail the entire clinical practice day.
>
> ***Look at the Ethical Dilemma and Examine the Outcomes While Reflecting on the Ethical Decision***
>
> As already indicated in the alternative review and analyses, the instructor could have asked them to leave clinical, review the virtual simulation, and return to the clinical unit later so that they would not fail the entire clinical practice day. It is the best immediate solution to the dilemma and is certainly safer than compromising patient care. As noted previously, the best long-term solution is to make sure that the educational institution supports the virtual simulation requirement and the faculty and students using this learning modality. The students should not feel that they can refuse to participate in required educational activities such as virtual simulation. This Application Byte, applying the ETHICAL Model, demonstrates the authors' perspective on this dilemma and the resulting ethical decision that was supported. Your decision might not match our perspective. You might have reached a different decision when you applied the ETHICAL Model based on your own background, assessment, viewpoint, and perspective. Even though you reached a different ethical decision, it does not make either decision right or wrong. Each ethical decision should reflect the best decision one can make given appraisal, review, consideration and reflection, and critical thinking about this particular situation.
>
> As you explore virtual simulation and the resulting educational dilemmas, apply the ETHICAL Model to each as it arises. You should be able to engage in thoughtful discussion and deliberation of these dilemmas with other faculty, administrators, and students. Everyone should receive the ETHICAL Model and be provided with the same information. Remember, if your decision is challenged, do not feel personally attacked, but instead explain how you used the model to analyze the dilemma and provide the details that led you to your ethical decision. Do not hesitate to question anyone's analysis or perspective during the process because this provides for an interactive dialogue and promotes the sharing of diverse viewpoints and perceptions.

KEY POINTS

- It is important to know technology integration trends.
- You must understand the terminology and learning impact associated with virtual simulation.

- The underpinning of learner-centered events is a constructivist approach reflecting on the DIKW pathway.
- We must be prepared to address ethical dilemmas using the ETHICAL Model for Ethical Decision Making.

SUMMARY

As educators and administrators, we have a collective responsibility to ensure that educational activities we associate ourselves with are conducted to the highest ethical standards. The convenience, the potential for innovation, and the opportunities to expand education in new and exciting ways are all temptations for falling into the trap of justifying the means with the ends. Throughout this text, you are challenged to reflect on your learning setting and learning tools. It is important to continually assess how we approach teaching and learning so that we can explore and integrate new instructional technologies. As technologies emerge and administration and faculty pioneer, the learning landscape will continue to change dynamically.

REFLECTIVE QUESTIONS

1. Think of a clinical experience or personal situation where you had to make decisions and analyze them using the DIKW pathway.
2. Identify an ethical dilemma arising from an educational situation and apply the ETHICAL Model for Ethical Decision Making to it.
3. How do administrators and faculty gain the knowledge, experience, and skill necessary to effectively select, implement, and evaluate virtual simulation technologies? Elaborate on the details in your answer.
4. Think of a learning episode that needs to be enhanced. Revise this learning experience to reflect a learner-centered, constructivist approach.
5. If you could implement virtual simulation today, what would your first virtual simulation learning experience look like? Describe in detail how this learning experience would be developed, enacted by learners, and assessed using constructivism and the DIKW pathway.

REFERENCES

Debabi, W., & Bensebaa, T. (2016). Using serious game to enhance algorithmic learning and teaching. *Journal of e-Learning and Knowledge Society, 12*(2), 117–140. doi:10.20368/1971-8829/1125

Dhuha International School. (2016). 9 educational trends that will rule in 2016. Retrieved from https://www.linkedin.com/pulse/9-educational-technology-trends-rule-2016-dhuha-international-school

Gordon, R. (2017). Debriefing virtual simulation using an online conferencing platform: Lessons learned. *Clinical Simulation in Nursing, 13*(12), 668–674. doi:10.1016/j.ecns.2017.08.003

Horn, M. (2016). Unbundling and rebundling: The lasting impact of alternative credentialing on higher ed. Retrieved from http://evolllution.com/managing-institution/higher_ed_business/unbundling-and-rebundling-the-lasting-impact-of-alternative-credentialing-on-higher-ed

International Council of Nurses. (2006). The ICN code of ethics for nurses. Geneva, Switzerland: Author.

Kelly, R. (2016). 9 ed tech trends to watch in 2016. Retrieved from https://campustechnology.com/articles/2016/01/13/9-ed-tech-trends-to-watch-in-2016.aspx

McGonigle, D., & Mastrian, K. (2018). *Nursing informatics and the foundation of knowledge.* Burlington, MA: Jones & Bartlett.

Miller, D., & Dousay, T. (2015). Implementing augmented reality in the classroom. *Issues and Trends in Educational Technology, 3*(2), 1–11. Retrieved from http://works.bepress.com/tadousay/15

Petrucco, C., & Agostini, D. (2016). Teaching cultural heritage using mobile augmented reality. *Journal of e-Learning and Knowledge Society, 12*(3), 115–128. Retrieved from https://www.learntechlib.org/p/173477

Ricciardi, F., & De Paolis, L. (2014). A comprehensive review of serious games in health professions. *International Journal of Computer Games Technology, 2014,* 1–11. doi:10.1155/2014/787968

Wang, R., Demaria, S., Goldberg, A., & Katz, D. (2016). A systematic review of serious games in training health care professionals. *Journal of the Society for Simulation in Healthcare, 11*(1), 41–51. doi:10.1097/SIH.0000000000000118

Faculty Administrators Students Technology Strategic Integration Model©

RANDY M. GORDON

LEARNING OBJECTIVES

Upon completion of this chapter, the reader will be able to:
- Assess the key comsponents of the Faculty Administrators Students Technology Strategic Integration Model© (FAST SIM) conceptual model.
- Explore the relationship between faculty, administrators, students, technology, and curriculum integration strategies.

KEY TERMS

Faculty Administrators Student Technology Strategic Integration Model© (FAST SIM)
Educational technology
Simulation
Technology
Technology integration
Virtual learning environment (VLE)

The integration of technology with healthcare is more than a trend. Numerous textbooks illuminate the need to transform nursing education to include technology as a fundamental educational tool. A still pervasive question is not whether to use technology in the nursing curriculum, but rather how to integrate it into the nursing curriculum. The infusion of technology into higher education is a complex and increasingly necessary process. Nursing educators and administrators need resources that reflect integration strategies, especially when a curriculum is already in place. Faculty, administrators, and students often explore technology for personal and professional use; however, the process for integrating innovative educational technology into the nursing curriculum is not intuitive. Integration strategies are not easily found in the literature or lack specificity. Therefore, the editors of this textbook created a conceptual model intended to impart a richer understanding of the relationships between integration influences when contending with the process of developing thoughtful and well-planned strategies.

PURPOSE OF THE FAST SIM©

One underlying purpose of the **Faculty Administrators Students Technology Strategic Integration Model© (FAST SIM)** is to provide a framework from which to guide the process of technology integration into the nursing curriculum. The

FAST SIM© may be used to bridge pedagogical approaches to curriculum design and development with the tools educators have at their disposal. The development of a common language and conceptual framework for communication and for guiding curriculum development is fundamental to sound progress in any nursing program (Spross, 2014, p. 27). This model is intended to help nursing educators articulate and organize concepts, as well as provide a basis for further development of knowledge. It also serves as a tool that can be used during evaluation after simulation integration.

MODEL DESCRIPTION

Faculty, administrators, and students are represented equally as key components of the FAST SIM© (Figure 2.1). The creators of the model believe that the influence and contribution from faculty, administrators, and students are integral and essential to achieving successful integration of technology into the curriculum. Throughout this text, the authors may use the words *faculty*, *teacher*, or *educator* synonymously. Likewise, the terms *students* and *learners* are used interchangeably. Directional arrows represent the continual relationship between faculty, administrators, and students in an unbroken circle. Technology is represented by a mechanical gear in the center of the model, which is "driven" by faculty, administrators, and students. Administrators and faculty determine the use of technology within the curriculum; faculty and student needs drive the type and use of technology that is integrated into the teaching/learning process during curriculum development and revision.

The definition of **technology** varies in the context in which it used. In the broadest sense, technology deals with the creation and use of technical means and their interrelationship with life, society, and the environment. **Educational technology** is as the study and ethical practice of facilitating learning and improving performance by creating, using, and managing appropriate technological processes and resources

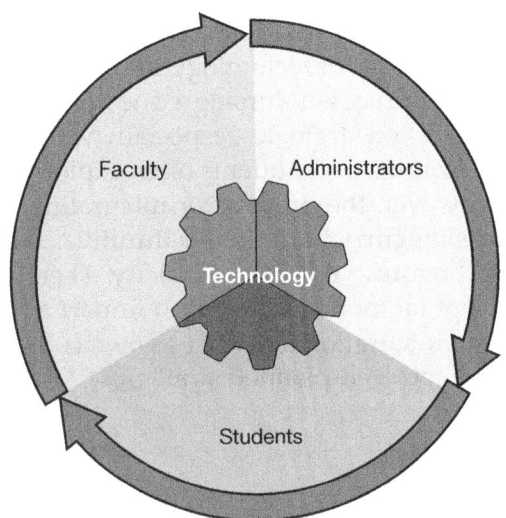

FIGURE 2.1 Components of the FAST SIM© (Faculty Administrators Students Technology Strategic Integration Model).

> **BOX 2.1 Educational Technology Resources**
>
> Computers/laptops
> Network-based communication systems
> Electronic products, software, and mobile devices
> Education-based apps (iOS and Android)
> Infrastructure

(Robinson, Molenda, & Rezabek, 2008). Educational technology resources include, but are not limited to, computers and specialized software, network-based communication systems, electronic products, software, and devices, as well as infrastructure (Box 2.1).

Integration refers to combining or incorporating into one. The authors of this textbook broadly define **technology integration** as the use of any technology to enhance and support the educational environment. A **virtual learning environment (VLE)** is a web-based platform for the digital aspects of courses of study, usually within educational institutions. VLEs typically allow participants to:

- Be organized into cohorts, groups, and roles
- Present resources, activities, and interactions within a course structure
- Have some level of integration with other institutional systems (Laurillard, 2013)

Technology and *simulation* are terms often used interchangeably. Discordant definitions of simulation illuminate the fact that a shared understanding of what constitutes simulation has not been developed in higher education. Gore and Thomson (2016) defined **simulation** as "a pedagogy using one or more typologies to promote, improve, or validate a participant's progression from novice to expert" (p. 88). Simulation is a teaching technique used for experiential learning, which allows students to practice in a safe environment, improve communication skills, and develop the ability to think and act as an advanced practice nurse. Simulation may or may not require the inclusion of technology. For example, simulation may include practicing intramuscular or subcutaneous injections on oranges or fellow classmates, using basic manikins to practice insertion of indwelling catheters, or role-playing to practice assessment and communication skills. Simulation may also include simulators or virtual patients that simulate real-life clinical scenarios in which the learner acts as a health care provider obtaining a history, doing a physical examination, and making diagnostic and therapeutic decisions. Regardless of the modality, simulation helps learners in bridging the gap between knowledge and practice through deliberate application of skills and reflective debriefing. As the use of simulation in nursing education increases, more regulations, guidelines, and standards are being developed to assist nursing programs in obtaining best outcomes (Gore & Thomson, 2016).

Integrating technology into nursing education requires an educator who is prepared to facilitate an effective learning experience. Faculty explore, select, and propose the technology to administration. The faculty's use of technology can enhance intrinsic motivation and instill the lifelong need to seek technology support. Faculty must be prepared to use available resources, have access to needed support, and develop competency for using resources and support throughout the curriculum. In Box 2.2, Tagliareni and Forneris (2016) shared their expert opinions regarding simulation and curriculum development. Dr. Tagliareni was

---

BOX 2.2 Expert Exemplar

M. Elaine Tagliareni, EdD, RN, CNE, FAAN
Chief Program Officer Director, Center for Excellence in the Care of Vulnerable Populations

Susan Gross Forneris, PhD, RN, CNE, CHSE-A
Excelsior Deputy Director, NLN Center for Innovation in Simulation and Technology

- The interface between curriculum and simulation should ideally be seamless. However, to achieve this, integration planning must be purposeful and thoughtful.
- Curriculum designers should set clear objectives and expected outcomes for each simulation-based experience, which must be communicated to students prior to each simulation activity.
- Learning outcomes for simulation must be clearly linked to course and program outcomes.
- Student performance in simulation should inform educators about how other facets of the curriculum are preparing students to be successful in the simulated learning activity.
- To best evaluate student learning, quantitative measures must be used.
- Simulation evaluation must go beyond mere satisfaction with the simulation experience.
- With regard to curriculum and simulation integration, educators and curriculum planners should consider the following:
    - Total number of anticipated simulations
    - Evaluation of student learning
    - Evaluation of simulation experience
    - Evaluation of simulation program
    - Staffing plan and available resources
    - Faculty development (roles and responsibilities)
    - Evaluation of faculty facilitation (incorporation of best practices and faculty performance)

(continued)

> **BOX 2.2 Expert Exemplar (*continued*)**
>
> - The simulation should begin with the end in mind and build evaluation plans during the inception of simulation integration in order to better understand the effectiveness of simulation activities.
> - Evaluation of student confidence, performance, and competency, as well as satisfaction, should be used to assess all simulation experiences.
>
> *Source:* Tagliareni, E., & Forneris, S. (2016, August 26). Curriculum and simulation: Are they related? [Webinar]. In *NLN Nursing Education Speaker Series Fall 2016*. Retrieved from https://edsaleslww.webex.com/edsaleslww/lsr.php?RCID=24f72fad4c0ca9e858308a952dfc222f

president of the National League for Nursing (NLN) from 2007 to 2009. Her work continues to shape a more diverse and educated nursing workforce. In today's technology-rich environments, nurse educators need to be up to date on the latest innovations in simulation, e-learning, telehealth, and the integration of informatics into curricula. The NLN is renowned as an advocate for simulation and technology, has created simulation scenarios for use across curricula, and has pioneered nursing education webinars, as well as established an annual technology conference to support incorporating technology into all its initiatives. Dr. Forneris has expertise in simulation development and debriefing, combining her research on critical thinking with the development and implementation of simulation education. She is actively engaged in simulation research and has several publications focused on the development and use of reflective teaching strategies and the use of simulation.

In most institutions, nursing education administrators provide the foundation for technology exploration and integration by creating an institutional culture that embraces the use of technology. Infusion of technology as a tool to enhance learning should be supported as part of ongoing curriculum development. The process to integrate technology requires administrators who endorse ongoing faculty development, as well as involvement and support for the use of technology as a pedagogical tool.

Students are the end users of technology in the nursing curriculum. Effective technology integration is achieved when students are able to satisfy course and program outcomes through the direct use of technology tools. These tools must facilitate analysis and synthesis of information and help them apply what they have learned to their professional practice role. The technology should become an integral part of the learning process throughout the curriculum.

KEY POINTS

- This chapter offers an introduction to and understanding of a new conceptual model from which well-developed strategies for the integration of technology into nursing curricula can be framed.
- Administrators and faculty determine the use of technology within the curriculum; faculty and student needs drive the type and use of technology that is integrated into the teaching/learning process during curriculum development.

- Faculty, administrators, and students influence the FAST SIM©.
- To achieve successful integration of technology into the nursing curriculum, the FAST SIM© posits that equal attention must be paid to faculty, administrator, and student influences.

SUMMARY

A growing trend in nurse educator literature is the need to transform nursing education to include technology as a fundamental educational tool. The literature lacks specific integration strategies to assist with incorporating virtual learning technologies into nursing education, which are necessary when attempting the integration process. Conceptual models, such as the FAST SIM©, provide a framework for the development of effective communication as well as guidance for the technology integration process. To achieve successful integration of technology into the nursing curriculum, the FAST SIM© posits that equal appreciation and recognition must be given to faculty, administrators, and students as significant contributors to the technology integration process.

REFLECTIVE QUESTIONS

1. How would you describe the FAST SIM©? How might it be used to inform nursing curriculum development?
2. Think of the relationship between faculty, administrators, and students and reflect on the key influences in the FAST SIM©. How might greater or lesser emphasis on one or more of these contributing influences impact the integration of technologies with the nursing curriculum?
3. Reflect on the current state of technology integration in your academic institution. What are some of the major stumbling blocks that might preclude successful technology integration?

REFERENCES

Gore, T., & Thomson, W. (2016). Use of simulation in undergraduate and graduate education. *AACN Advanced Critical Care, 27*(1), 86–95. doi:10.4037/aacnacc2016329

Laurillard, D. (2013). *Rethinking university teaching: A conversational framework for the effective use of learning technologies* (2nd ed.). Abingdon-on-Thames, UK: Routledge.

Robinson, R., Molenda, M., & Rezabek, L. (2008). Facilitating learning. In A. Januszewski & M. Molenda (Eds.), *Educational technology: A definition with commentary* (pp.15–48). New York, NY: Routledge.

Spross, J. (2014). Conceptualizations of advanced practice nursing. In A. B. Hamric, C. M. Hanson, M. F. Tracy, & E. T. O'Grady (Eds.), *Advanced practice nursing: An integrative approach* (5th ed., pp. 27–66). St. Louis, MO: Elsevier.

Tagliareni, E., & Forneris, S. (2016, August 26). Curriculum and simulation: Are they related? [Webinar]. In *NLN Nursing Education Speaker Series Fall 2016*. Retrieved from https://edsaleslww.webex.com/edsaleslww/lsr.php?RCID=24f72fad4c0ca9e858308a952dfc222f

CHAPTER 3

Application of the Faculty Administrators Students Technology Strategic Integration Model© as the Basis for Integrating Virtual Educational Technologies

RANDY M. GORDON

LEARNING OBJECTIVES

Upon completion of this chapter, the reader will be able to:
- Explore factors that influence success and failure of technology integration strategies.
- Assess ways in which the Faculty Administrators Students Technology Strategic Integration Model© (FAST SIM) facilitates technology integration.
- Identify reasons and opportunities for integrating simulation into the nursing curriculum.

KEY TERMS

Active engagement
Assimilate technology
Asynchronous learning methods
Implementation
Interactive technology
Synchronous instruction
Technology integration

Success or failure of **technology integration** is largely dependent on factors beyond the technology. Integration should be seamless, efficient, and effective in supporting curriculum goals and purposes. The goal of flawless technology integration is a challenge for a myriad of reasons, not the least of which is that technology evolves and curricula develop. Application of the Faculty Administrators Students Technology Strategic Integration Model© (FAST SIM) does not guarantee a successful integration experience. The process of technology integration is one of continuous change, learning, and improvement. Furthermore, the manner by which the faculty and their institutional setting adapts to these changes plays a pivotal role in success.

FAST SIM© APPLICATION

It is sometimes difficult to describe how technology can impact learning because the term *technology integration* is a broad umbrella that covers many varied tools and practices; there are many ways technology can become an integral part of the learning process. The authors of this book define *technology integration* as the use of any technology to enhance and support the educational environment. Some might argue that the goal of technology integration is to completely redefine how we teach and learn and to do things that we never could before the technology was available (Puentedura, 2014). The FAST SIM© provides a framework for guiding the process of technology integration with the nursing curriculum. This chapter provides an overview of the key contributors to the technology integration process. It also offers suggestions as to how faculty, administrators, and students influence the process and identify opportunities to apply the FAST SIM©. Table 3.1 provides the reasons, as well as the opportunities, for incorporating technology in a nursing curriculum relevant to each contributing influence to the FAST SIM©.

Emphasis and appreciation for the importance and contribution from faculty, administrators, and students underpin the most significance tenet of the FAST SIM©. As stakeholders, faculty, administrators, or students may find relevance in applying the model from their own perspective or needs. Failure to recognize the significance of one or more of these contributors may jeopardize the success of a technology integration plan or strategy for learning. Figure 3.1 offers possible roles that faculty, administrators, and students may play in the integration process.

TABLE 3.1 Reasons and Opportunities for Integrating Technology Into the Nursing Curriculum

	Reasons and Opportunities for Technology Integration
Faculty	Increase in student engagement Improvement in the quality and variety of learning modalities Improvement in consistency among student experiences Methods of collecting/recording data Improvement in clinical judgment and decision making Opportunities for expressing understanding via multimedia Deliberate practice Healthcare technologies Team training Quality and safety Delegation Therapeutic and interprofessional communication
Administrators	Creation of partnerships with other institutions and clinical agencies Alignment of outcomes across programs and curriculum Development of simulation teams Support of the development of simulation leaders among faculty Reputation as a champion in the industry for innovation in education
Students	Improvement in communication between students and faculty Fostering of collaboration between students Social networking Support of the transfer of knowledge to practice Maximization of skills Access to up-to-date, primary source material

3: FAST SIM© AS THE BASIS FOR INTEGRATING VIRTUAL EDUCATIONAL TECHNOLOGIES 33

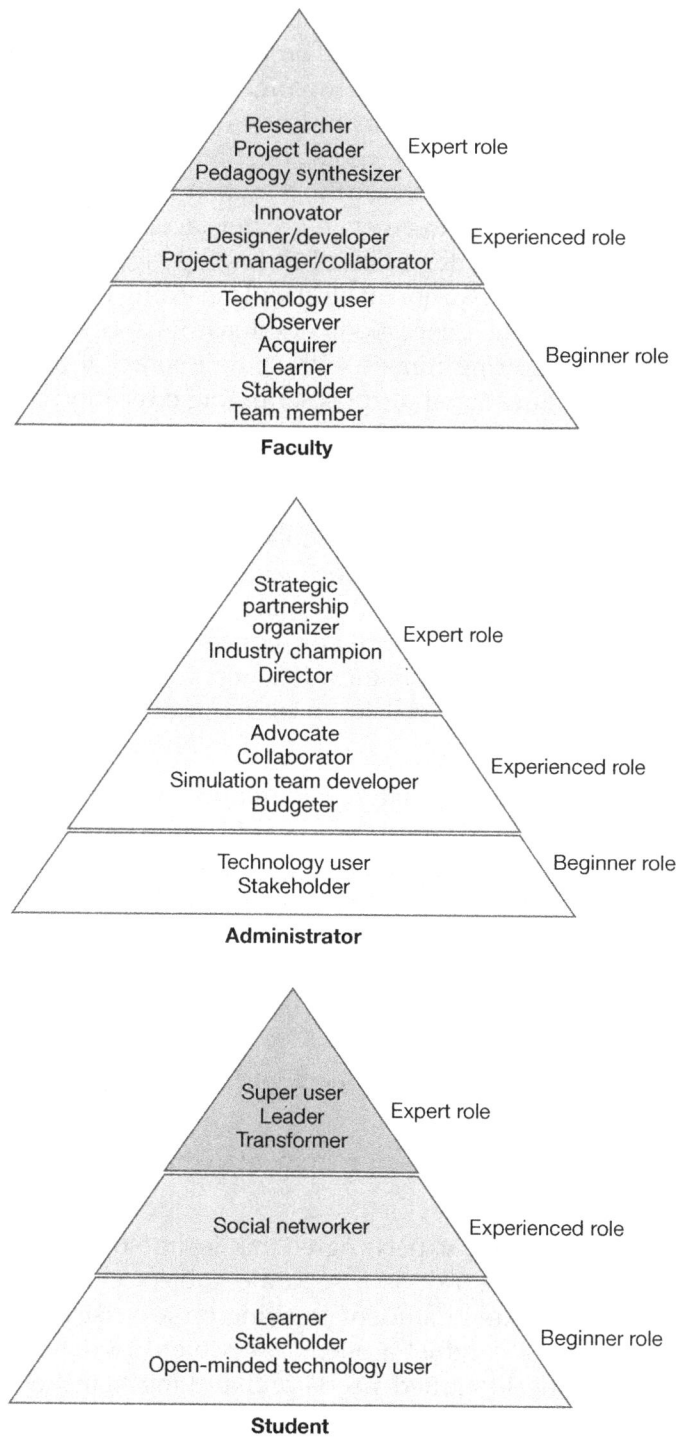

FIGURE 3.1 Faculty, administrator, and student roles.

FACULTY INFLUENCE

Nursing educators recognize that it is imperative to **assimilate technology** and education or risk becoming obsolete. For nurse educators, the learning environment paradigm must merge pedagogy, content, and technology to facilitate learning in the classroom (Wright & Davis, 2016). The need for technological fluency and competency among nursing educators is growing. This need coincides with a myriad of other issues in nursing education, including an educator shortage. The efforts needed to address shortage-related concerns, together with the burdens and stresses of learning a new technology, can increase the dissatisfaction with the nurse educator role and, in turn may contribute to an even greater faculty shortage. Nevertheless, arguments for supporting the integration of technology into teaching and learning are credible. With the rapid expansion of electronic learning environments, the need to bridge the gap between the generations of educators and learners is critical. By equipping and training aspiring nurses with contemporary technology and using clinical simulations for educational purposes, nursing education can help influence outcomes for the next generation. As new technologies emerge, instructional designers and educators have unique opportunities to foster interaction and collaboration among learners, thus creating a true learning community. With the impetus to expand the use of technology, faculty must be prepared to use available resources, have access to needed support, and develop competency for using resources and support throughout the curricula.

With regard to curriculum development, educators should have overarching goals for simulation integration strategies. Rea and Haas (n.d.) recommended the following overarching strategies relating to undergraduate and graduate nursing curricula:

- Enhance and promote patient safety and quality health care by advocating the use of simulation in the clinical education of healthcare professionals.
- Enhance the clinical competency of healthcare professionals.
- Assess and demonstrate the competency of undergraduate and graduate health care providers.
- Maintain the continuing competency of healthcare providers by using clinical simulation for continuing education.
- Improve the productivity and efficiency of healthcare professionals in clinical settings.
- Encourage research leading to improvement in the clinical education of healthcare providers.

Most educational technology experts agree that technology should be integrated across a program curriculum, not as a separate subject or ancillary activity, but as a tool to promote and extend student learning on a consistent basis (Wright & Davis, 2016). Faculty must conduct a needs assessment to determine appropriate solutions for meeting the identified needs and pulling stakeholders together to discuss their proposed integration strategy. After the adoption decision is made, they must prepare not only other faculty, but also students for its integration into the curriculum. The challenge, of course, is to find ways to use technology so as to not distract or detract students from essential topics. Technologies should provide opportunities to improve the quality and variety of teaching and learning that are not being achieved using current methods. Table 3.2 provides suggestions for technology tools that can be integrated with courses. This list is not inclusive.

TABLE 3.2 Technology Tools and Learning Advantages

Technology Tool	Advantages and Opportunities	Example
Online collaboration tools	Allows students and faculty to share documents online, edit them in real time, and project them on a screen. This gives students a collaborative platform in which to brainstorm ideas and document their work using text and images.	Google Apps
Presentation software	Enables instructors to embed high-resolution photographs, diagrams, videos, and sound files to augment text and verbal lecture content.	PowerPoint
Tablets	Tablets can be linked to computers, projectors, and the cloud so that students and instructors can communicate through text, drawings, and diagrams.	iPad
Learning/course-management tools	Allow instructors to organize all the resources students need for a class (e.g., syllabi, assignments, readings, online quizzes), provide valuable grading tools, and create spaces for discussion, document sharing, and video and audio commentary.	Canvas
Clickers, smartphones, and tablets	Provide a mechanism for surveying students during class, such as instant polling, which can quickly assess students' understanding and help faculty adjust pace and content.	Socrative
Lecture-capture tools	Allow instructors to record lectures directly from a computer, without elaborate or additional classroom equipment. Recorded lectures can be posted so that students may review them at their own pace.	Panopto

The use of web-based **synchronous instruction** has been shown to increase student engagement compared with exclusively **asynchronous learning methods**. Increased student engagement may improve learning outcomes and expand educational opportunities for students in the safety of a controlled environment versus a live clinical setting or classroom simulation. Table 3.3 provides examples of synchronous and asynchronous tools. Commonly used synchronous tools include:

- Audio and video conferencing for lectures, discussions, presentations, and meetings concerning complex issues
- Chat programs and instant messaging for quick communications and discussions of lesser complexity
- Whiteboard and application sharing wherein teams may develop ideas and create documents pertinent to group projects

Enhancing these methods with asynchronous tools can help sustain collaboration and intragroup dialogue while keeping resources available at all times despite students' differing schedules (Aebersold & Tschannen, 2013). Asynchronous methods include:

TABLE 3.3 Virtual Learning Tools

Synchronous	Asynchronous
Audio-video conferencing	Discussion forums
Online chat rooms	Blogging platform
Instant and text messaging	Podcasts/audio files
Whiteboards and screen sharing	Instructional videos
Webcasts	Prerecorded training modules
Virtual learning environments	Web-based coursework and lessons
	Virtual learning environments

- Discussion forums and emails that can track communication occurring over a longer time
- Blogging platforms where students can keep personal or group blogs
- Streaming media, such as podcasts or video, for instructors to communicate with students or students to communicate with one another
- Web-based training courses that can be useful and even popular for students with self-discipline and that include webbooks, document libraries, and a variety of media

Virtual learning environments (VLEs) may be used for both synchronous and asynchronous learning activities. VLEs are often used for the digital aspects of courses of study and allow participants to be organized into cohorts, groups, and roles; present resources, activities, and interactions within a course structure; provide for the different stages of assessment; report on participation; and have some level of integration with other institutional systems. A VLE may include some of the following elements:

- Course syllabus
- Administrative information about the course: prerequisites, credits, registration, payments, physical sessions, and contact information for the instructor
- Notice board for information about the ongoing course
- Basic content of some or all of the course; the complete course for distance learning applications, or some part of it, when used as a portion of a conventional course, normally including material such as copies of lectures in the form of text, audio, or video presentations, and supporting visual presentations
- Additional resources, either integrated or as links to outside resources, typically consisting of supplementary reading or innovative equivalents for it
- Self-assessment quizzes or analogous devices, normally scored automatically

- Formal assessment functions, such as examinations, essay submission, or presentation of projects, which now frequently includes components for supporting peer assessment
- Support for communications, including e-mail, threaded discussions, chat rooms, Twitter, and other media, sometimes with the instructor or an assistant acting as moderator, with additional elements including wikis, blogs, RSS, and three-dimensional virtual learning spaces
- Links to outside sources—pathways to all other online learning spaces linked via the VLE

VLEs may also provide a platform for the following functions:

- Management of access rights for instructors, their assistants, course support staff, and students
- Documentation and statistics as required for institutional administration and quality control
- Authoring tools for creating the necessary documents by the instructor, and, usually, submissions by the students
- Provision for the necessary hyperlinks for creating a unified presentation to the students.

A VLE may or may not be designed for a specific course or subject. It may be capable of supporting multiple courses over the full range of the academic program, giving a consistent interface within the institution or with other institutions using the system. The VLE supports an exchange of information between users and the learning institute they are enrolled in through digital mediums such as e-mail, chat rooms, web 2.0 sites, or a forum, thereby helping convey information to any part of the world with just a single click (Seale, 2009).

A particular type of VLE used to engage students is the simulation environment, which has also been referred to as "game-play." Although simulated environments have a longer history in aviation, the military, and the nuclear power industry, simulation is becoming an important part of nursing instruction at the novice level and continues to provide enrichment to career nurses as well (Aebersold & Tschannen, 2013). Aebersold and Tschannen reported improvement in patient outcome, safety culture, and self-assessment across key learning themes such as clinical techniques, diagnostic factors, safety techniques, and other areas. Simulation in virtual environments is continuing to prove effective as a teaching modality, and the results of some studies have demonstrated practical application. One example of a VLE is Second Life®, an open-access virtual environment used by nurse educators to develop competencies related to leadership and management skills. Box 3.1 provides an example of a feasibility pilot project conducted by graduate nursing program faculty to explore adding a VLE activity to the curriculum.

ADMINISTRATOR INFLUENCE

Nursing education administrators generally endorse ongoing faculty development and involvement in the area of distance education and the use of technology in the

> **BOX 3.1 Competency and Student Satisfaction With Problem-Based Learning in a Virtual Learning Environment**
>
> The aim of this pilot project was to assess feasibility and **implementation** of an innovative teaching tool in a nursing practitioner course. Students were asked to rate their perceived level of competency using a rating scale ("very poor," "poor," "fair," "good," and "very good") by completing a survey before and immediately following the Virtual Learning Environment (VLE) immersion learning activity. Students rated their perceived competency with obtaining pertinent patient data, communicating with intra/interprofessional team members, with using appropriate communication skills to interact with a patient, and with demonstrating clinical judgment and knowledge with respect to a list of differential diagnoses. All respondents rated their perceived competency to obtain pertinent patient information as "good" before and after the learning activity. Interestingly, although students rated their ability to use appropriate communication skills to interact with the patient as "good" or "very good" before the learning activity, respondents indicated their perceived competency as only "fair" or "good" following the learning activity in Second Life. Similarly, the students' rated their perceived competency to demonstrate clinical judgment and knowledge to establish appropriate patient diagnoses as "fair," "good," or "very good" before the learning activity; however, they changed their rating to "fair" or "good" after the immersion intervention.
>
> The Creighton Competency Evaluation Instrument (C-CEI) was developed for use as the evaluation instrument for both simulation and traditional clinical training experiences. Reliability and validity testing were established. The students were observed during an interactive patient learning activity and individual performance was rated using the C-CEI. In addition, the students completed a VLE satisfaction questionnaire to assess satisfaction with the virtual learning technology, Second Life, as well as their overall satisfaction with the learning experience. All respondents agreed that the VLE was user-friendly, useful in the course, aroused learning interest, and was effective in gaining knowledge.
>
> The findings suggested that some students reevaluated their level of competency or preparedness as a result of their performance during the learning activity. It should be noted that each student's performance met the evaluation score for competency with assessment and communication skills as observed by one of the researchers. This finding supports a possible discordance between the students' perceived and observed level of competency, which warrants further investigation.
>
> *Source:* Gordon, R., & Meeks, D. (2016, July). *Competency and student satisfaction with problem-based learning in a virtual learning environment.* Poster session presented at the International Nursing Association for Clinical Simulation and Learning Conference, Grapevine, TX.

teaching–learning processes. The nurse administrator's role is to ensure that technological systems are transformed effectively and that financial, ethical, and legal implications are considered (Ford, 2012). Technologies should reduce the administrative burden on teachers, thus allowing them to manage their workload more efficiently and give more time to the individual student's educational needs.

The National League for Nursing (NLN, 2015) promotes simulation as a teaching methodology to prepare nurses for practice across the continuum of care in today's complex health care environment. In *A Vision for Teaching with Simulation*, the NLN offered the following strategies to administrators of nursing programs:

- Create strategic partnerships with schools and clinical agencies to capitalize on shared simulation resources.
- Ensure an adequate number of dedicated simulation faculty with training and expertise in the pedagogy of simulation.
- Include operational support staff as a part of the simulation team.
- Budget annually for faculty development in simulation pedagogy and theory-based debriefing.
- Support the development of simulation leaders among the faculty (NLN, 2015, p. 6).

In addition to these strategies, administrators must inform student services, advisers, marketing, faculty, and students about the simulation goals and rationales for integration strategies.

STUDENT INFLUENCE

As educators seek to improve the quality of their curriculum and enhance the opportunities for improved educational activities, they face the challenge of meeting the needs of a diverse population that is more mobile and technology-savvy than any previous generation. The 21st-century learner requires educational opportunities that are not bound by time or place and that allow for interaction with the instructor and peers. Voice and video conferencing, virtual worlds, whiteboards, live presentation tools, application sharing, chats, and emails are just a few of the many tools available for interaction and collaboration. Blogs, wikis, and podcasts, as well as social software, are emerging technologies that foster the sense of connectedness between the members of a group.

From a student perspective, it is important to consider the balance of educational opportunities and the transferable skills intended to be gained by using a technology. Technologies should be specifically selected to maximize learning and skills development. As mentioned, the new generations of students have learning styles that are different from those of previous generations; therefore, integrating **interactive technology** helps meet the needs of students who are technology-savvy, cooperative team players and who gravitate toward group activities. Learning activities conducted using interactive technologies, including multiparticipant VLEs, promote **active engagement** and preferred learning experiences (Wright & Davis, 2016).

The student perspective is an integral influence on the FAST SIM© and may drive technology integration into the curriculum. One important factor in terms of success or failure of curricular integration of virtual technologies is student opinion. For example, if the users' expectations do not match the curricular use envisaged by the faculty or the options offered by the application itself, the possibility of a successful integration of virtual technologies in a nursing curriculum is limited (Botezatu, Hult,

& Fors, 2010). In one study, researchers posited that medical students must embrace learning with simulated patients for this teaching modality to be adopted successfully. Study results indicated that the complexity of the virtual patients used in this study appeared to be particularly well suited for learning and assessment purposes for early medical students who had not had significant clinical contact (Gesundheit et al., 2009). In another study conducted with nursing students, researchers sought to determine the student's perception of using a virtual patient-based assessment as a learning experience. Students reported that the virtual patient cases were realistic and engaging, which the researcher concluded was indicative of a high level of acceptance for this assessment method (Forsberg, Georg, Ziegert, & Fors, 2011). Other factors that influence how students perceive the use of simulated patients are encouraging students to be open-minded about their learning experiences, paying attention to the goals of the activity and providing a rationale for choosing the delivery modality for a particular learning activity.

Emerging technologies provide opportunities for student–student collaboration. Educators must acknowledge the need to foster social interaction through collaboration for the purpose of knowledge construction. By providing the opportunity for enhanced social interaction, pedagogical approaches are adjusted and new teaching modalities emerge. Learning activities that integrate technologies (such as blogs or wikis) may afford more learner control and thus may be more effective at delivering instructional strategies that support knowledge construction. Today's learners desire more control of the learning experience, as well as when and how they use it, which encourages educators to change outdated practices that no longer serve the needs of highly mobile students.

Mobile devices provide learners additional opportunities to collaborate, discuss content with classmates and instructors, and create new meaning and understanding (Hoffman, 2009). Furthermore, social media provides for collaborative and engaging opportunities for students (Pang, 2009). Cochrane and Bateman (2010) identified how the use of mobile devices can facilitate social constructivist pedagogies and engage students in learning opportunities. In this study, a sense of connectivity between students and instructors was developed by encouraging students to maintain constant connection to the Internet to blog about work progress, share photos, and communicate immediately using instant or text messaging. The inclusion of social media tools allowed students to collaborate and share with one another while learning. When integrated effectively into the curriculum, mobile devices can support a collaborative, constructivist approach to learning (Cochrane & Bateman, 2010; Liaw, Hatala, & Huang, 2010).

KEY POINTS

- The process of technology integration is one of continuous change, learning, and improvement, the success or failure of which depends on numerous factors.
- Equal emphasis and appreciation for the important influence of faculty, administration, and students underpin the most significant tenet of the FAST SIM©.
- Influence from faculty, administration, and students impacts the success of a technology integration plan or strategy.

- Educators should choose to use technologies to provide opportunities to improve the quality and variety of teaching and learning that are not being achieved using current methods.
- Administrators should create strategic partnerships that capitalize on shared simulation resources, ensure an adequate number of dedicated and appropriately trained simulation faculty, provide operational support staff, budget annually for faculty development in VLEs, and support the development of simulation leaders among the faculty.
- Students who are familiar with technology and thrive in a technology-rich culture are particularly equipped to be successful in simulation-based learning environments.
- The student perspective is an integral influence of the FAST SIM© and may drive technology integration into the curriculum, as well as its success or failure.

SUMMARY

The process of technology integration is continually shifting. Successful integration of technology into the nursing curriculum is contingent on a myriad of contributing factors, not the least of which is that technology and curriculum continue to develop. The FAST SIM© provides faculty, administrators, and students a foundation from which well-developed strategies for the integration of technology into a nursing curriculum can be framed. As stakeholders, faculty, administrators, or students may find relevance in applying the model from their individual perspective and particular needs. Paying particular attention to the influence and contribution from faculty, administrators, and students plays a significant role in the success of a technology integration plan or strategy.

REFLECTIVE QUESTIONS

1. Reflect on the growing reliance on technology in our daily lives and in the healthcare industry. Think of how technology in general is meant to enhance and improve our lives and healthcare. With regard to curriculum development, what are three reasons to integrate technology into the nursing education?
2. Technologies should provide opportunities to improve the quality and variety of teaching and learning that are not being achieved using current methods. What technologies might be better than current methods at providing opportunities for learning?
3. In what way might virtual learning technologies reduce the administrative burden on educators and why?
4. In today's technology-laden culture, for what reasons do you think students might be driven toward learning in a virtual environment? Conversely, what might detract students from learning in these environments?

REFERENCES

Aebersold, M., & Tschannen, D. (2013). Simulation in nursing practice: The impact on patient care. *Online Journal of Issues in Nursing, 18*(2). doi:10.3912/OJIN.Vol18No02Man06

Botezatu, M., Hult, H., & Fors, U. G. (2010). Virtual patient simulation: What do students make of it? A focus group study. *BMC Medical Education, 10*(1), 91–98. doi:10.1186/1472-6920-10-91

Cochrane, T., & Bateman, R. (2010). Smartphones give you wings: Pedagogical affordances of mobile Web 2.0. *Australasian Journal of Educational Technology, 26*(1), 1–14. doi:10.14742/ajet.1098

Ford, J. (2012). Facilitating the transformation of information technology: Strategies for nurse administrators. *Kentucky Nurse, 60*(3), 3–4.

Forsberg, E., Georg, C., Ziegert, K., & Fors, U. (2011). Virtual patients for assessment of clinical reasoning in nursing: A pilot study. *Nurse Education Today, 31*(8), 757–762. doi:10.1016/j.nedt.2010.11.015

Gesundheit, N., Brutlag, P., Youngblood, P., Gunning, W. T., Zary, N., & Fors, U. (2009). The use of virtual patients to assess the clinical skills and reasoning of medical students: Initial insights on student acceptance. *Medical Teacher, 31*(8), 739–742. doi:10.1080/01421590903126489

Gordon, R., & Meeks, D. (2016, July). *Competency and student satisfaction with problem-based learning in a virtual learning environment*. Poster session presented at the International Nursing Association for Clinical Simulation and Learning Conference, Grapevine, TX.

Hoffman, E. (2009). Social media and learning environments: Shifting perspectives on the locus of control. *In Education, 15*(2), 23–38. Retrieved from http://journals.uregina.ca/ineducation/article/view/54/532

Liaw, S., Hatala, M., & Huang, H. (2010). Investigating acceptance toward mobile learning to assist individual knowledge management: Based on activity theory approach. *Computers in Education, 54*, 446–454. doi:10.1016/j.compedu.2009.08.029

National League for Nursing. (2015). A vision for teaching with simulation. Retrieved from http://www.nln.org/docs/default-source/about/nln-vision-series-(position-statements)/vision-statement-a-vision-for-teaching-with-simulation.pdf?sfvrsn=2

Pang, L. (2009). A survey of web 2.0 technologies for classroom learning. *International Journal for Learning, 16*(9), 743–759.

Puentedura, R. (2014, December 12). Technology in education: An integrated approach [Web log post]. Retrieved from http://www.hippasus.com/rrpweblog/archives/000141.html

Rea, G., & Haas, B. (n.d.). *Simulation in nursing schools: Integrating simulation into nursing curriculum* [PowerPoint slides]. Retrieved from http://www.laerdal.com/in/usa/sun/pdf/indianapolis/rea_haas.pdf

Seale, J. (2009). Digital inclusion. Retrieved from http://www.tlrp.org/docs/DigitalInclusion.pdf

Wright, V. H., & Davis, A. (2016). Integrating technology in nurse education: Tools for professional development, teaching, and clinical experiences. In V. C. X. Wang (Ed.), *Handbook of research on advancing health education through technology* (pp. 23–38). Hershey, PA: IGI Global. doi:10.4018/978-1-4666-9494-1.ch002

Technology's Impact on Society and Culture

MICHAEL H. REITZEL

LEARNING OBJECTIVES

Upon completion of this chapter, the reader will be able to:
- Explore the integration of a virtual environment into a real-world classroom activity.
- Describe how to prepare learners for entering and enacting in the virtual environment of Second Life® (SL).
- Assess how virtual environments can be used to facilitate team-based assignments.

KEY TERMS

Avatar
Cyberspace simulation or cyber simulation
Face-to-face
Second Life® (SL)
Three-dimensional (3D)
Virtual environment
Virtual worlds

This chapter is an explanation and illustration of how the **Second Life® (SL)** virtual environment was used to provide a rich learning experience. In a general capstone course focused on *technology, society,* and *culture,* the description explained that the course investigates the connection among culture, society, and technology. The activities in the course help the student explore the cultural, social, political, ethical, environmental, and economic effects of integrating technologies into nursing curricula. Students must also identify concerns and deal with many appealing aspects of the impact technologies have on our culture and society. To engage students, instructors discuss many topics such as political impact, historical events that can be related to the integration of new ideas, concepts, or technologies, and the ethical dilemmas resulting from various technologies. These topics can be expanded to include art and other areas of interest to students to enhance their participation in the topics and the course; an especially pertinent portion of a course such as this could deal with technology and identity.

Students could be given a team project to be enacted and completed in SL. The subject of their project can vary from team to team, but it could serve to motivate the team to explore various aspects of the SL world and interact with the other people who inhabit that world.

RELATION TO THE FAST SIM©

The Faculty Administrators Students Technology Strategic Integration Model© (FAST SIM) is a conceptual model intended to impart a richer understanding of the relationships between key components when contending with the process of developing thoughtful and well-planned integration strategies. This chapter deals with the use of the SL **cyberspace or cyber simulation** to allow faculty to take students beyond the simulators owned by a college and explore the larger world in the SL environment. The intention is to show how the use of the broad world of the SL environment can add richness to the learning experience and can reveal the advantages of the **virtual environment**.

CONCEPTS OF A TYPICAL CAPSTONE COURSE

Some basic concepts should run through capstone courses as themes. These are touched on in various ways, depending on the subject being covered. This course could deal with the impact of technology on society, ethics, and culture in history and in the future.

The world has gone through many revolutions—political, economic, social, and cultural. Until now, there have been only two great technological revolutions that, in hindsight, were truly revolutionary: agricultural and industrial. Experts now talk of a third revolution in how we do things: the knowledge or information revolution.

Our relationship to technology is complex and ambivalent. Much of this is illustrated by the Prometheus mythology. The titan Prometheus stole fire from the gods and brought it down to Earth to give to humans. For this act, Prometheus was chained to a rock for all eternity, and an eagle would come daily to eat his liver, providing ongoing and eternal punishment for providing humans with fire. Technology represents fire here. The moral of the story is technology is a double-edged sword that cannot only bring benefits but also turn on us to harm or destroy us. This is captured by Mary Shelley's book, *Frankenstein, or the Modern Prometheus,* set in the 19th century, in which Dr. Frankenstein created a monster that turned on and destroyed him (Shelley, 1881). For a major part of the novel, the doctor and the monster are locked in a paranoid struggle for supremacy that ultimately leads to their mutual destruction. This represented the fear during the Industrial Revolution and the anticipation that humans' hubris in dealing with industrialization would result in their own demise. If we take this to be a statement about technology, it expresses both our ambition and our fear. It also expresses our distrust of our own creations. Genetically modified organisms (GMOs) are widely used in agriculture. When the anti-GMO movement wanted to come up with a particularly provocative name for genetically altered foods, they decided on "Frankenfoods," at once a reference to the story and recognition of its implications.

Another theme could be that the power of technology to solve our problems is an object of faith; since the dawn of the Enlightenment and the Industrial Revolution, technology, along with science, has in many ways displaced religion as the central belief system of Western culture. This is illustrated in history by the arrest of Galileo for heresy because he challenged the religious organization's pronouncement that the Earth is the center of the universe; today, science has declared global warming a fact, and it is modern "heresy" to question it.

One theme of this course must be that as our needs change, so does our technology, which, in turn, ultimately changes our way of thinking about life. How we use technology can vary and reflects our different perspectives and priorities. Technologies link all aspects of our lives together in a web of dependency. We are forever altered by our technology. How we are changed could be emphasized in this course.

STANDARD DELIVERABLES OF A CAPSTONE COURSE

In a capstone course, students should be divided into teams. Each team selects a technology and should be tasked to explore and research how that technology has or could impact society, ethics, and culture. In the traditional brick-and-mortar course, students could research these technologies and document their impact.

Each team identifies and explores an emerging technology. The technology may already exist but drew attention because of new applications, anticipated impacts, or potential controversies. Examples could include nanotechnology in manufacturing, GMOs, remote or robotic surgery, and wireless electricity. The teams would explore the technical, social, cultural, moral, and ethical issues presented by the technology. The project team could research a cultural or an ethical outcome of an adopted technology, a potential cultural or ethical outcome of a future technology, the general impact of a technological system on a part of society, or any combination of these; the research could emphasize not how the technology worked and all the things it could do, but how and to what degree our lives are or might be affected by it. The major deliverables in the course should involve a team presentation and a final team report.

INCORPORATING SL INTO A CAPSTONE COURSE

Courses such as this have always been intellectually stimulating and enlightening by opening a student's view of culture in unexpected ways. As an example, in one class, we discussed an article by Sherry Turkle titled, "Cyberspace and Identity" (Turkle, 1999), and a student prepared an excellent presentation discussing Turkle's assertion that the computer is a "second self" and that in this transformative identity, we can catch sight of our own images in the machine. In cyberspace, she discussed how we can step into **virtual worlds** that include other people who are also in their own virtual identity. One student demonstrated that the SL platform is a real example of Turkle's model. In that class, it became clear that students could experience other cultures by immersion in the SL virtual environment.

Once a student logs into SL, many new and otherwise inaccessible cultures can be experienced. People from around the world enter SL with their own avatar. People from business cultures log in. Sweden even has a virtual embassy, and many universities and corporations have space in the SL virtual environment. However, the largest opportunities for many organizations is the use of SL as a learning and collaborative tool. It uses technology to open a multitude of possibilities for students to learn how other cultures live and to provide a chance to gather their views as they work on their projects.

The addition of a course modification, adding SL activities, was presented to and approved by campus administrators. This innovative approach, and rich addition to the learning environment, was encouraged and integrated into the course. It was necessary to have the IT department install the SL viewer on the classroom computers and to train students on how to create avatars and to operate their avatars in the orientation area. Experience showed that it took 60 to 90 minutes in the first classroom meeting to get through this phase.

Instead of teaching this course as a traditional lecture/discussion, during the first week of the course, students were asked to register in SL and create avatars. For the instructions provided to students, refer to Table 4.1.

Students were given notice of what the SL virtual world is like. It is much like any online environment with some safe areas and some seedy areas. Students were instructed not to use money or register their names as adults. This kept them away from adult-oriented portions of SL that are not appropriate for

TABLE 4.1 Student Instructions for Entering Second Life

1. Go to www.secondlife.com and register for an avatar. Your avatar should have professional attire and behave appropriately at all times, which includes actions toward others.
2. You may download the Second Life (SL) Viewer or go to www.firestormviewer.org to get a better viewer.
3. By Week 3:
    a. Sign into SL.
    b. Go through orientation to learn how to operate in that environment.
    c. Never use any real money; this is a free service.
    d. Do not register as an adult.
    e. Behave appropriately at all times.
    f. Work as a team and locate and visit some areas in SL that are relevant to your group's overall topic.
    g. Gather information from those areas and talk to the people there.
4. In Week 5, your team will provide a report on your progress and discuss at least three areas of interest your team has located.
5. By noon on the day of scheduled class in Week 8, turn in a PowerPoint presentation of up to 10 slides that documents your visits and discussions. Turn this into the assignment drop box in Week 8.
6. In Week 8, we will NOT meet in our assigned campus classroom but will gather in SL to review these presentations. At this time, each team member should be prepared to explain a portion of the team's findings.

educational purposes. This is a **three-dimensional (3D), virtual world** where users are known as residents and choose avatars to represent themselves. An **avatar** is a graphical representation of the resident or user. The residents interact with each other and the environment using their avatars. On the basic level, an avatar can walk, run, sit, stand, and fly. It can also teleport or digitally change locations. Space can be rented and users may buy or develop virtual objects. This international playground has language translators. Think of it as a virtual platform for simulations that we can manipulate for our learners. As a virtual world or simulated environment, SL contains adult content and commercial and noncommercial solicitations, and the avatars might be guided by annoying or even offensive people.

It is possible for students to interact in a totally controlled simulator, without the threat or possibility of encountering dangerous people who may wish to interfere with the immersion experience. For this course, isolating students was not a viable option because we wanted them to explore and experience other technology-driven cultures. The best way to maintain safety was to instruct students not to use money and to avoid designation as an adult, which protected them from sordid environments.

Students are asked to behave appropriately at all times, including actions toward others and the attire chosen for their avatars. Because they were students, their avatars were expected to be professional. After they were divided into teams, students were strongly encouraged to work together and help one another as they created and became more skillful with their avatars. The professor acted as a mentor, but the teams of students formed rapidly, and those who were quickly adept at the SL technology were eager to help their team mates.

PRESENTATIONS IN SL

The teams of students finished the course by logging into SL in the last week of the course. The instructor and all the students met in a virtual classroom in SL, rather than in a real-world classroom. Each team of students created a 10-slide presentation that captured their experience in SL related to the technology of their team's assigned topic. The two exemplars presented in Boxes 4.1 and 4.2 illustrate student presentations.

KEY POINTS

- This chapter offers insight and perspective relating to technology's historical and projected future impacts on society, ethics, and culture.
- Training, guidance, specific instructions, and instructor and peer mentorships are effective strategies for improving student acclimation to virtual simulation, maintaining safety, and bolstering a positive learning experience.
- Once integrated with a capstone nursing course, virtual simulation was demonstrated to have enhanced the delivery of course content, added richness to the learning experience, and revealed the advantages of the virtual environment.
- Virtual simulation is an effective environment for team-based course assignments.

BOX 4.1 Technology and the Ethics of Surveillance in Second Life

Overview: One team of students examined the technology of surveillance and their experiences in the Second Life (SL) virtual environment.

Student Learning Experience: A team of five students was formed in Week 1 of the course, as would be done no matter how the course was being delivered. They were instructed to choose a technology to examine in the course, and this team chose surveillance. The team used the college library, the Internet, and other forms of secondary research as they prepared. They also worked individually and as a team in SL. One of the team members struggled with the technology and complexity of creating and operating her avatar, but in this small team environment, her team members successfully engaged and helped her. This is an intended element of small teams because it is well documented that such teams create cohesion and members form strong bonds that can lead to high performance (Dyaram & Kamalanabhan, 2005; Greenberg, Greenberg, & Antonucci, 2007; Levi, 2017). Members of strongly cohesive groups are more inclined to participate readily and to stay with the group (Dyaram & Kamalanabhan, 2005; Greenberg et al., 2007; Levi, 2017).

As the team explored SL, they learned more about surveillance technology, both in the real world and in the SL virtual world. They visited the SL homes of Sun Microsystems (Sun was acquired by Oracle in 2010 and has created Java, which a lot of applications need to run properly today), IBM, and Advanced Micro Devices (AMD; ranked eighth among semiconductor manufactures in revenue and the second-largest global supplier of microprocessors). It was clear that privacy concerns were real; even these companies were concerned about various governments and organizations stealing real-life conversations and private information.

Computer hard drives hold massive amounts of data and multiple file types; everything from pictures to chat logs can be stored. Chats between friends on a phone can be monitored or stored for later use. Text messages can be tracked and used as evidence in a trial. Computers are a huge part of our society. Granted, not everyone spends a lot of time on an actual computer, but people not on the computer are using other portable computer-based devices such as cell phones; even runners use distance calculators or GPS navigation devices while they run.

The team was a bit surprised how easy conversation had become in SL and continued their quest. In their travels, the team encountered an avatar and discussed surveillance with him.

The following is a short excerpt of a chat log conversation:

- *Team:* What do you think of surveillance and its national application in major cities and locations around the United States?
- *Avatar:* I find it strange that the government would allow this type of monitoring. I would think it is against the Constitution.

(continued)

> **BOX 4.1 Technology and the Ethics of Surveillance in Second Life (*continued*)**
>
> - *Team:* I see, but there are positives to having cameras and recorders in bigger areas. Like being able to catch criminals is easier with the use of cameras.
> - *Avatar:* Yeah, that is a good point, but how far will it go, where will it end?
> - *Team:* I understand what you are saying. When will a line be drawn between what is needed by the police and the right to privacy? What do you think of Surveillance in SL?
> - *Avatar:* I have heard stories of it going on. I just haven't seen any around.
> - *Team:* What if I told you it is being used the same way in SL as it is used in real life. To monitor people and to read their chat logs. As well as to gain access to other SL businesses.
> - *Avatar:* Wow. I was unaware it was being used like that in SL.
>
> The team visited SL vendors of surveillance technology. They discovered many surveillance tools. One vendor was the Thomas Conover group, which offered many products (www.thomas-conover.com/index.html).
>
> The team discovered TGS SECURITY CAMERA III. This realistic camera follows visitors and guests. It has a built-in alarm, can show a laser beam, and is controllable by a dialogue menu. When TGS SECURITY CAMERA III is touched by someone else, that person will get a warning in instant message (IM) and the alarm will activate. It can be used in and around the office. Cameras are everywhere. No privacy. The team exposed a surveillance tool that secretly tracks and records avatars.
>
> **Conclusion:** The team came to some conclusions: Real-life surveillance is used in almost all facets of society. It is used by businesses to control employees and customers. It is used by corporations to steal ideas and products from other corporations. Surveillance exists in several forms; examples are information surveillance, where information is taken from a secure or nonsecure part of a group, and physical surveillance, which are cameras or video recorders built to record photos or audio from locations. SL surveillance, much like real-life surveillance, is used by groups or companies to get information from other agencies. It is used to monitor customers to figure out items that are being purchased the most to maximize cash flow. It is used on a much smaller scale, for the most part, in SL, which mostly uses bugs, much like a real-life wire is used to obtain information (video and text).
>
> The team also had some overall observations about SL. Although the game is made up of computer parts, there are very few computers around. It seems that in SL people are almost more primitive. Fewer people are walking around talking on phones or sitting alone typing on computers. Nearly everyone is conversing, dancing, or flying around together. It is very strange to think about how the people, who are on the computer playing or are obviously attached to an electronic device, conduct themselves during immersion in SL.

(continued)

> **BOX 4.1 Technology and the Ethics of Surveillance in Second Life (*continued*)**
>
> It is the way people would behave in the real world if they were not continuously connected to a device.
>
> The team found the experience of being in SL change from difficult and unfamiliar at first to more natural and stimulating as they grew accustomed to the virtual environment. They felt that the surveillance in SL helped to make clear the real-world concerns. It also raised the question: Is SL a precursor of what might come about in real life? There is no simple causal chain. We construct our technologies, and our technologies construct us and our times. Turkle (1999) stated, "Our times make us, we make our machines, our machines make our times. We become the objects we look upon but they become what we make of them" (p. 643). Can the avatars we create and become in SL show who we are becoming in the real world? Is the polynational, technology-driven, fast-paced culture in SL indicative of how our world will look in the future? Is it clear that this rich environment can lead to a rich learning experience and show what areas might be best for something like SL?

> **BOX 4.2 Exploring and Discussing Technology and the Environment in Second Life**
>
> **Overview:** Another team of students aimed to conduct conversations with residents of Second Life (SL) about climate change and whether or not it is caused by humans. During the analysis phase of their experience, students recognized one of the course precepts that science has become our new religion.
>
> **Student Learning Experience:** This team of students was organized by the course faculty. Students had a range of experience and opinions, which made for an interesting team. They selected as their subject "Technology and the Environment." As expected, they became a cohesive team and had few issues preparing for their exploration of technology and the environment and their foray into SL. They realized that most of the team members were strong believers in climate change caused by humans, but a couple of team members did not hold that view. With this varied background, the team began their research and logged into SL.
>
> The first place the team found was Etopia Island. It is an Educational EcoVillage modeling a sustainable community, renewable energy, and organic products; it is located at http://maps.secondlife.com/secondlife/Etopia%20Island/170/84/23. This island is a showcase of environmentally friendly technologies and the businesses that specialize in them in the real world. All structures on the island are designed to be energy efficient, and the village also shows off public transportation ideas such as a light-rail train and a gondola. In addition, the island is a learning center on energy and environmental subjects. It showcases many sustainable

(continued)

> **BOX 4.2 Exploring and Discussing Technology and the Environment in Second Life** (*continued*)

approaches, including waste-water handling, mirrors for heat in third-world environments, and wind energy. One insight students gained from Etopia was that technology and the environment should work together and not adversely. To show this insight, students cited a poem by Emily Dickinson (n.d.) about how a train runs through the countryside.

The next island the team found was One Climate Island. This island was broken into five themes: earth, water, air, fire, and spirit. Each of these themes discussed environmental facts and issues, as well as alternative energy sources and the ways that they work. The island had links to other islands and websites on the same subject. The most exciting aspect of this island was a house of horrors that showed how much energy people waste. If a user clicked on the washing machine, for example, they were given a ride in it. Another island students found was Friends of the Earth Scotland (www.foe-scotland.org.uk)—Climate Change Island. This environmental group in Scotland helped pass the Climate Change (Scottish) Act.

A quote that was viewed as very valuable to students in this learning experience was by Janet Sawin (2003), who said, "Resistance to change is inevitable, but the world cannot afford to be held back indefinitely to those who are wedded to energy systems of the past" (p. 88). The team was asked to list choices for renewable energy. They named the following:

- Petroleum—limited resources
- Coal—but they questioned whether it was good for the atmosphere
- Nuclear power plants—Are they trouble or have they had bad press?
- Bio fuels
- Natural gas
- Wind energy
- Solar energy
- Geothermal energy
- Nanotechnology energy concepts

Conclusion: There was no agreement about whether climate change is caused by humans or is natural, although all team members concluded that the world has been warming. The team members in favor of human causes pointed to the report by the Intergovernmental Panel on Climate Change (IPCC) and its acceptance broadly in the world, including the Kyoto protocol (United Nations, 2014). Those who did not agree pointed to information from The Green Agenda (n.d.). This information demonstrated how the earth was much warmer in the past and that the warming trend began hundreds of years ago, before human-made carbon dioxide was in abundance. However, all team members agreed that there is an attitude about climate change that sounds like a religious tenet.

(*continued*)

> **BOX 4.2 Exploring and Discussing Technology and the Environment in Second Life** (*continued*)
>
> If someone admits in public they have questions, they are called *climate deniers* and can be harassed and punished much like they have committed a heresy. This was a realization that as technology has become a large part of our society; it is believed that these advances have replaced the church as the undeniable truth and that if anyone dares question the technology doctrine, they will suffer and be ostracized.
>
> The team also reflected on some SL experiences not directly related to technology and the environment. The three women liked to dress up and show off their avatars and explored many fashion places in SL. They said that SL is a three-dimensional (3D) world where everyone you see is a real person and every place you visit is built by people just like you and me. They explored many other interesting places, such as the Instituto Español, another educational arena; it displays various cultural articles of clothing and contains various artifacts, architectural designs, and sculptures (e.g., Cuba, Mexico). The Instituto Español even contains an area where meetings or various shows can be held. They visited the American Cancer Society sim. An interesting note is that this forum has embedded videos of personal stories and contains cancer facts on their documented walls. There is even an area where meetings and group sessions can be conducted. This demonstrates how engaged these students were in the environment. They were immersed and wanted to experience more than what was required for their assignment. One interesting place was the Louisiana State University (LSU) Science Center. This area represents LSU's Health Science Center in New Orleans that specializes in providing training and various medical simulations. They also discovered classrooms and forums where simulated presentations and medical procedures were presented for training purposes.
>
> SL brings an alternate virtual reality where students can visit and learn about other educational environments without being there physically. It also provides a space for learning, socialization, exploration, and creativity. Students eagerly share their perspectives on SL. This virtual world provides a rich and varied environment for students to learn in and explore. It is an entertaining and social source of experiences and exposure to other cultures. The students learned and had fun. Is it possible that the many exposures to other people's avatars and their cultures and differing points of view may have hastened and enriched the experience for the team of students? How remarkable is it that the team could not agree on whether climate change is caused by humans yet still came to conclusions that were valuable and insightful?
>
> The following student perspectives were shared:
> - Best and most challenging course
> - SL should be considered for all online courses
> - SL wa s difficult at first for students who did not know how to use computers but still a good experience

(continued)

> **BOX 4.2 Exploring and Discussing Technology and the Environment in Second Life** (*continued*)
>
> - Liked exploring the virtual world of SL and discovering great sites
> - Will continue to go into SL after the course ends
> - Did not like SL but see the benefits

SUMMARY

The SL experience added another dimension that further engaged the students. There is a learning curve, and some students are more adept than others. Students more comfortable in the SL virtual environment willingly assisted others who needed help in becoming comfortable with their avatars and the virtual world. It was evident that they were able to work together easily as a team and gained a wealth of information from exploring and discovering within the SL platform.

In this author's experience, students learn in a number of ways, but student–student interaction is one of the keys to excellent learning. That is an advantage of onsite classes with good faculty–student ratios but can be missing from online offerings, which can simply be many students doing individual studies where, except for a bit of discussion, they do not interact over the major course assignments.

Using a virtual environment like SL allows students to be remotely located and still have a **face-to-face** interaction. It requires simultaneous interaction, as opposed to the normal asynchronous online environment, but brings in the richness of student–student learning as well as an opportunity for a deep experiential experience from remote locations. Students have found this learning environment to be intriguing and enriching.

The world has become fast-paced and interconnected. Project teams at work are now starting to look like movie production teams, formed and launched, often to attack immediate, urgent, and important cross-functional issues. This is why we have aggressively incorporated a rich collaborative environment built on leading-edge technology to encourage creativity and grow a sense of responsibility in our students. This allows them to increase their interpersonal teamwork skills and helps them not only learn from the textbook and professor, but also share and learn from one another, which provides a deeper, richer, more durable learning experience.

> **REFLECTIVE QUESTIONS**
>
> 1. Consider the exemplars and determine how these activities could be enhanced and expanded.
> 2. How could you incorporate the personal excursions the students took to broaden their exploration of SL and go beyond the assignment outcomes?
> 3. Review the approach that was taken to incorporate SL into this course. Is this something that could occur at your institution?

a. If not, what are the barriers?

   b. If so, what would influence you to consider adding technology to your courses?

4. If you have explored integrating technology into your curriculum, how would you advise a new faculty member to approach the administrators and prepare themselves and students?

REFERENCES

Dickinson, E. (n.d.). I like to see it lap the miles. Retrieved from https://www.poetryfoundation.org/poems/56019/i-like-to-see-it-lap-the-miles-383

Dyaram, L., & Kamalanabhan, T. J. (2005). Unearthed: The other side of group cohesiveness. *Journal of Social Sciences, 10*(3), 185–190. doi:10.1080/09718923.2005.11892479

The Green Agenda. (n.d.). What about Greenland? Retrieved from http://green-agenda.com/greenland.html

Greenberg, P., Greenberg, R., & Antonucci, Y. (2007). Creating and sustaining trust in virtual teams. *Business Horizons, 50*(4), 325–333. Retrieved from http://onlineprograms.widener.edu/sites/wid/files/creating-and-sustaining-trust-in-virtual-teams_00_0.pdf

Levi, D. (2017). *Group dynamics for teams* (5th ed.). Los Angeles, CA: Sage. Retrieved from http://home.ubalt.edu/tmitch/650/Levichapters.htm#C5

Sawin, J. (2003). Charting a new energy future. *State of the World 2003.* New York, NY: W. W. Norton.

Shelley, M. (1881). *Frankenstein, or the modern Prometheus.* London, UK: Lackington.

Turkle, S. (1999). Cyberspace and identity. *Contemporary Sociology, 28*(6), 643–648. Retrieved from http://www.jstor.org/stable/2655534

United Nations. (2014). Framework convention on climate change: Kyoto protocol. Retrieved from http://unfccc.int/kyoto_protocol/items/2830.php

SECTION II

FACULTY PERSPECTIVE—PEDAGOGICAL APPLICATIONS AND SPECIFIC INTEGRATION STRATEGIES

Faculty are key components in the learning landscape. They are on the front lines dealing with students and their expectations, learning styles, literacy, and learning goals. Teachers must explore and recognize technology-based learning opportunities. Innovative faculty design technology-rich, learner-centered, authentic educational solutions that transforms the practice of education. In Section II, nine chapters address the influence faculty have in the Faculty Administrators Students Technology Strategic Integration Model© (FAST SIM) and the integration of instructional technologies (Figures II.1 and II.2).

In Chapter 5, the authors discuss the use of virtual simulation in nursing education and the incorporation of a methodology that provides consistent educational experiences and feedback in an affordable, accessible manner. The education of nurses and nursing students is enhanced through the integration of virtual technology in a number of ways, including the use of clinical practicum hours, clinical experience consistency, standardized feedback, virtual patient (VP) assessment, and deliberate practice of clinical skills. Opportunities for the use of virtual simulation in nursing education are vast, and the advantages for this teaching pedagogy are clear.

Chapter 6 describes educational technologies that provide opportunities to bridge the gap between theory and practice; however, integration comes with challenges. This chapter explores factors that can negatively impact the adoption of educational technologies, especially virtual simulation. Barriers related to faculty, administrators, students, and the technologies themselves are examined, and exemplars provide examples of successful and unsuccessful integrations of simulation technologies with lessons learned. Faculty and student buy-in can make or break an integrative technology strategy.

Chapter 7 describes an online graduate program that supports students in their executive practicum within Second Life® (SL), a virtual learning platform, to gain real-life experiences to prepare them to be nursing leaders. Faculty developed the content for this course and are involved with students throughout the completion of their practicum. The inclusion of SL as an alternative practicum site was specifically intended to assist students who resided in remote areas or places where a qualified mentor was not available to assist them in completing their practicum course. The integration of a virtual learning environment (VLE) for graduate virtual world practicum (VWP) students has been a success based on student, faculty, and mentor feedback.

Chapter 8 describes how to prepare the instructional environment to teach with simulation. The key components of the FAST SIM© are examined in terms of the challenges they faced and the ways to educate or train through successful engagement in virtual simulation. Legal, financial, and infrastructure issues are identified, and ways to manage them are explained.

Chapter 9 presents information for educational designers, faculty, and staff who endeavor to introduce game-based teaching and learning into the curriculum; it has an introduction to how and why game-based learning provides motivation for learners and evaluation for educators as well as a framework for its implementation. This chapter briefly reviews traditional experiential learning theory to support nursing education and, more discretely, simulation-based teaching and learning within nursing and other forms of clinical education as an anchor for the introduction of contemporary theory specifically envisioned to support the integration of game-based teaching and learning into nursing curricula. The authors also address evaluation as it relates to student and curriculum outcome.

Chapter 10 describes virtual gaming simulation (VGS) as a novel pedagogical approach that combines virtual simulation and serious gaming. Learners are immersed in safe, interactive, and simulated experiences that resemble real life to enrich and deepen learning. In this chapter, an overview of VLEs and tools are provided, followed by discussion of two VGS exemplars, including challenges encountered in design, resolution considerations, and lessons learned. Empirical work helps establish best practice guidelines and standards for the use of this novel educational strategy.

Chapter 11 reviews the games have been used for education in the past to create a climate of fun and excitement, encouraging students' sense of competitiveness and curiosity. Today, with advanced technology and various devices becoming popular even in developing countries, serious games (SGs) are an upcoming trend. An updated systematic review of the literature combines outcome information related to SGs or games for learning (the terms are used interchangeably). Researchers using virtual games recognize that player characteristics, game features, and the context of the play variable all influence game outcomes and require further development. In addition, studies examining skill-acquisition outcomes were more common with higher-quality randomized controlled trials (RCTs) in health. SGs are educational games that use *fun* to engage students while also incorporating entertainment components, as animated and motivating resources, to support the learning experience. Advantages include that once created, SGs can be reused and that students have an opportunity to make mistakes in a safe environment.

In Chapter 12, the authors discuss the use of LVLEs for simulation. Two learning experiences that pertain to nursing education and technology integration are addressed in this chapter. The first learning experience in a virtual world addresses triage, and the second concerns assessment of environments. Simulation in nursing is one of many methods used for teaching students. Teaching and learning in a VLE has many advantages for administrators, faculty, and students. One of the advantages includes use of other disciplines to help create or participate in a VLE. Virtual worlds provide faculty with a way of presenting possible real-life scenarios without risk of injury to participants. Flexibility in creating learning experiences in a virtual world also has the advantage of providing variation for students.

Chapter 13 reminds us that clinical simulation has changed significantly over the last three decades. The emergence of resuscitation manikins in the 1960s led to increasingly complex, high-fidelity equipment able to mirror aspects of the clinical world. However, scenarios and simulations need to integrate the myriad of complex and demanding aspects of a clinical setting, taking into account the technical and nontechnical aspects of healthcare. The introduction of virtual simulation programs enables safe repetition of practice in standardized scenarios that, if rigorously developed, can support validity and reliability. It is importantly to realize that this form of delivery is increasingly feasible with web-based access and may reduce face-to-face instructor time. In this chapter, the authors focus on enhancing rigor across five stages of development of virtual simulation programs, drawing on our experience of developing a patient deterioration management program known as Feedback Incorporating Review and Simulation Techniques to Act on Clinical Trends (FIRST2ACT) and a web-based simulation version called FIRST2ACTWeb. Each scenario is based on a video recording of a simulated patient.

The faculty influence in the FAST SIM© is reflected in this section. While reviewing chapters in this section, readers should reflect on how faculty influence in the model can be applied to the integration of technology in their specific teaching and learning context.

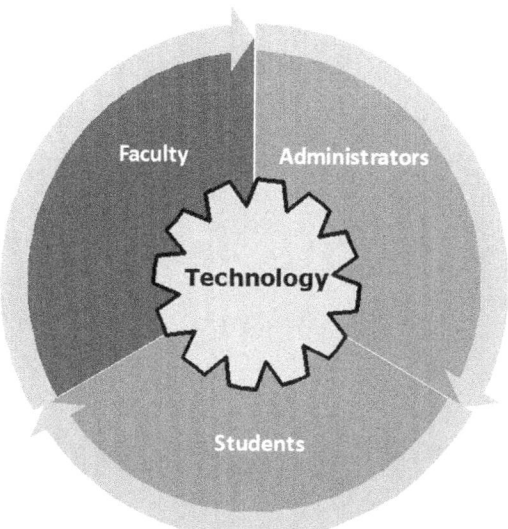

FIGURE II.1 Components of FAST SIM© (Faculty Administrators Students Technology Strategic Integration Model).

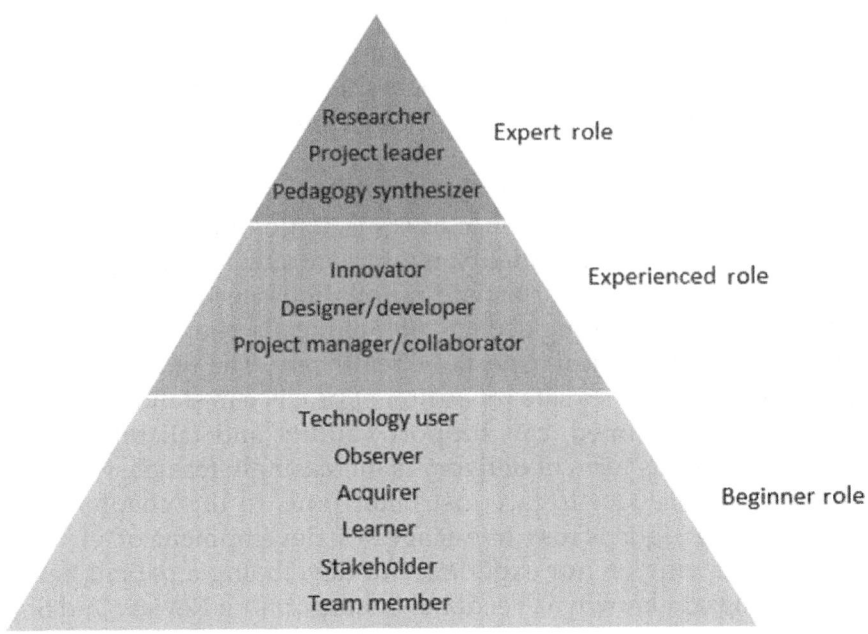

FIGURE II.2 Faculty roles.

CHAPTER 5

Opportunities and Advantages With Virtual Technology Integration

MEGAN KEISER AND CARMAN TURKELSON

LEARNING OBJECTIVES

Upon completion of this chapter, the reader will be able to:
- Assess the advantages of virtual technology integration for nursing education.
- Explore opportunities for the use of virtual technology in nursing education.

KEY TERMS

Deliberate practice
Feedback
Interprofessionalism
Nursing education
Simulation

Standardized feedback
Technology-enhanced healthcare simulation
Virtual learning environment (VLE)
Virtual patient (VP)
Virtual simulation

The use of virtual simulation in nursing education has been increasing in the past decade, but the evaluation of advantages of and opportunities for virtual technology integration and **technology-enhanced healthcare simulation** has only been explored in a fragmented manner as educators publish their own experiences with this educational pedagogy. The use of virtual simulation in nursing education incorporates a methodology that provides consistent educational experiences and feedback in an affordable, accessible manner. The education of nurses and nursing students is enhanced through the integration of virtual technology in a number of ways, including the use of clinical practicum hours, clinical experience consistency, standardized feedback, **virtual patient (VP)** assessment, deliberate practice of clinical skills, remote collaboration, interprofessional education, and **interprofessionalism**. The use of virtual strategies for educating nursing students provides experiences for them to integrate theory and practice and also provides safe, effective, enjoyable, and cost-effective experiential learning opportunities that are consistent with the learning styles of the millennial generation (Bonnel, Fletcher, & Wingate, 2007; Foronda & Bauman, 2014; Verkuyl, Hughes, Tsui, Betts, St-Amant, & Lapum, 2017). This chapter explores the opportunities and advantages of virtual simulation and the integration of virtual technology in nursing education.

RELATION TO THE FAST SIM©

The Faculty Administrators Students Technology Strategic Integration Model© (FAST SIM) was presented in Chapter 2 as a framework for guiding technology integration in **nursing education**. At the center of the model is technology. This chapter focuses on the opportunities and advantages of virtual technology integration for nursing education, so support is provided as to the importance of technology as the center point of the FAST SIM©. The definition of *educational technology* within the FAST SIM© is the study and ethical practice of facilitating learning and improving performance by creating, using, and managing appropriate technological processes and resources (Robinson, Molenda, & Rezabek, 2007). This definition guides the exploration of technology integration into nursing education because it informs the importance of how and why technology should be integrated. By providing information and evidence related to the advantages of virtual technology integration in nursing education, as well as exploring the many opportunities for its integration, this chapter strengthens the position of technology as an integral part of the FAST SIM© and as an appropriate pedagogical method in nursing education.

CLINICAL PRACTICUM HOURS

One of the many advantages of **virtual simulation** is in its ability to create and manage a scenario similar to that which nursing students are exposed to in a traditional clinical setting. Obtaining clinical sites for student practicums has become progressively more challenging due to increased enrollments and a larger pool of academic nursing programs (Foronda & Bauman, 2014). Online options in virtual worlds are becoming more appealing as nursing programs struggle to provide quality clinical practicum hours in the face of decreased availability of clinical sites. The National Council of State Boards of Nursing (NCSBN) commissioned a study, which took place from Fall 2011 through Spring 2013, that assessed nursing students for whom **simulation** was used as a substitute for traditional clinical practicum hours. This study examined whether the time and activities in a simulation laboratory could effectively substitute for traditional clinical hours in the prelicensure nursing curriculum (Hayden, Smiley, Alexander, Kardong-Edgren, & Jeffries, 2014). The study provided "strong evidence supporting the use of simulation as a substitute for up to 50% of traditional clinical time" (Hayden et al., 2014, p. S36). However, all simulation activities reported in this landmark study were in a simulation laboratory with no virtual simulation activities being evaluated.

As a result, to justify the use of virtual simulation activities as a substitute for traditional clinical practicum hours, one must turn to evaluating exemplars in the literature. Foronda and Bauman (2014) reviewed strategies to incorporate virtual simulation. They suggested many ways to integrate virtual simulation into nursing education, including web-based instruction, augmentation of lectures, formative assessments, high-stakes testing, high-risk situations, documentation, and clinical practicum. They also suggested that virtual simulation can be developed for all clinical experiences, including community health and leadership. One example can be seen in Ross and Crusoe's (2014) creation of a virtual health system to be used for leadership clinical experiences. Although the only data presented was in the form of narrative comments on course evaluations, the virtual health system was felt to represent a viable option for leadership clinical practicum hours (Ross & Crusoe, 2014). Another example of the use of virtual simulation as a substitute for clinical practicum hours was provided by Tilton, Tiffany, and Hoglund (2015) as they explored the use of virtual simulation to prepare students to care for the chronically ill. The authors used the virtual reality (VR) environment of Second Life® (SL) in a mixed-methods study and concluded that "virtual simulation has good potential for addressing and closing the gap in clinical nursing education associated with learning about chronic care management in community-based settings" (p. 395).

Aebersold, Tschannen, Stephens, Anderson, and Lei (2012) provided another example describing virtual simulation using SL as a strategy for learning in a "clinical arena" and highlighting the "opportunity to simulate emergent, complex situations in a nonthreatening, safe environment" (p. e469). This exemplar is presented in greater detail in Box 5.1. One important finding from this exemplar was that students felt that their experience in the **virtual learning environment (VLE)** was as good as or better than their experiences with high-fidelity simulators in the simulation laboratory. This more recent research suggests that virtual simulation may be as effective as laboratory-based simulation (Aebersold et al., 2012; Youngblood et al., 2008) and that a high level of fidelity can be established through virtual experiences (Irwin & Coutts, 2015).

CLINICAL EXPERIENCE CONSISTENCY

An unfortunate reality of the traditional clinical environment (e.g., hospital, health care agencies) is that faculty cannot control the experiences that nursing students will be exposed to in their clinical practicums. Although most nursing clinical faculty plan ahead as to which patients students are assigned, unforeseen events often happen that prevent students from getting the planned clinical experience or skills. Simulation allows nursing faculty to control the experiences and clinical skills that students are exposed to during their clinical practicum hours. In addition, both laboratory and virtual simulation clinical experiences can be delivered with consistency, facilitating the evaluation of clinical skills and performance. In fact, virtual gaming simulation (VGS) has been used to expose students to a consistent clinical experience in mental health nursing that involves interpersonal violence assessment and intervention (Verkuyl et al., 2017). This experience was felt to be best presented in a virtual environment because of the unpredictable nature of the exposure students will have to this topic in a traditional clinical setting, as well as the potential volatile nature of the scenario. The VGS was felt to represent a much-needed consistent clinical experience, and it was determined that VGS was a safe and effective method of nursing education (Verkuyl et al., 2017).

Further research has shown that virtual simulation can optimize the ability of nursing students to consistently apply theoretical knowledge to a clinical scenario. Georg and Zary (2014) developed a learning activity with VPs that supported nursing students in applying scientific knowledge ane integrating theory and practice into clinical situations. They concluded, "Virtual patients that are adapted to the nursing paradigm can support nursing students' development of clinical reasoning

> **BOX 5.1 Using Second Life as an Educational Strategy**
>
> - The University of Michigan School of Nursing designed and implemented a virtual hospital unit in Second Life (SL) to integrate virtual simulation into the curriculum.
> - The hospital was named Wolverine Hospital and the unit that the students were in for their clinical experience had eight beds.
> - Three virtual simulations were developed and were completed by senior nursing students.
>   - Safety issues with medication and adverse events—scenario involved an intravenous antibiotic that was infused on the wrong patient.
>   - Difficulty with interprofessional communication—scenario involved an altercation with a physician over a patient who was fed despite the fact that he was supposed to be NPO for a procedure.
>   - Priority setting—scenario involved assessing four different patients, prioritizing their needs, and delegating appropriate tasks to assistive personnel.
> - Student performance was evaluated using a standardized tool.
> - The students felt that the experience in the virtual environment was as good as or better than their experiences with high fidelity simulators in the simulation laboratory.
> - The students reported some struggles with the speed of the text chat function when in the virtual environment because it was slow especially for students with poor typing skills—students wanted the ability to talk to each other as well as with the other avatars in the simulation.
> - The main recommendation from this study is that "the SL platform may also provide avenues for learning in the clinical arena for a multitude of health care professionals" (p. e474).
>
> *Source:* Aebersold, M., Tschannen, D., Stephens, M., Anderson, P., & Lei, X. (2012). Second Life®: A new strategy in educating nursing students. *Clinical Simulation in Nursing*, 8(9), e469–e475. doi:10.1016/j.ecns.2011.05.002

skills" (Georg & Zary, 2014, para 5). They stated that these skills must be consistently taught in the context of clinical and experiential learning. Cant and Cooper (2014) reiterated that one of the main advantages of virtual simulation (e-simulation) is that it enables controlled and predictable outcomes, which keeps the clinical experience consistent over time for all students. Bryant, Miller, and Henderson (2015) also reported that "virtual patients permit a standardized clinical simulation environment with a consistent experience to practice and assess skills" (p. 438). There is growing support in the literature that virtual simulation, through a variety of virtual technology platforms, can provide consistent clinical experiences for nursing students, which in turn creates a consistent method for evaluating the clinical skills and performance of students.

STANDARDIZED FEEDBACK

The support for consistency of simulation-based learning experiences (SBLE) for students also extends to the **feedback** that students receive. Simulation-based instruction typically provides students with specific feedback related to their performance (Söderström, Häll, Nilsson, & Ahlqvist, 2015). "Feedback provides learners with information about their performance with the goal of improving their performance" (Hatala, Cook, Zendejas, Hamstra, & Brydges, 2014, p. 252). Many virtual simulation platforms offer **standardized feedback** on completion of the SBLE. One example is Digital Clinical Experience™, which allows students to view a report page containing information as to which clinical findings were identified or missed by the student (Bryant et al., 2015). Another example is vSim® for Nursing™, which allows students to interact with VPs and receive direct feedback and a score on their individual performance (Foronda et al., 2016).

One potential issue with standardized feedback is that it often provides only feedback as to what students did right or wrong and does not delve into the "why" or the reflective process that is recommended following simulation by the International Nursing Association for Clinical Simulation and Learning (INACSL) Standards of Best Practice: Simulation℠ Debriefing (INACSL Standards Committee, 2016). Although standardized feedback is seen as an advantage of virtual simulation, debriefing must also occur following the simulation experience to offer participants the opportunity to reflect on their virtual clinical experience. The debriefing should be carried out by a trained debriefer and should also be based on a theoretical framework for debriefing that is structured and purposeful (INACSL Standards Committee, 2016). This debriefing can be accomplished face-to-face or in a virtual setting such as Skype™ or GoToMeeting™. Standardized individual feedback within the virtual simulation platform, coupled with group debriefing, assists in optimizing the student's learning.

ACCESSING AND ASSESSING VPs

One of the most appealing features of virtual simulation platforms is their accessibility. In this technological age, online options for the assessment of VPs are seen as favorable, especially by the generation of college students known as millennials. Ellaway and colleagues defined a VP simulation as "an interactive computer simulation of real-life clinical scenarios for the purpose of health care and medical training, education or assessment" (Ellaway, Poulton, Fors, McGee, & Albright, 2008, p. 173). VPs allow participants to complete potentially dangerous activities in a manner that is not only safe, but also accessible (Kidd, Knisley, & Morgan, 2012). High-risk activities are best performed in simulation to prevent harm to patients as students learn the skills required. One example is a study performed by Kidd and colleagues (2012), who used Second Life to teach nursing students how to perform mental health assessment. The patients were readily accessible in this virtual world and faculty did not have to worry that students would say the wrong thing to an emotionally fragile patient during their assessment. These researchers concluded that "SL simulation has real potential as an effective tool for mental health nursing education—accessible, convenient, and safe for skills experimentation" (Kidd et al., p. 37). It has also been demonstrated that assessing VPs who were adapted to the nursing paradigm supported the development of clinical reasoning skills by nursing students (Forsberg, Ziegert, Hult, & Fors, 2016; Georg & Zary, 2014). As a result of the accessibility of VPs, students can be exposed to more clinical scenarios than they would be in a traditional clinical setting with real patients. This allows students to assess a large number of patients in a readily accessible, safe, and controlled environment (Georg & Zary, 2014; Kononowicz et al., 2016).

DEVELOPING PROFICIENCY WITH CLINICAL SKILLS

To become proficient in performing hands-on clinical skills, nursing students require many opportunities for **deliberate practice**. Once considered optimal for practice of clinical skills, task trainers are now being compared to VR simulation for skills training. "Virtual reality (VR) based training is an efficient and effective methodology for learning manual skills" (Choi, He, Chiang, & Deng, 2015). For example, researchers have studied a VR-based simulator for learning nasogastric tube (NGT) placement. The VR training system was perceived positively by nurses who felt that the computer-generated forces were similar to those experienced in NGT placements on actual patients (Choi et al., 2015). As such, this VR trainer could be used to train nursing students on NGT placement prior to them attempting this skill on actual patients.

In another study, a randomized trial was performed comparing methods of teaching intravenous (IV) cannulation (also known as *IV starts*) using a VR/haptics IV simulator vs. an IV arm task trainer vs. the IV arm with the IV simulator. The researchers concluded that although there was no difference in skill acquisition among the groups, the group that was able to practice with the VR/haptics IV simulator before demonstrating the skill on the IV arm had the best outcomes (Jung et al., 2012). These examples further support the idea that VR allows for safe and repetitive (deliberate) practice (Georg & Zary, 2014), which has been shown to facilitate skill acquisition.

VR has also been used to train nursing students for clinical situations that they may encounter. Ulrich, Farra, Smith, and Hodgson (2014) used VR to teach decontamination in a disaster situation. Using qualitative data, these researchers demonstrated that a "VR simulation decontamination experience was a positive, fun, and safe way to learn the skill of decontamination" (Ulrich et al., 2014, p. 552). Kalisch and colleagues used virtual simulation to improve nursing teamwork. Teamwork and communication are most certainly skills that nursing students must learn prior to entering the workforce as RNs. The three scenarios developed using SL included avatars representing different health care providers (e.g., staff nurse, charge nurse, nursing assistant) who are placed in situations requiring teamwork to manage a patient care issue. Although the participants' actual knowledge of teamwork principles did not improve, the witnessed teamwork behaviors did (Kalisch, Aebersold, McLaughlin, Tschannen, & Lane, 2015). Each of these examples lends further support to the idea that virtual simulation allows for accessible, safe, and deliberate practice of nontechnical skills such as disaster training and teamwork.

REMOTE COLLABORATION AND INTERPROFESSIONAL SIMULATION

Tthe accessibility of virtual simulation makes it a valuable tool for facilitating remote collaboration and opportunities for interprofessional education (IPE). Using virtual simulation removes many of the barriers that exist when attempting to provide opportunities for experiential learning to online students, as well as to an interprofessional group of students (Foronda & Bauman, 2014). Virtual simulation can also reduce or eliminate the geographical barriers for students in online education programs, as well as for those who do not live close to campus. It also allows for the participation of groups of students who may not live close to one another (Duff, Miller, & Bruce, 2016). Breen and Jones (2015) explored the use of a virtual community with community health nursing students in an RN-to-BSN program. Students were asked to complete three scenarios: clinical reasoning, disaster nursing, and coalition building for homeless veterans. "The primary goal of the activities was for the students to demonstrate a broader knowledge base to include abilities in leadership, health policy, system improvement, research and evidence-based practice, teamwork, collaboration, and a greater orientation toward community-based care" (Breen & Jones, 2015, p. 32). The researchers concluded a virtual community to facilitate experiential learning was an effective strategy for the use of technology to support learning and practice in nursing (Breen & Jones, 2015). Attempting to create opportunities for experiential learning for students in online education programs is challenging. The use of virtual simulation platforms has been shown to be a viable option for experiential learning with online students.

Interprofessional simulation in a virtual environment allows students from various healthcare programs to come together for the purpose of interprofessional collaboration while caring for the same VP situation. Research on the use of virtual simulation for interprofessional healthcare education is presented as an exemplar in Box 5.2. Caylor, Aebersold, Lapham, and Carlson (2015) used virtual simulation and a modified Team Strategies and Tools to Enhance Performance and Patient Safety (TeamSTEPPS) training program to provide IPE for nursing, pharmacy, and medicine students. SL and Skype were theplatforms used by interprofessional student teams to collaborate, communicate, and provide care for a patient who had been exposed to a medical error (Caylor et al., 2015). Again, students in this study felt SL provided an effective mechanism for interprofessional learning with multiple users (Caylor et al., 2015). Furthermore, students felt that using the virtual platform reduced stress, was realistic, and offered a convenient option for learning (Caylor et al., 2015).

Similarly, SIMULATIONiQ™ IPE from Education Management Solutions (EMS) has the unique ability to replicate interprofessional delivery of patient care over time by allowing multiple learners from different healthcare professions to participate in virtual team practice. SIMULATIONiQ IPE operates using a web-based, multiuser virtual environment that allows learners access anywhere, anytime, from their personal computers, tablets, or phones, as often as they would like, potentially expanding the audience and increasing the frequency of team training. SIMULATIONiQ IPE also enables the faculty to create individual role-based cases, establish evaluation criteria, assign teams, create assignments, and review the progress of learners. Learners are able to engage with team members at a time convenient for the team, communicate and collaborate through a discussion

> **BOX 5.2 Use of Virtual Simulation for Multiprofessional Education**
>
> - Students from medical, nursing, and pharmacy programs participated in a virtual simulation in Second Life (SL) using a modified TeamSTEPPS training program.
> - Team Strategies and Tools to Enhance Performance and Patient Safety (TeamSTEPPS) was developed by the Agency for Healthcare Research and Quality (AHRQ) to integrate teamwork and communication practices into healthcare teams with the goal of improving the quality, safety, and efficiency of healthcare.
> - The objectives of this project were (a) to examine the usefulness and effectiveness of SL in multiprofessional education, (b) to evaluate the student attitudes and perceptions toward teamwork and communication in multiprofessional education, and (c) to evaluate an evidence-based training program as the foundation of the multiprofessional curriculum for students working in interprofessional teams (p. 165).
> - Student participants independently completed an online modified TeamSTEPPS training module as a pre-simulation activity.
> - Student teams were then formed with representation from students in each discipline.
> - The scenario focused on communication rather than discipline specific skills to promote interaction from all team members.
> - At the beginning of the simulation each student was provided with a virtual notecard providing discipline specific information about the patient situation.
> - Each discipline received different information to deliberatelyencourage communication and collaboration among the team members.
> - The students were instructed to meet in SL using their avatars to represent themselves. After introductions were made, the team had 5 minutes to review their patient case prior to going to the patient room to address the patient and family.
> - After the simulation was completed, a debriefing was completed with the team and the faculty.
> - Overall, this pilot project was a successful learning opportunity that is likely to be beneficial to many of the participants. Students indicated that they enjoyed interacting and learning with other health disciplines. This learning experience positively impacted student attitudes related to multiprofessional learning and working in teams (p. 169).
>
> Source: Caylor, S., Aebersold, M., Lapham, J., & Carlson, E. (2015). The use of virtual simulation and a modified TeamSTEPPS™ training for multiprofessional education. *Clinical Simulation in Nursing, 11*(3), 163–171. doi:10.1016/j.ecns.2014.12.003

forum, and participate in a team debriefing session, sharing critical reflections after completion of the patient case scenario. Through the use of the virtual simulation platform SIMULATIONiQ IPE, students can log into the system from any location and complete the deliberate practice activities as assigned. Deliberate practice opportunities using virtual simulation provide reinforcement for the process of diagnostic reasoning, collaboration, communication, and teamwork required for the clinical practice of nursing and other health professions (Duff, Miller, & Bruce, 2016).

KEY POINTS

- This chapter explored the opportunities and advantages of virtual simulation and the integration of virtual technology in nursing education.
- The use of virtual simulation in nursing education has been increasing in the past decade, and there is emerging evidence supporting the numerous benefits of this creative pedagogical approach in nursing education.
- Because of variations in virtual simulation strategies and research, there is a need for rigorous, high-quality implementation studies to further validate this innovative approach.

SUMMARY

Opportunities for the use of virtual simulation in nursing education are vast, and the advantages for this teaching pedagogy are clear. The use of virtual simulation for clinical practicum hours, clinical experience consistency, standardized feedback, VP assessment, deliberate practice of clinical skills, remote collaboration, and IPE has been explored and is supported. Virtual simulations in nursing education use technology to provide safe and realistic SBLEs for nurses and nursing students. These virtual SBLEs may be used to learn new skills that may require both high-order thinking and psychomotor elements. They may also be used to assess skill competency, as well as to assess low-volume, high-risk skills. Virtual simulation is a creative approach that provides interactive, engaging instruction. Virtual simulation, VPs, and virtual worlds are all valid tools applicable to nursing education in both the academic and practice setting (Schwartz, 2017). Although evidence supports ease of use, interactivity, accessibility, and cost-effectiveness, further study is needed to solidify virtual simulation as a teaching pedagogy in nursing education.

REFLECTIVE QUESTIONS

1. How may virtual simulation be used to substitute for traditional clinical experiences?
2. What are some of the advantages of using virtual simulation in this way?
3. What should be included in feedback received by students after virtual simulation experiences, and how should it be delivered?
4. How would the use of virtual simulation permit remote collaboration and enhance interprofessional clinical experiences?

REFERENCES

Aebersold, M., Tschannen, D., Stephens, M., Anderson, P., & Lei, X. (2012). Second Life®: A new strategy in educating nursing students. *Clinical Simulation in Nursing, 8*(9), e469–e475. doi:10.1016/j.ecns.2011.05.002

Bonnel, W., Fletcher, K., & Wingate, A. (2007). Integrating geriatric resources into the classroom: A virtual tour example. *Geriatric Nursing, 28*(5), 301–305. doi:10.1016/j.gerinurse.2007.02.004

Breen, H., & Jones, M. (2015). Experiential learning: Using virtual simulation in an online RN-to-BSN program. *Journal of Continuing Education in Nursing, 46*(1), 27–33. doi:10.3928/00220124-20141120-02

Bryant, R., Miller, C. L., & Henderson, D. (2015). Virtual clinical simulations in an online advanced health appraisal course. *Clinical Simulation in Nursing, 11*(10), 437–444. doi:10.1016/j.ecns.2015.08.002

Cant, R. P., & Cooper, S. J. (2014). Simulation in the Internet age: The place of Web-based simulation in nursing education. An integrative review. *Nurse Education Today, 34*(12), 1435–1442. doi:10.1016/j.nedt.2014.08.001

Caylor, S., Aebersold, M., Lapham, J., & Carlson, E. (2015). The use of virtual simulation and a modified TeamSTEPPS™ training for multiprofessional education. *Clinical Simulation in Nursing, 11*(3), 163–171. doi:10.1016/j.ecns.2014.12.003

Choi, K. S., He, X., Chiang, V. C. L., & Deng, Z. (2015). A virtual reality based simulator for learning nasogastric tube placement. *Computers in Biology and Medicine, 57*, 103–115. doi:10.1016/j.compbiomed.2014.12.006

Duff, E., Miller, L., & Bruce, J. (2016). Online virtual simulation and diagnostic reasoning: A scoping review. *Clinical Simulation in Nursing, 12*(9), 377–384. doi:10.1016/j.ecns.2016.04.001

Ellaway, R., Poulton, T., Fors, U., McGee, J. B., & Albright, S. (2008). Building a virtual patient commons. *Medical Teacher, 30*(2), 170–174. doi:10.1080/01421590701874074

Foronda, C. L., & Bauman, E. B. (2014). Strategies to incorporate virtual simulation in nurse education. *Clinical Simulation in Nursing, 10*(8), 412–418. doi:10.1016/j.ecns.2014.03.005

Foronda, C. L., Swoboda, S. M., Hudson, K. W., Jones, E., Sullivan, N., Ockimey, J., & Jeffries, P. R. (2016). Evaluation of vSIM for Nursing™: A trial of innovation. *Clinical Simulation in Nursing, 12*(4), 128–131. doi:10.1016/j.ecns.2015.12.006

Forsberg, E., Ziegert, K., Hult, H., & Fors, U. (2016). Assessing progression of clinical reasoning through virtual patients: An exploratory study. *Nurse Education in Practice, 16*(1), 97–103. doi:10.1016/j.nepr.2015.09.006

Georg, C., & Zary, N. (2014). Web-based virtual patients in nursing education: Development and validation of theory-anchored design and activity models. *Journal of Medical Internet Research, 16*(4), e105. doi:10.2196/jmir.2556

Hatala, R., Cook, D. A., Zendejas, B., Hamstra, S. J., & Brydges, R. (2014). Feedback for simulation-based procedural skills training: A meta-analysis and critical narrative synthesis. *Advances in Health Sciences Education, 19*(2), 251–272. doi:10.1007/s10459-013-9462-8

Hayden, J. K., Smiley, R. A., Alexander, M., Kardong-Edgren, S., & Jeffries, P. (2014). The NCSBN national simulation study: A longitudinal, randomized, controlled study replacing clinical hours with simulation in prelicensure nursing education. *Journal of Nursing Regulation Education, 5*(2), S3–S40. Retrieved from http://mtcahn.org/wp-content/uploads/2015/12/JNR_Simulation_Supplement-2015.pdf

International Nursing Association for Clinical Simulation and Learning Standards Committee. (2016, December). INACSL standards of best practice: Simulation^SM debriefing. *Clinical Simulation in Nursing, 12*(Suppl.), S21–S25. doi:10.1016/j.ecns.2016.09.008

Irwin, P., & Coutts, R. (2015). A systematic review of the experience of using Second Life® in the education of undergraduate nurses. *Journal of Nursing Education, 54*(10), 572–577. doi:10.3928/01484834-20150916-05

Jung, E. Y., Park, D. K., Lee, Y. H., Jo, H. S., Lim, Y. S., & Park, R. W. (2012). Evaluation of practical exercises using an intravenous simulator incorporating virtual reality and hapics device technologies. *Nurse Education Today, 32*(4), 458–463. doi:10.1016/j.nedt.2011.05.012

Kalisch, B. J., Aebersold, M., McLaughlin, M., Tschannen, D., & Lane, S. (2015). An intervention to improve nursing teamwork using virtual simulation. *Western Journal of Nursing Research, 37*(2), 164–179. doi:10.1177/0193945914531458

Kidd, L. I., Knisley, S. J., & Morgan, K. I. (2012). Effectiveness of a Second Life® simulation as a teaching strategy for undergraduate mental health nursing students. *Journal of Psychosocial Nursing and Mental Health Services, 50*(7), 28–37. doi:10.3928/02793695-20120605-04

Kononowicz, A. A., Woodham, L., Georg, C., Edelbring, S., Stathakarou, N., Davies, D., . . . Zary, N. (2016). Virtual patient simulations for health professional education (protocol). *Cochrane Database of Systematic Reviews, 2016*(5). doi:10.1002/14651858.CD012194

Robinson, R., Molenda, M., & Rezabek, L. (2007). Facilitating learning. In A. Januszewski & M. Molenda (Eds.), *Educational technology: A definition with commentary* (2nd ed., pp. 15–48). London, UK: Routledge

Ross, A. M., & Crusoe, K. L. (2014). Creation of a virtual health system for leadership clinical experiences. *Journal of Nursing Education, 53*(12), 714–718. doi:10.3928/01484834-20141120-03

Schwartz, L. (2017). Virtual simulations: A creative, evidence-based approach to develop and educate nurses. *Creative Nursing, 23*(1), 29–34. doi:10.1891/1078-4535.23.1.29

Söderström, T., Häll, L., Nilsson, T., & Ahlqvist, J. (2015). Computer simulation training in health care education: Fueling reflection-in-action? *Simulation & Gaming, 45*(6), 805–828. doi:10.1177/1046878115574027

Tilton, K. J., Tiffany, J., & Hoglund, B. A. (2015). Non-acute-care virtual simulation: Preparing students to provide chronic illness care. *Nursing Education Perspectives, 36*(6), 394–395. doi:10.5480/14-1532

Ulrich, D., Farra, S., Smith, S., & Hodgson, E. (2014). The student experience using virtual reality simulation to teach decontamination. *Clinical Simulation in Nursing, 10*(11), 546–553. doi:10.1016/j.ecns.2014.08.003

Verkuyl, M., Hughes, M., Tsui, J., Betts, L., St-Amant, O., & Lapum, J. L. (2017). Virtual gaming simulation in nursing education: A focus group study. *Journal of Nursing Education, 56*(5), 274–280. doi:10.3928/01484834-20170421-04

Youngblood, P., Harter, P. M., Srivastava, S., Moffett, S., Heinrichs, W. L., & Dev, P. (2008). Design, development, and evaluation of an online virtual emergency department for training trauma teams. *Simulation in Healthcare, 3*(3), 146–153. doi:10.1097/SIH.0b013e31817bedf7

Challenges and Disadvantages With Virtual Technology Integration

REBECCA A. BURHENNE, KRISTIN A. KERLING, AND RANDY M. GORDON

LEARNING OBJECTIVES

Upon completion of this chapter, the reader will be able to:
- Analyze the challenges of integrating educational technologies into nursing education associated with faculty, administrators, and students.
- Examine practical and philosophical barriers related to technology integration.
- Explore challenges unique to the adoption of virtual simulation.

KEY TERMS

Cybersickness
Digital divide
Technological resistance
Technological solutionism
Technostress

Healthcare is in a state of rapid change. Although practice environments have become more complex, educational delivery methods have remained stagnant (Scully, 2011). Both the American Association of College of Nursing (AACN; 2015) and the Institute of Medicine (IOM; 2011) have encouraged nursing programs to explore the expanded use of innovative educational approaches, especially simulation. Innovative technologies provide opportunities to enhance nursing student learning and help nursing programs become more responsive to changes in the practice environment; however, obstacles may hinder successful implementation.

RELATION TO THE FAST SIM©

Each facet of the Faculty Administrators Students Technology Strategic Integration Model© (FAST SIM) provides a window to potential challenges. Faculty characteristics and beliefs play a role in whether or not technologies are accepted and used to the optimal extent. Even when faculty support the use of educational technologies, administrative backing is crucial to success. Concerns about cost, staffing, or the fit of the technology to the program's culture may inhibit administrative support. Students may lack the interest or resources necessary to engage with nontraditional teaching strategies. The rapid pace of technological change, as well as the absence of research support for some educational technologies, may lead to hesitation about the adoption of technological tools, particularly virtual simulation. This chapter explores some of the general challenges associated with the integration of innovative educational technologies, as well as some challenges unique to virtual simulation.

FACULTY

"Innovative curricula, with a focus on concepts rather than content, technology, simulation, and flexible pathways are critical to answering the call for curriculum reform" (Phillips et al., 2013, p. 1). Nursing faculty buy-in is crucial to the successful integration of educational technologies. Innovations offer new opportunities for nursing education to respond to changes in healthcare; however, gaining faculty buy-in for curriculum revision and technology integration can be problematic. Nurse educators, especially those with training in curriculum development, are in short supply (AACN, 2017). Many nurses who enter nursing education are expert clinicians but lack formal preparation to teach or participate in scholarship. The increased use of part-time faculty and decreased availability of full-time faculty positions puts more pressure on existing full-time faculty, making the process of technology integration more challenging (Nardi & Gyurko, 2013). Lack of faculty time and the sense of already being overwhelmed with other obligations contribute to delays in the adoption of new technologies (Fiedler, Giddens, & North, 2014). Many part-time faculty juggle multiple positions at several institutions, which may lead to limited investment in one particular college or university or limited availability for training in the use of new technologies. Faculty may struggle to justify the time commitment required to incorporate new technologies or virtual learning tools into courses that are already written, are not undergoing revision, or are being taught successfully using traditional methods.

If technologies are not integrated thoughtfully, with an eye on best practices, they could become more of a distraction than a tool. Tacy, Northam, and Wieck (2016) noted that faculty make use of new technology when they perceive it as easy to use and useful for teaching. Unfortunately, most faculty lack expertise in the selection and application of appropriate hardware and software. Some faculty members also lack confidence in the effectiveness of educational technologies. Faculty struggle to engage with teaching modalities when they feel unsupported by administration or peers (Box 6.1).

ADMINISTRATORS

Although faculty buy-in is critical to be successful, technology integration must have sufficient organizational support. Adoption of new pedagogies requires congruence

---

BOX 6.1 Tips to Overcoming Technology Integration Challenges for Faculty

- Ensure appropriate time for learning.
- Provide sufficient administrative support.
- Identify faculty champions to assist with buy-in.

with institutional mission and philosophy, as well as accrediting body requirements. Organizations with traditional leadership or models of instruction may struggle to provide the support and approval necessary for success. When faculty have strong administrative support, they are empowered to take on the commitments associated with the integration of innovative curriculum; however, in today's educational climate, organizations face competing demands for resources (Phillips et al., 2013). Owing to rising costs and increased demands for fiscal responsibility, tremendous economic pressure exists in higher education (Altbach, Gumport, & Berdahl, 2011). Innovation is expensive. Whereas the use of some social media platforms are free, most other educational technologies are not. Purchase of products developed by outside vendors could be costly and may incur contractual fees. Once technologies are selected, organizations must ensure that internal resources can support the change. Additional faculty with expertise in technology or simulation may be needed. Expansion of information technology (IT) services could be necessary to provide faculty and student support. Students and faculty require training in the use of technologies. Some products include training modules, but the development of additional modules may be necessary. Faculty need time to become proficient with new tools. Administrators may need to provide coverage for regularly contracted teaching responsibilities. Even with strong administrative support, with the speed of technological change, there is a risk that technologies will become obsolete before full integration (Box 6.2).

STUDENTS

Student factors may be a barrier to the successful curricular integration of educational technologies. Not all students demonstrate the same technological aptitude or interest. Generational differences may affect student desire to engage with apps or social media for educational purposes. Urso and Fisher (2015) noted the appeal of educational technologies to Millennial and Generation X learners but pointed out that older students may have a difficult time embracing nontraditional methods of instruction. Another consideration is the increased proportion of nontraditional students enrolled in postsecondary education. According to the National Center for Education Statistics (2017), up to 80% of students enrolled in 4-year undergraduate programs in 2016 were considered nontraditional students. Nontraditional students often have more responsibilities outside of the classroom than traditional students, leaving them little time to learn new technologies. Students may have financial constraints or challenges with computer literacy that limit their desire to use technologies (Zayim & Ozel, 2015). With the addition of multiple learning modalities, student overload could occur. Students may experience behavioral or psychological consequences because of increased exposure to information and

---

BOX 6.2 Tips to Overcoming Technology Integration Challenges for Administrators

- Advocate for innovation.
- Provide faculty support for empowerment.
- Explore strategies for cost containment.

> **BOX 6.3 Tips to Overcoming Technology Integration Challenges for Students**
> - Consider student workload and technology savviness.
> - Assess potential impact of the digital divide.
> - Provide skill assessment and support for students.

communication technologies (Lee, Son, & Kim, 2016). Faculty need to be sensitive to the time constraints students may feel and weigh the benefits and burdens of new educational technologies.

Technologic specifications of educational technologies may pose problems for students. In 1999, the United States Department of Commerce (USDoC) identified a concern related to disparities in access (USDoC, 1999). The USDoC described a **digital divide** between those with and without access to new technologies. Factors involved in the divide included location, family income level, level of education, and ethnicity. Although some communities have made progress in reducing the digital divide, ongoing gaps remain between urban and rural populations (USDoC, 2016). Rural residents are less likely to use the Internet from home or own Internet-compatible devices. Broadband services may be cost prohibitive or unavailable. Faculty may assume that all students have the same level of access, but students may not have the ability to participate, especially in virtual technologies. Before initiating technology-based approaches to teaching, faculty must consider whether students have the resources to participate (Box 6.3).

TECHNOLOGY

The selection of the right technology is essential for successfully meeting learning outcomes (Decker, Sportsman, Peutz, & Billings, 2008). Faculty and administrators must assess the proposed technology's compatibility with existing educational delivery methods. The impact of technology integration on those involved must be considered prior to execution (see Table 6.1). Lack of thoughtful implementation sabotages success.

Extreme philosophies related to the use of educational technologies may create barriers to innovation. Some educators display **technological resistance** owing to the uncertainty about appropriate applications for technological resources or lack of research support for the value of technology in education (Howard, 2013). Even when research support exists, some faculty resist the use of educational technology, feeling that it is superfluous and detracts from learning. Fears of students' multitasking or engaging in off-task activities during learning time may impede acceptance of new modalities. At the other extreme, the indiscriminate inclusion of educational technologies can be detrimental. **Technological solutionism** is the belief that every problem has a technology-based solution and that technological advances will save society (Morozov, 2013). Faculty who embrace technological solutionism may implement a wide variety of modalities without considering whether they are appropriate to meet learning outcomes or whether there is enough research to support the technologies.

Even when faculty and students support innovation, overstimulation from technostress may still occur. Weil and Rosen (1997) define **technostress** as an adaptation

> **TABLE 6.1 Factors That Influence Successful Implementation of Education Technology**
>
> - The degree to which faculty can make sense of the need for the innovation
> - The innovation's fit with current curriculum
> - The organization's priorities
> - Organizational support at the time of the innovation and following

Source: Iriti, J., Bickel, W., Schunn, C., & Stein, M. K. (2016). Maximizing research and development resources: Identifying and testing "load-bearing conditions" for educational technology innovations. *Educational Technology Research and Development, 64,* 245–262. doi:10.1007/s11423-015-9409-2

problem in which individuals struggle to cope with adjustments to and use of technology. People experiencing technostress are unable to adapt to the use of technology in a healthy manner (Tacy et al., 2016). Technostress occurs when users are intimidated by a technology or do not receive sufficient orientation or support. Faculty experiencing technostress exhibit lower levels of job satisfaction and are less likely to pursue adoption of innovative technologies in the future (Tacy et al., 2016). Glitches may occur during the integration of new educational technologies. When technological applications are not intuitive or technical support is lacking, the resulting stress may lead to abandonment of the change. Excitement may be replaced by withdrawal or dissatisfaction if the user becomes frustrated by a technology (Harder, Ross, & Paul, 2013). Faculty and students may also disengage if there is no clear connection between educational technologies and outcomes.

VIRTUAL SIMULATION

In 2014, a study by National Council of State Boards of Nursing Simulation supported the replacement of up to 50% of traditional clinical experiences with simulation in prelicensure nursing education (Hayden., Smiley, Alexander, Kardong-Edgren, & Jeffries, 2014). Many programs are moving toward the use of simulation, including virtual simulation, to replace a percentage of required traditional face-to-face clinical experiences. Although research support exists for the inclusion of virtual simulation in prelicensure nursing education, support for its use is limited in advanced nursing education. A concern with existing research is study design. Hansen and Bratt's review of the literature (2015) noted that studies demonstrated simulation-related increases in student knowledge, self-efficacy, confidence, and satisfaction; however, results relied on students' self-assessments. Self-assessments may not be congruent with actual performance. Further research must be conducted using objective methods of clinical performance assessment. Adamson and Kardong-Edgren (2012) noted three reliable, validated evaluation instruments that could be used to assess student learning outcomes in human patient simulation (HPS)—the Lasater Clinical Judgement Rubric, the Seattle University Evaluation Tool, and the Creighton Simulation Evaluation Instrument. In virtual reality simulations, some platforms have built-in reliable, validated clinical evaluation tools. For example, the Student Performance Index in Shadow Health collects data regarding certain aspects of student performance during virtual simulations, which decreases the amount of subjectivity in clinical educator assessments (Jiminez, Kleinheksel, & Kotranza, 2015). A gap exists in the nursing literature related to whether attainment of competence within simulation translates to better patient care and outcomes (Adamson & Kardong-Edgren, 2012; Decker et al., 2008). Even with research support, some faculty believe that simulation cannot replace hands-on experience with live patients. Dunnington (2014) noted that no matter how high fidelity a simulation is, human responses are more complex and qualitatively different than simulated experiences.

The virtual learning environment poses unique challenges. Users may resist the use of virtual environments due to lack of computer skills, lack of desire to participate in a world that is not "real," time constraints, resistance to change, and unwillingness to learn new technologies (Hermanns & Kilmon, 2012). Wiederhold and Wiederhold (2014) noted potential unintended consequences of the use of virtual reality in the treatment of anxiety, including postural instability, visual fatigue, and **cybersickness.** LaViola (2000) described cybersickness as a collection of motion sickness–type symptoms experienced by people using virtual reality (see Table 6.2). Symptoms may last for hours or days. Some organizations use virtual reality to practice disaster preparedness or trauma training. Students with exposure to comparable events may experience distress or trauma when participating in simulated scenarios. Box 6.4 offers suggestions to overcome virtual simulation integration challenges surrounding technology.

TABLE 6.2 Symptoms of Cybersickness
• Eye strain
• Headache
• Pallor
• Sweating
• Dryness of mouth
• Fullness of stomach
• Disorientation
• Vertigo
• Ataxia
• Nausea
• Vomiting

Source: LaViola, J. J. (2000). A discussion of cybersickness in virtual environments. *SIGCHI Bulletin*, 32, 47–56. Retrieved from https://www.deepdyve.com/lp/association-for-computing-machinery/adiscussion-of-cybersickness-in-virtual-environments-AweEgZm4sG

BOX 6.4 Strategies to Overcoming Virtual Simulation Integration Challenges
• Develop strategies to reduce technostress.
• Participate in professional organizations that promote simulation, such as the International Nursing Association for Clinical Simulation and Learning (INASCL).
• Engage in simulation research.

KEY POINTS

- Curricular innovation is necessary for responding to changes in health care.
- Barriers exist to the integration of educational technologies
- Factors critical to success include the following:
  - Faculty and student buy-in
  - Administrative support and resources
  - Appropriate technology selection
  - Adequate time for implementation and training
- Ongoing research regarding the uses and efficacy of educational technologies is required.

SUMMARY

With the increasing complexity of today's health care environment, innovations in nursing curricula are necessary. Both the AACN (2015) and the IOM (2011) support the expanded use of educational technology; however, integration is multifaceted. Boxes 6.5 and 6.6 provide examples of challenges faced by nursing programs. Consideration of the following challenges are essential for increasing the likelihood of successful integration:

- **Faculty:** Absence of faculty buy-in to the adoption of new technologies because of lack of skills, resources, or interest makes effective use of educational technologies unlikely.
- **Administrators:** Cost, staffing constraints, and level of organizational commitment impact the administrative support available for integration of innovative educational technologies.
- **Students:** Students' lack of skill, equipment, access, or interest related to educational technologies impact the effectiveness of technologies.
- **Technology:** Philosophical barriers inhibit adoption; expense, rapid pace of change, and lack of research support may dampen enthusiasm for virtual simulation.

REFLECTION QUESTIONS

1. How do nursing programs select appropriate educational technologies?
2. What steps could be taken to secure faculty and student buy-in?
3. What can faculty and administrators do to improve the likelihood of a successful integration of educational technologies?
4. What types of organizational support are needed?

> **BOX 6.5 Exemplar 1—Faculty Technology Trial**
>
> ### ABSTRACT
>
> The infusion of technology into higher education is a complex and increasingly necessary process. As mentioned in this chapter, several barriers preclude new technology integration into curricula, especially if courses are operating well without the new technology. Forceful inclusion of new virtual learning technologies without thoughtful consideration and evidence to support their benefit often fail. This exemplar details a strategy to trial two technologies prior to further consideration for adoption to an online family nurse practitioner (FNP) program.
>
> ### INTRODUCTION
>
> A *technology trial* was proposed for evaluating two web-based virtual learning environments (VLEs), Shadow Health and i-Human. The purpose of this trial was to determine individual and comparative user evaluations for Shadow Health and i-Human VLEs. In lieu of piloting these technologies directly in courses with students, FNP faculty members posed as students who were using each technology to complete a course assignment for the first time. The advantages of this approach were the ability to gauge how each technology functions from the student perspective and to collect faculty feedback and preference. Access to both technologies was donated by the respective companies for the trial. The technology with the highest summative evaluation score would receive further consideration for integration with the FNP curriculum.
>
> ### METHODS
>
> Full-time and visiting professors volunteered to participate in the technology trial. Instructions for the trial were provided and participants received access information via email directly from the individual technology companies. Learning activities per technology platform were limited to a time constraint of no more than two hours and the mandatory content requirement of at least one case study module. As long as these minimum requirements were met, any additional content and orientation/training (including prerecorded or live webinars) were determined by the technology company. Access to the technology learning platforms remained open for 14 consecutive days, followed by seven days to complete the post-trial survey.
>
> ### SETTING
>
> This trial was conducted entirely online. Communication was conducted via secured email. Trial activities were conducted using Shadow Health's and i-Human's web-based virtual learning platforms. Qualtrics statistical software was used to collect and analyze survey results.

(continued)

> **BOX 6.5 Exemplar 1—Faculty Technology Trial (*continued*)**

RESULTS

Of the 76 ($N = 76$) faculty who responded to the trial invitation, 60 participants began the trial; 40 ($n = 40$) completed the post-trial survey. Descriptive analysis using Qualtrics software was conducted on survey questions that incorporated a 5-point Likert rating scale. Free-text written responses aimed to increase response rates, elaborate responses to closed questions, and allow respondents to identify other feedback not captured in the closed questions, were reviewed and analyzed by the researcher.

Navigation, Understanding, and Functionality in the VLE

The ability to seamlessly navigate a VLE is fundamental to student success. Respondents reported that difficulty with navigating or understanding the learning platform was the greatest weakness for Shadow Health and i-Human (65% and 87%, respectively). However, the ability to navigate (move in or progress through the learning platform) using Shadow Health was preferred by 73% of participants compared with i-Human. Regarding functionality or the quality of having a practical use, 68% of respondents preferred Shadow Health. Likewise, when asked about the ability to understand (comprehend) the learning platform, 75% preferred Shadow Health to i-Human.

Engagement, Critical Thinking, and Clinical Reasoning

Participants were asked to rate their level of agreement with statements regarding whether participation in the learning activities promoted user engagement; allowed students to reflect on their performance, skills, and assumptions in a meaningful way; and assisted with learning critical thinking and clinical reasoning skills necessary for nurse practitioners in the clinical environment. All respondents (100%) answered in the affirmative (agreed or strongly agreed) regarding learning activities and the Shadow Health platform. Thirty-six percent (36%) disagreed, strongly disagreed, or were neutral with respect to their level of agreement with the same statements and the i-Human learning platform.

Health History, Physical Examination, Documentation, and Feedback

The mechanism for obtaining a health history, performing a physical examination, and documenting subjective and objective findings varied between technologies. Respondents preferred their experience with Shadow Health's digital patient with regard to collection of the health history, physical examination, documentation method, and performance feedback. The manner in which information for the health history was solicited in Shadow Health was preferable to i-Human by 65% of participants. Similarly, the simulated physical

(continued)

> **BOX 6.5 Exemplar 1—Faculty Technology Trial (*continued*)**
>
> examination was preferred by 68% of respondents, and 55% preferred Shadow Health's ability to compose a history & physical (H&P) and write a SOAP (subjective data – objective data – assessment – plan) note. Regarding the richness of the automatically generated student performance feedback following the learning activities, 58% preferred Shadow Health.
>
> *Overall Virtual Learning Experience Quality and Preference*
>
> Regarding the overall quality (high level of value or excellence) of the learning experience, 63% of respondents preferred Shadow Health. When asked to select one virtual learning technology platform for further consideration and integration into the curriculum, nearly two thirds (62.5%) of the trial participants preferred the Shadow Health digital patient experience to i-Human.
>
> *Technical Support*
>
> Technical support was provided by both technology companies. Feedback regarding participant's experience with technical support, including prompt and efficient telephone or email response, was similar.
>
> *Additional Comments*
>
> Participant comments and feedback not captured in the post-trial survey were analyzed for common words, phrases, and themes. Difficulty navigating the i-Human platform was a common theme. A respondent added that navigating i-Human might get easier with practice, but Shadow Health was "easier to use from the start." The different method of collecting health history information between the two technologies prompted several comments. One participant favored the dropdown list of interview questions with i-Human more than the free-text input method with Shadow Health. However, the same respondent noted that the long list of interview questions seemed cumbersome and off-putting. It was posited that the free-text input method may help students retain information, foster independence, and assist with critical thinking skills versus the dropdown method, but typing questions was time consuming compared to using an "interpreter."
>
> Several participants suggested that a talk-to-text input method for gathering subjective information to complete the health history would be preferable to both data-collection methods. Regarding the physical assessment, the use of real photographs rather than simulated graphics for assessment data was suggested. Shadow Health provided more in-depth rationales during performance feedback. With regard to product development, a participant suggested that the ability to interact in learning scenarios with multiple users might simulate collaborative practice between providers and add additional

(continued)

> **BOX 6.5 Exemplar 1—Faculty Technology Trial** (*continued*)
>
> interpersonal learning experience. Another enhancement might be adding the ability to control the degree of difficulty in the case study scenario to appropriately suit the learner's level of need.
>
> ## SUMMARY/LIMITATIONS/DISCUSSION:
>
> Survey results clearly demonstrated a strong affinity for Shadow Health as the preferred virtual learning platform. Participants were surveyed regarding the overall quality of the VLE, the ability to navigate the learning platform, the ability to comprehend the learning environment, and the degree to which the learning activity in the learning environment supported student engagement in the activity, the development of patient assessment skills, and critical thinking and clinical reasoning skills. Shadow Health was preferred over i-Human with respect to graphic design, the ability to obtain a health history, simulation of the physical examination, ability to document a patient encounter, and richness of performance feedback.
>
> Although both technology platforms offer students the ability to conduct interviews with virtual patients to collect the subjective health history, the method of soliciting information from the avatar is vastly different. Using a natural language-conversation engine, students in Shadow Health engage in open-ended conversations to gather subjective data and practice patient-centered communication. The virtual patient replies to over 70,000 questions about medical history and family background. This method of data collection promotes transformative learning and fosters clinical reasoning. However, to facilitate a transformative learning experience, virtual patient simulations must allow students to explore the history of the presenting illness as well as the past medical history, beyond superficial clinical findings (Kleinheksel, 2014). Conversely, i-Human offers the student a dropdown list of interview questions or key word search for questions from a question bank. Students must select appropriate questions from the prewritten questions provided.
>
> One limitation of this technology trial was the inability to demonstrate all the capabilities of each technology to participants beyond the required learning activities for the sake of the trial. The 12 case study simulations and 4 concept labs in Shadow Heath allowed students to practice interview and assessment skills without the need of a synchronous faculty or preceptor. Students perform tests and use instruments to gather and then record objective patient data. Students synthesize their findings and compare their work to an exemplar's model note. When selecting treatment interventions, students must provide rationales for clinical decisions throughout the simulation, specifically in the Clinical Decision Making assignment.
>
> Shadow Health uses a validated framework to measure six discrete components of clinical reasoning: Therapeutic Communication, Subjective Data
>
> (*continued*)

> **BOX 6.5 Exemplar 1—Faculty Technology Trial** (*continued*)
>
> Collection, Objective Data Collection, Information Processing, Documentation, and Self-Reflection. These components of clinical reasoning are assessed as students interact with virtual patients and are used to provide automatic scores of each student's clinical reasoning ability. Shadow Health incorporates postsimulation questions and self-reflective journaling. Automatic scoring and feedback is preformatted and standardized, immediate, and timesaving for faculty if used for a graded assignment (i.e., documentation shows a "Model Note"). The various layers of feedback allow faculty to see the growth of individuals, as well as compare individual student performance against an aggregate of students. Also, feedback can be modified to suit the needs of the student or emphasize specific content. Students engage in debriefing immediately following every assignment and are given feedback on the discrete components of clinical reasoning measured by the validated Student Performance Index tool.
>
> Published research indicates overall student and faculty satisfaction with the use of Shadow Health in graduate curricula, as well as improved documentation, communication, assessment techniques, and transferability of skills to actual clinical practice. The implications of this trial support Shadow Health as an effective learning platform in meeting student learning outcomes for practicum experiences.

> **BOX 6.6 Exemplar 2—Unsuccessful Integration of a Simulated Electronic Medical Record**
>
> ### ABSTRACT
>
> An attempt was made to integrate a web-based simulated electronic medical record (EMR) into an established prelicensure nursing program curriculum. The implementation was rushed and did not have the necessary faculty or administrative support to be successful. The technology was not intuitive, and training was insufficient. Students resisted the use of the simulated EMR. Integration was ultimately unsuccessful.
>
> ### INTRODUCTION
>
> Faculty may have the best intentions when attempting to integrate educational technology into the curriculum; however, if not done carefully, efforts may be unsuccessful. Faculty at one campus of a multisite, prelicensure associate degree nursing program in the Midwest were concerned about ensuring student competence in relation to documentation using EMRs. Clinical sites associated with the program were beginning to restrict student access to electronic patient records, limiting students' ability to practice documentation

(continued)

> **BOX 6.6 Exemplar 2—Unsuccessful Integration of a Simulated Electronic Medical Record (*continued*)**

skills. During a visit, a textbook representative mentioned the availability of a web-based simulated clinical documentation system designed to complement the textbooks already in use in the program. The system contained case studies that would allow students to practice skills such as documentation of medication administration, assessments, and nursing notes. The representative arranged a demonstration and described the product, training resources, and technical support that was available to faculty and students. With the adoption of the product, faculty would receive free access to the product and training; students would pay a fee for access.

Faculty met to discuss the pros and cons of integrating the product into the skills laboratory for each clinical course in the curriculum. Pros included discounted book fees for students; alternate means for students to attain competence with electronic clinical documentation; reasonable cost; and reinforcement of course content using a case study–based approach. The school agreed to provide the laboratory space and laptops necessary for the simulated charting experience. The only drawback appeared to be that faculty would be required to train students. However, implementation proved to be more difficult than anticipated.

CHALLENGES

Faculty decided to adopt the simulated EMR at the end of the spring semester with implementation scheduled for the following fall. By the time classes started, however, several of the most outspoken supporters of the technology had left the organization to pursue other opportunities. Remaining faculty were ambivalent about the product and the short time frame for implementation. Vacant positions had been filled with new faculty who were expert clinicians but had limited teaching experience. Between teaching and clinical requirements, committee participation, accreditation visit preparation, and mentoring of inexperienced instructors, seasoned faculty experienced overload. There was not sufficient time to determine the most advantageous application of the technology to course content. To accommodate the simulated EMR, skills laboratory lesson plans required modification. Part-time skills laboratory staff were not invested in redesigning lessons. The product training provided by the textbook company was limited, consisting of one brief session. Because faculty had limited experience with educational technologies, the training was insufficient. Faculty spent more time than anticipated learning to navigate the system on their own so that they would feel comfortable training skills laboratory staff and students.

Although administration supported the idea of curricular innovation, practical considerations proved to be a barrier. A web-enabled computer was required to access the simulated chart. The physical space in the skills laboratory was not designed to accommodate desktop computers. No nearby classroom space with computers was available. The organization decided to purchase two

(continued)

> **BOX 6.6 Exemplar 2—Unsuccessful Integration of a Simulated Electronic Medical Record** (*continued*)
>
> laptop computers with wireless connections for use in the laboratory. Wi-Fi access in the laboratory was inconsistent. Two laptops were not sufficient to allow an entire group of 10–15 students to use the simulated EMR. Students were not permitted to complete assignments using the product outside of scheduled skills laboratory time. The university was unable to provide technical support for the product due to lack of access to and experience. The administration did not provide any type of release from scheduled load for faculty to implement the curricular change.
>
> Students expressed dissatisfaction for several reasons. Since the nursing program was offered at a commuter campus of a larger university, nontraditional students composed the majority of the student population. Many students displayed technological resistance, which was compounded by the fact that the product was not intuitive. Training did not go smoothly. Faculty provided the training for the simulated EMR during scheduled class time, which reduced the amount of time available to cover course content. Students also expressed frustration with the limited number of computers and available time in the skills laboratory, as well as the inability to complete assignments in the simulated EMR on their own time. With limited opportunities to use the documentation system, students felt the product was not worth the money they were required to pay for the subscription.
>
> **RESOLUTION**
>
> Although there was initially some enthusiasm for the simulated EMR, over time, the technostress experienced by faculty and students led to dissatisfaction. Elected student representatives attended a faculty meeting in which they expressed concern that the product was detracting from their learning and overall satisfaction. Faculty agreed and discontinued required use of the product.
>
> **SUMMARY AND LESSONS LEARNED**
>
> The attempted integration of the simulated EMR led to several lessons learned. First, learning outcomes should drive the selection of technology, not vice versa. When the decision was made to adopt the product, faculty did not research alternative options. Other technologies may have been a better fit for the program needs and resources. Consideration of an organization's mission, philosophy, delivery methods, and available resources is necessary to ensuring a good fit. It is also important to consider the population who will use the technology. Faculty and student buy-in can make or break an endeavor. Once a technology is selected, sufficient time should be allowed so that the implementation is not rushed.

REFERENCES

Adamson, K., & Kardong-Edgren, S. (2012). A method and resources for assessing the reliability of simulation evaluation instruments. *Nursing Education Perspectives, 33,* 334–339. doi:10.5480/1536-5026-33.5.334

Altbach, P. G., Gumport, P. J., & Berdahl, R. O. (2011). *American higher education in the twenty-first century.* Baltimore, MD: Johns Hopkins University Press.

American Association of Colleges of Nursing. (2015). Re-envisioning the clinical education of advanced practice registered nurses [White paper]. Retrieved from http://www.aacnnursing.org/Portals/42/News/White-Papers/APRN-Clinical-Education.pdf

American Association of Colleges of Nursing. (2017). Nurse faculty shortage. Retrieved from http://www.aacnnursing.org/News-Information/Fact-Sheets/Nursing-Faculty-Shortage

Decker, S., Sportsman, S., Peutz, L., & Billings, L. (2008). The evolution of simulation and its contribution to competency. *Journal of Continuing Education in Nursing, 39,* 74–80. doi:10.3928/00220124-20080201-06

Dunnington, R. M. (2014). The nature of reality represented in high fidelity human patient simulation: Philosophical perspectives and implications for nursing education. *Nursing Philosophy, 15,* 14–22. doi:10.1111/nup.12034

Fiedler, R., Giddens, J., & North, S. (2014). Faculty experience of a technological innovation in nursing education. *Nursing Education Perspectives, 35*(6), 387–391. doi:10.5480/13-1188

Hansen, J., & Bratt, M. (2015). Competence acquisition using simulated learning experiences: A concept analysis. *Nursing Education Perspectives, 36,* 102–107. doi:10.5480/13-1198

Harder, B. N., Ross, C. J., & Paul, P. (2013). Instructor comfort level in high-fidelity simulation. *Nurse Education Today, 33,* 1242–1245. doi:10.1016/j.nedt.2012.09.003

Hayden, J. K., Smiley, R. A., Alexander, M., Kardong-Edgren, S., & Jeffries, P. R. (2014). The NCSBN National Simulation Study: A longitudinal, randomized, controlled study replacing clinical hours with simulation in prelicensure nursing education. *Journal of Nursing Regulation, 5*(2 Suppl.), s3–s40. doi:10.1016/j.ecns.2012.07.070

Hermanns, M., & Kilmon, C. (2012). Second Life® as a clinical conference environment: Experience of students and faculty. *Clinical Simulation in nursing, 8,* e297–e300. doi:10.1016/j.ecns.2011.04.002

Howard, S. K. (2013). Risk-aversion: Understanding teachers' resistance to technology integration. *Journal of Technology Pedagogy and Education, 22,* 357–372. doi:10.1080/1475939X.2013.802995

Institute of Medicine. (2011). *The future of nursing: Leading change, advancing health.* Washington, DC: National Academies Press.

Iriti, J., Bickel, W., Schunn, C., & Stein, M. K. (2016). Maximizing research and development resources: Identifying and testing "load-bearing conditions" for technology innovations. *Educational Technology Research and Development, 64,* 245–262. doi:10.1007/s11423-015-9409-2

Jiminez, F., Kleinheksel, A. J., & Kotranza, A. (2015). *The student performance index.* Gainesville, FL: Shadow Health.

Kleinheksel, A. J. (2014). Transformative learning through virtual patient simulations: Predicting critical student reflections. *Clinical Simulation in Nursing, 10*(6), e301–e308. doi:10.1016/j.ecns.2014.02.001

LaViola, J. J. (2000). A discussion of cybersickness in virtual environments. *SIGCHI Bulletin, 32,* 47–56. Retrieved from https://www.deepdyve.com/lp/association-for-computing-machinery/a-discussion-of-cybersickness-in-virtual-environments-AweEgZm4sG

Lee, A. R., Son, S. M., & Kim, K. K. (2016). Information and communication technology overload and social networking service fatigue: A stress perspective. *Computers in Human Behavior, 55,* 51–61. doi:10.1016/j.chb.2015.08.011

Morozov, E. (2013). *To save everything, click here: The folly of technological solutionism.* New York, NY: Public Affairs.

Nardi, D. A., & Gyurko, C. C. (2013). The global nursing faculty shortage: Status and solutions for change. *Journal of Nursing Scholarship, 45,* 317–326. doi:10.1111/jnu.12030

National Center for Education Statistics. (2017). Characteristics of postsecondary students. Retrieved from https://nces.ed.gov/programs/coe/indicator_csb.asp

Phillips, J. M., Resnick, J., Boni, M. S., Bradley, P., Grady, J. L., Rulund, J. P., & Stuever, N. L. (2013). Voices of innovation: Building a model for curriculum transformation. *International Journal of Nursing Education* Scholarship, *10,* 1–7. doi:10.1515/ijnes-2012-0008

Scully, N. J. (2011). The theory-practice gap and skill acquisition: An issue for nursing education. *Collegian, 18*(2), 93–98. doi:10.1016/j.colegn.2010.04.002

Tacy, J. W., Northam, S., & Wieck, K. L. (2016). Understanding the effects of technology acceptance in nursing faculty: A hierarchical regression. *Online Journal of Nursing Informatics, 20*(2). Retrieved from http://www.himss.org/library/understanding-effects-technology-acceptance-nursing-faculty-hierarchical-regression

United States Department of Commerce. (1999). Falling through the net: Defining the digital divide. Retrieved from https://www.ntia.doc.gov/legacy/ntiahome/fttn99/introduction.html

United States Department of Commerce. (2016). The state of the urban/rural digital divide. Retrieved from https://www.commerce.gov/news/blog/2016/08/state-urbanrural-digital-divide

Urso, P., & Fisher, L. R. (2015). Education technology to service a new population of elearners. *International Journal of Childbirth Education, 30*(3), 33–36. Retrieved from https://search.proquest.com/openview/66501ab645e55cf29484c8b207012d2f/1?pq-origsite=gscholar&cbl=32235

Weil, M. M., & Rosen, L. D. (1997). *Technostress: Coping with technology@ work@ home@ play*. Hoboken, NJ: Wiley.

Wiederhold, B. K., & Wiederhold, M. D. (2014). Virtual reality for posttraumatic stress disorder. In B. K. Wiederhold & S. Bouchard (Eds.), *Advances in Virtual Reality and Anxiety Disorders* (pp. 211–233). New York, NY: Springer.

Zayim, N., & Ozel, D. (2015). Factors affecting nursing students' readiness and perceptions toward the use of mobile technologies for learning. *Computers, Informatics, Nursing, 33*(10), 456–464. doi:10.1097/CIN.0000000000000172

CHAPTER 7

Faculty Role in Integrating Virtual Simulations

DEE McGONIGLE, RANDY M. GORDON, AND DIANA MEEKS

LEARNING OBJECTIVES

Upon completion of this chapter, the reader will be able to:
- Assess how virtual simulation relates to executive practicum nursing students.
- Evaluate the use of Second Life® (SL) in the practicum course.
- Examine the role of faculty in integrating virtual simulation into nursing courses and curriculum.
- Explore the process for debriefing following immersion in a simulated practicum environment.

KEY TERMS

Debriefing	Real-world practicum (RWP)
Executive specialty practicum	Second Life (SL)
Immersed	Scenario
Journal club	Virtual learning environment (VLE)
Mentor	Virtual simulation
Pre-brief	Virtual world practicum (VWP)

In a graduate-level executive course at a large nursing university, students have a choice of practicum experience with a mentor—a **real-world practicum (RWP)** or a **virtual world practicum (VWP)**. The practicum is designed to provide students with experience in enacting the role they are preparing for, in this case, the role of the nurse executive. The addition of a VWP resulted from a need to provide access to quality experiences for all graduate nursing students. Some students in remote areas had difficulty securing qualified mentors who were master's prepared and working in an executive role. In addition, some areas have a limited number of master's prepared nurses, and securing a practicum site with a mentor who met the required qualifications was occasionally a challenge. To support our students and avoid delay in completion of their degree, a VWP option was developed. This chapter highlights some aspects of the faculty's role in the integration of this virtual simulation into a nursing practicum course, specifically in the executive specialty.

RELATION TO THE FAST SIM©

The Faculty Administrators Students Technology Strategic Integration Model© (FAST SIM) is a framework underpinning curriculum development to support integration strategies. By providing a VWP option, students in remote and other areas were able to complete their graduate nursing degree. The content of this chapter aligns with the student and faculty integration components of this model. When students can complete course and program outcomes in a satisfactory manner through the use of technology, effective technology integration is attained. In addition, our virtual simulation use has been highly supported by the administrators of the program.

VIRTUAL SIMULATION AND THE EXECUTIVE VWP NURSING STUDENT

The impetus to include **virtual simulation** in the nurse **executive specialty practicum** started as a strategy for helping students in remote areas who had difficulty securing qualified mentors with whom they could complete their practicum course. However, as students and faculty began discussing their experiences in the VWP, it attracted the interest of many other students who wished to participate in this virtual simulation experience. In addition, some graduate students were challenged to identify and secure practicum placement agreements with master's prepared qualified mentors, even in settings that were not considered to be remote. Student satisfaction increased when the nursing program offered this as an option to these students, only after they had exhausted all alternatives in their geographic location. A practicum coordinator also worked closely with the students to ensure that the VWP was offered only if all options were exhausted and there were no practicum sites with qualified mentors available. This led to the opportunity to choose the VWP.

The **Second Life (SL) virtual learning experience (VLE)** is a rigorous VWP course that was developed by faculty experts in the nurse executive specialty (Box 7.1). This VWP course met the same standards as the usual RWP course for students. The VWP students completed the same threaded discussions in the class with the other students. The opportunity for students to share their perspectives as they discussed their practicum experience and developed their practicum projects provided a lot of exciting and stimulating dialogue between students and faculty members. As a result of this robust interaction and the success of the VWP option, all students are now introduced to virtual simulation in the core courses.

SL USE IN THE VWP COURSE

As mentioned, because of the lack of a qualified mentor and/or a RWP site for select students, a VWP was developed by experienced nurse faculty who specialized in healthcare leadership. Just as in the RWP, VWP students were assigned to a mentor. Therefore, students completing the practicum course interacted with their faculty member for the course and a mentor for the practicum regardless of it being an RWP or a VWP. Faculty and mentors also collaborated concerning learning outcomes, student progress, or issues or concerns that arose during the practicum. SL allowed the students and mentors to communicate with one another in real time. The learning platform also allowed students to interact with other students within their course, as well as with students enrolled in other specialty areas within the graduate nursing program. The specialty areas included executive students, nursing informatics students, education students, and healthcare policy students. One exciting project that was developed was a virtual journal club in which all specialty area students and mentors came together in SL to discuss pertinent topics of interest. The journal club is presented as Exemplar 1 (Box 7.2). In addition, students shared ideas regarding their final VWP projects and had the opportunity to share and request information from other students and faculty mentors within their own area, as well as those in other areas (Box 7.3).

In the nurse executive area, students had weekly case **scenarios** in which they met with different members of the virtual healthcare leadership team. Some of the roles they encountered included the chief executive officer, chief nursing officer, chief financial officer, director of nursing, staffing coordinator, and others. Prior to these weekly meetings within SL, students prepared questions and researched the role of the person with whom they were meeting that week. Each week, students collected information to help them complete their final VWP project, which was to develop an outpatient cardiac care unit. Students gathered information regarding staffing needs for the intended unit, budgeting proposals, collaboration among various departments and key leaders of the organization, communication with other disciplines, and input from the community in the form of focus groups and windshield surveys. Students felt that the scenarios depicted the reality of the role for which they were preparing, and in certain RWP settings, students may never have an opportunity to meet with someone in some of the specific roles due to scheduling and availability or to deal with an impaired employee. After each weekly scenario, students participated in 30-minute **debriefing** sessions and received feedback from their mentors. A **mentor** is a faculty member with expertise in the specialty who is also prepared to mentor in the VLE VWP. Mentors must complete the virtual world mentoring course. They do not always teach the practicum course and may be responsible only for the VWP component. In addition, students were asked to provide feedback and comments by completing an end-of-course survey. Mentors also completed surveys to provide feedback on their experience and offer insights. Feedback from students indicated that they had had an excellent experience; many felt that they would never have an opportunity to develop a unit and meet with so many different persons in their roles and that the collaborative efforts with other students and their mentors was supportive. The feedback from mentors indicated that most of the students participated fully and were well prepared for their weekly meetings and scenarios.

FACULTY ROLE IN VIRTUAL SIMULATION

Faculty were integral to ensuring the success of the executive specialty area students within the SL VWP. Faculty were involved in the development of the curriculum during every step. The faculty and mentors collaborated with the VLEs team who designed and developed the SL setting that brought the faculty-developed experiences to life. The faculty were responsible for the course content, the mentors for the VWP activities, and the VLE team for the design and development of the virtual world based on the learning outcomes. Faculty mentors oriented the students to the VWP activities and expectations. The virtual learning experiences team oriented students to the virtual world of SL, their avatars, and the navigation and interactive skills necessary to be able to fully participate in VWP learning activities and become **immersed** in the simulation. The mentors met each week with students and participated in the scenarios by assuming various roles; their immersion into the scenarios helped them assess students in relation to the learning outcomes. Mentors completed preparation that involved researching the role of the person they were representing in the scenario; they took a role in the virtual simulation and interacted with their students. Mentors also had to plan how they could offer input into the student's final project as students acquired the necessary data and information to develop their final projects during the scenario. Mentors **prebrief** the students during the meeting prior to that week's activities, and they were also involved in the debriefing sessions and collaborative efforts with other specialty areas' mentors. Mentors met with students each week to ensure their VWP success and answered questions regarding their course. However, the threaded discussions section of the practicum course was led by the faculty member teaching the course; both the RWP and VWP students interacted in the weekly threaded discussions, in which the students responded to the question for the week posted by the faculty and also communicated with their peers in the discussion of the required weekly topic.

Technical support was provided to the students by the VLE team, who has the necessary SL expertise; the support specialists oriented the students to the virtual world and the skills necessary to successfully complete their virtual simulation. As additional scenarios and groups were developed in SL, mentors were intimately involved in each step and offered consultation, input, and feedback. The mentors collaborated with the VLE team to ensure that the virtual simulations facilitated student learning.

One of the major strengths of the VWP is that the faculty and mentors have control over the learning experience. In a RWP, the students are subject to the personnel and experiences available to them while they are in attendance. In the VWP, faculty and mentors can design the exact learning activities they want the students to experience. There are experiences, such as dealing with an impaired employee, that the students cannot enact in a RWP due to ethical and legal issues. In the VWP, nurse executive students can remove an impaired employee from a patient's room, call the institution's human resources department (who is part of the virtual simulation), and then remove the employee from the facility. VWP students can interact with community focus groups in communities that are economically challenged while remaining in the safe environment of the virtual world. Sometimes in the RWP, students shadow nurse executives, whereas in the VWP, they become the nurse executive and enact the role.

DEBRIEFING

At the end of each weekly case scenario, the mentors would ask students to share their experience for that week. Some discussion topics and questions included:

- Were there any challenges in preparing for this week's scenario?
- Discuss feedback regarding the assignments.
- Provide input or recommend changes.
- Discuss your thoughts on collaborating with other students this week.

The weekly debriefing session was very informal, and students shared information verbally with their mentor, by email to the course faculty, or through an anonymous survey completed within SL. Faculty who oversaw the executive area course reviewed all feedback and made any necessary changes based on the feedback and their expertise of how to enhance the course. The goal of receiving feedback was to improve the course each week; to enhance clarity, ensuring students were clear regarding their roles and the expectations of the assignments; and to improve the overall experience for future students. For suggestions regarding implementation strategies for faculty, refer to Box 7.1.

BOX 7.1 Tips for Faculty and Mentors Working in Second Life

- Faculty
  - Collaborate with virtual world practicum (VWP) mentors to facilitate student success in achieving course outcomes through their VWP learning activities.
  - Establish expectations for students in the course and VWP:
    - Students collaborate with their mentors to mutually develop the learning agreement that defines the learning outcomes for the VWP.
    - Students schedule a conference call with their faculty and mentors to mutually agree on the learning outcomes established for the VWP.
    - Students must actively participate in the course and submit all assignments on time while completing their VWP activities with their mentors.
- Mentor
  - Collaborate with the course faculty.
  - Prepare for the mentoring role by completing the VWP mentoring course.
  - Review all VWP materials.
  - Actively participate in the prebrief, enactment, debrief, assessment (PEDA).
  - Establish expectations for students in VWP—students must:
    - Collaborate with their mentors to develop learning agreements that define the learning outcomes they will achieve from their VWP.

(continued)

> **BOX 7.1 Tips for Faculty and Mentors Working in Second Life (*continued*)**
>
> - Actively participate in the VWP orientation process.
> - Successfully complete the VWP orientation process.
> - Prepare for each Second Life activity as prebriefed by their mentor.
> - Establish a quiet environment within which to enter Second Life.
> - Enter Second Life 15 minutes before the established time to complete their virtual simulation so that they were ready to begin on time.
> - Enact the Second Life activity.
> - Actively participate in the debriefing process.
> - Review the assessment. Self-assess based on their perception of the learning outcomes and on how they met them or why they did not.

KEY POINTS

- Virtual simulation offers students the opportunity to successfully complete executive practicum hours and overcome the obstacle of the lack of qualified or available practicum mentors.
- Using virtual simulation and a virtual learning platform, faculty and mentors can design the exact learning activities they want students to experience, thus providing standardization and control over the learning experience.
- Faculty share various roles with regard to virtual simulation integration, including assisting with curriculum development, serving as course leaders, and playing the role of mentors in virtual simulation environments.
- Offering students various options for debriefing following immersion in virtual simulation has a positive impact on students' and faculty's satisfaction with the VLE.
- Students who enacted their future role as nurse executives using virtual simulation while completing executive practicum hours reported a greater satisfaction with their experience than students who completed practicum hours with traditional real-world mentors.

SUMMARY

Overall, the integration of a VLE for graduate VWP students has been a success based on faculty, mentor, and student feedback. SL helped provide students with the opportunity to complete their practicum without any delays, which would have been the case of a lack of qualified mentors or appropriate on-ground practicum placement sites. Student, mentor, and faculty feedback on this option for students completing their practicum has been positive. Mentors working in SL have been instrumental in support of this option for students and dedicated their area through the development of scenarios and other aspects of the VWP component. VWP students enact their future role as nurse executives and experience more than RWP students. In Exemplar 2, Virtual World Practicum Project Development, you will explore how the graduate nursing students are facilitated throughout their practicum course as they develop a virtual healthcare unit as their final practicum project. We constantly continue to seek ways to enhance our program.

REFLECTIVE QUESTIONS

1. Reflect on the challenges faced by academic institutions and students regarding the national shortage of available or qualified practicum mentors. What are the advantages and disadvantages of using virtual simulation to achieve practicum goals?
2. Should virtual simulation replace RWP experiences, or augment these experiences? Discuss your thoughts in detail.
3. Aside from a satisfaction survey, what are other modalities for evaluating the student's experience using virtual simulation?

BOX 7.2 Exemplar 1—Developing a Virtual Journal Club

ABSTRACT

A journal club was developed to promote research and expand knowledge within a virtual platform to engage learners and promote critical thinking and evidence-based practice with graduate nursing students. The virtual world practicum (VWP) students in all specialty areas had the opportunity to collaborate via the journal club.

INTRODUCTION

A virtual journal club was developed by a multidisciplinary team of nursing faculty mentors to engage their students and promote critical thinking by reviewing and critiquing current research literature pertinent to their respective specialty areas in their nursing program.

Faculty mentors wanted to bring all nursing students from four different specialty areas (executive, education, nursing informatics, and healthcare policy) to review, critique, and share research in an open forum. Each week, one of the four specialty areas was assigned to present an article with the other students and faculty. The chosen article was emailed to all faculty, who shared it with their respective students. The students were provided with an outline regarding how to critique an article. The specialty area students chosen to present for the week would share their presentation of each of the critique points. Each specialty area rotated the presentation of the research articles for all the attendees. The research article critique presentations were held in the nursing auditorium within Second Life. All students and faculty mentors could ask questions. At the end of each week's presentaion, a survey was sent to the students to inquire if the information shared was helpful and request future topics and feedback regarding the process. All students logged into the meeting with their avatars in the Second Life virtual platform. The results by students and faculty mentors was positive each week.

(continued)

> **BOX 7.2 Exemplar 1—Developing a Virtual Journal Club (*continued*)**
>
> ### CHALLENGES
>
> Occasionally, students had some difficulty directing their avatar to the auditorium within Second Life to attend the virtual journal club. In addition, occasional sound and technical issues occurred that delayed the start or components of the article presentation to the other attendees.
>
> ### RESOLUTIONS
>
> Students were provided with an in-depth orientation within Second Life. This orientation involved navigating their avatars and locating certain places for future reference. Students were also encouraged to log into the Second Life virtual learning platform well before the start time of the journal club to address any technical issues that may arise. A virtual learning environment (VLE) team member was available to provide technical support to students and faculty mentors.
>
> ### SUMMARY
>
> Each week the presentations and process received feedback from participating students and faculty mentors. All students had an opportunity to participate in the presentation of the research articles to their peers and faculty. Overall, the feedback was positive by all students and faculty mentors, and it was felt to be a very informative and worthwhile activity.
>
> ### LESSONS LEARNED
>
> Because many students had never or had not recently critiqued a research article, training was provided regarding how to do so. To avoid being late for the journal club, students were encouraged to engage in the Second Life virtual platform on their own and become familiar with moving their avatars and locating the auditorium. After the first journal club session, the students, rather than the faculty mentors, chose the article for the critiques. Students seemed to take ownership and mentor one another in this process.

> **BOX 7.3 Exemplar 2—Virtual World Practicum (VWP) Project Development**
>
> ### ABSTRACT
>
> In the executive area, graduate nursing students are facilitated throughout the course as they develop a virtual healthcare unit as their final practicum project.

(continued)

BOX 7.3 Exemplar 2—Virtual World Practicum Project Development (*continued*)

INTRODUCTION

The role of the nurse faculty is complex. Innovative teaching strategies must be developed to aid student learning. A virtual final practicum project to develop a cardiac outpatient center is developed by each nursing executive student by the time that they complete their practicum course. This final practicum project promotes critical thinking and incorporates various scenarios each week to facilitate each student in the development of the unit, as well as enable them to have real-life interaction with members of the executive healthcare team within the Second Life platform.

Faculty mentors wanted to engage nursing students in the executive area through weekly scenarios to facilitate the students as they work toward their final practicum project. Each week, the graduate nursing students in the executive area met with various healthcare team members to learn about the role of the persons they were meeting and develop questions to ask them to solicit information that would assist them in the development of their final practicum project. Some of the weekly healthcare team member meetings included the hospital administrator, chief nurse officer (CNO), chief financial officer (CFO), director of nursing, and staffing coordinator. Each weekly meeting involved the students reviewing a case study and researching the role of the healthcare worker with whom they were meeting.

At the end of each week's case study, a survey was completed by each student to solicit feedback regarding the scenario. Each student logged into a link within the Second Life virtual platform to complete the survey. The results were positive each week, and students felt that the scenarios were helpful in the development of their final project.

CHALLENGES

Occasionally, students had some difficulty directing their avatars to attend the meetings. In addition, occasional sound and technical issues occurred that delayed the start or components of the meetings.

RESOLUTIONS

Students were provided with an in-depth orientation within Second Life. This orientation involved navigating avatars and locating certain places for future reference. Students were also encouraged to log into the Second Life virtual learning platform well before the start of each meeting to address any technical issues that may arise. A virtual learning environment (VLE) team member, as well as their faculty mentor, was available to provide technical support to students.

(*continued*)

> **BOX 7.3 Exemplar 2—Virtual World Practicum Project Development (*continued*)**
>
> ### SUMMARY
>
> The students were able to build their final project through their weekly scenarios and activities within SL. During week 8, the final week of the session, they presented their practicum projects to their course mates in SL. Overall, the feedback from all of the students and faculty mentors was positive. The virtual world practicum (VWP) was viewed by most of the students as a more potent experience than they could have received in a real world practicum (RWP).
>
> ### LESSONS LEARNED
>
> The students were experiencing the virtual world for the first time and needed support for issues related to navigation as well as course content. The technical issues were addressed by the support staff in-world and course issues were handled by their mentors. We wanted to promote a collaborative environment for the students; they worked together, built relationships with each other, and collaborated when possible. These geographically dispersed students who would never have met in a real world practicum (RWP), began mentoring each other and they gained confidence in assuming their future nursing role in the process.

REFERENCE

Zulkosky, K. (2012). Simulation use in the classroom: Impact on knowledge, acquisition, satisfaction, and self-confidence. *Nursing Simulation in Nursing 8*(1), e25–e33. doi:10.1016/j.ecns.2010.06.003

CHAPTER 8

Preparing the Instructional Environment

JULIE McAFOOES

LEARNING OBJECTIVES

Upon completion of this chapter, the reader will be able to:
- Identify key stakeholders, including administrators, faculty, and students, who influence the simulation instructional environment.
- Describe the preparation of administrators, faculty, and students for supporting, teaching, and learning with simulation.
- Examine the financial, legal, faculty, and student issues related to simulation.
- Assess aspects of information technology/infrastructure and support that promote success in simulation.

KEY TERMS

Certifications
Hardscape simulation center
Information technology (IT)
Infrastructure
Instructional environment
Realism
Simulation
Simulation-based learning
Simulation-based learning environment
Stakeholder
Virtual simulation

Preparing the instructional environment is crucial to the success of simulation. Often, those new to simulation focus on the technologies that are the most visible part of the learning environment. Administrators and faculty may be concerned with how to find funds to buy the technology, how to purchase it, how to store it, and how to access it. It is easy to become wrapped up in the hardware and software that are part of virtual learning. It is just as important to consider the cognitive preparation for simulation. All members of the team must develop knowledge and understanding about simulation to turn the technology cog in the Faculty Administrators Students Technology Strategic Integration Model© (FAST SIM) that will generate the momentum to produce a well-planned simulation.

RELATION TO THE FAST SIM©

The mere presence of a **simulation-based learning environment** does not ensure that simulation will be used effectively. Successful **simulation** requires that the key people involved—administrators, faculty, and students—be adequately prepared to make sound decisions about simulation use. The FAST SIM© depicts the relationships between the technology and the people who are the major forces that push the success of **simulation-based learning**.

STAKEHOLDERS AND TEAM

The FAST SIM© identifies the major **stakeholders** in simulation. They are the faculty, administrators, and students. Each is examined in more detail in relationship to **instructional environment** and design.

Faculty

Faculty may be involved in almost every aspect of simulation planning and preparation. In smaller organizations, faculty may assume many roles, including technical support, but typically, faculty are responsible for determining how simulation is used for instruction that fits the needs of the curriculum. The vision of the faculty regarding simulation impacts how the instructional environment is designed and delivered.

Administrators

Administrative stakeholders are present at all levels of the organizational chart. The highest-level administrators, such as the college president or chief nursing officer, are focused on the vision and mission of the organization. Simulation can consume significant resources. Top administrative stakeholders must be able to make the connection between the simulation and these organizational drivers, or they may not support the effort.

Middle-level administrators, including deans and directors, usually oversee strategic planning and budgeting that dictate the direction of the instructional environment. These stakeholders must be willing to allocate resources to prepare and carry out simulation.

Front-line managers may have direct oversight of simulation-based learning experiences. Their power over how simulations are conducted makes them significant stakeholders.

Students

Students arguably have the highest stake in simulation because they benefit the most from well-prepared simulation or suffer the most if it is ill planned. Students pay the cost of simulation either directly or indirectly; therefore, they are also financial stakeholders.

Technology Experts

Technology is at the center of the FAST SIM©; therefore it stands to reason that technology experts, who may be employed by the organization, hired as consultants, or associated with the third-party vendors whose products are purchased, should be included as stakeholders. Technical experts must carry out the plans of

> **BOX 8.1 Technology Experts**
>
> | Technology Expert | Role and Responsibilities |
> |---|---|
> | Front-end developers | These experts develop the front-end (i.e., aspects of the system that are visible to the user). Experts include three-dimensional modeling programmers who build realistic objects, such as people and furniture, for the virtual environment. Graphic designers may draw the landscapes and scenery. |
> | Back-end developers | These experts, who possess data-programming skills, manage the back end (i.e., aspects of the system that are not visible to the user). The backend consists of the database, applications, and server that houses and delivers the virtual simulations. |
> | Technical support specialists | These experts support the users of simulation. They may install, configure, and troubleshoot the computer systems and applications for faculty, staff, and students. They staff the help desk for those seeking answers via email, chat, or phone. |
> | Simulation coordinators | These experts oversee the simulation operation and work with all team members to ensure smooth delivery of these learning experiences. |

the administrators and faculty who design and deliver the simulation and assist students who learn through simulation. See Box 8.1 for a list of technology experts and their respective roles and responsibilities in technology integration.

The Society for Simulation in Healthcare (SSH) offers three **certifications**, including one called the Certified Healthcare Simulation Operations Specialist (CHSOS; www.ssih.org/Certification/CHSOS). The CHSOS is an overarching term for simulation technology specialist, technician, and coordinator. These specialists are stakeholders who provide valuable insight to the simulation team.

Employers

Ultimately, the purpose of simulation-based learning is to ensure that nursing students are ready to participate in the workforce as nurses who possess the skills necessary to provide safe and effective care. Potential employers of graduates have a stake in how well the simulation prepares their staff to nurse patients in the real world.

Once stakeholders are identified, a process needs to be put into place to bring forth their insights and opinions that may be shared through information-collection approaches such as surveys, individual talks, and group meetings. Information needs to be gathered and carefully analyzed for decision makers to be informed of the priorities and expectations of all of the stakeholders.

ADMINISTRATOR PREPARATION

Administrators at different levels of the organization need different levels of preparation. The front-line manager, who must learn how to program the simulation, does not undergo the same preparation as the president who must study trends in simulation technology to make sound recommendations to the board of trustees, who approves expensive new initiatives. It is important to identify what needs to be understood to successfully fulfill that particular role on the simulation team.

Transformational leaders create a vision of innovation and change that can inspire those around them to engage in new endeavors such as simulation (Conrad, Guhde, Brown, Chronister, & Ross-Alaolmolki, 2011). Some administrators do not need to see simulation in action to grasp what advantages it offers, but many benefit from a demonstration of a simulation-based learning experience.

Simulation vendors who sell products may come to the educational facility to make presentations and demonstrate technology to administrators to give them a better perspective. Vendors may also demonstrate these online during web conferences if the simulation is an online learning experience. In both examples, the simulation comes to the administrator.

When administrators do not yet have the **infrastructure** in-house to see a demonstration of the simulation technology, they may attend conferences and conventions where simulation vendors exhibit their products and provide staff who can listen to the administrators explain their needs and suggest possible solutions. These face-to-face encounters may lead to follow-up visits and meetings with vendors who sell products that are a good fit.

Another way to become informed is to visit an established simulation center and speak with experts who are willing to share insights. The visit may be done by giving the administrator a guest login to the simulation environment. The host may give the administrator a tour of the virtual environment and emulate a typical student simulation experience. Even a glimpse can quickly open the mind to the many possibilities that simulation holds, and provide context when discussing how to approach simulation at one's own institution.

Financial Issues

Simulation can be an expensive proposition. Indeed, it may be the largest nonsalary, financial outlay that a nursing program can make. Some organizations make the mistake of not buying in at a high enough level to make a real impact. One simulation episode is one too many if the faculty and students require orientation and training that is longer than the learning experience itself.

There are different ways to finance simulation. Some organizations purchase products outright, whereas others sign a lease. A financial expert who understands the organization's situation should consider all options and advise the best course to pursue.

An organization may decide to forego developing and managing its own simulation environment and instead contract for the services of a vendor who offers ready-to-use simulations. Whether to buy off the shelf or make it yourself is a major decision. Using commercial products makes it easier to predict the cost of offering simulation to students. The downside to adopting such products is the loss of control over full customization of the simulation. A vendor may offer to partially modify its application to better fit the instructional needs of a particular program, albeit generally at an additional cost to the institution.

Totally online nursing programs may engage in **virtual simulation** conducted only in an online environment. They have no bricks-and-mortar or physical simulation centers. The financial responsibility may be put directly on the student who may be asked to pay an individual fee for a subscription to access Internet-based learning experiences.

An organization may apply for grants, seek sponsors, or collect donations to enable a large, initial investment into building the simulation infrastructure. This could include purchasing the technology necessary to develop, store, and deliver virtual simulation online.

A nursing program may decide to create an immersive virtual reality simulation environment. These very-high-fidelity simulations may require investment in physical spaces and technology in which "caves" or rooms with special projection, eyewear, or haptic devices can heighten the sense of **realism**. These simulations may require securing square footage; installing utility and network access; purchasing simulation equipment; and buying software, hardware, and other resources to help students suspend disbelief and feel that they are in a real-world situation.

The need for funds does not end once the hardware and software are purchased. Ongoing income is necessary to pay for the staff and the maintenance and upgrading of the technology. How to manage ongoing costs is critical to the success of the venture. Usually, students provide the money for simulation either directly through "simulation" fees that are tacked onto tuition or indirectly through increases to tuition itself. If continual funding is not considered, the once state-of-the-art simulations may become outdated and have to be abandoned.

One resource that must be calculated in the cost of providing simulation, and one that is frequently underestimated or overlooked, is time. The old adage that "time is money" holds true for simulation. Faculty need time to adequately plan, implement, and evaluate simulation-based learning. They may be paid under a separate contract or given workload credit to design and develop quality experiences. Salaries for staff who support the faculty, including simulation managers, technicians, and other personnel, need to be factored into the budget.

Legal Issues

There are legal issues that can present themselves when offering simulation-based learning experiences. It is important to prepare the organizational environment to avoid them.

Faculty who design and develop content for simulation may claim that it is their intellectual property. On the other hand, the organization may assert the simulation is its property because the faculty who created the simulation were compensated through their regular employment or additional contract. Organizational policy should make clear the extent to which the faculty own the simulation content they author. This includes whether they may sell it to a publisher. If existing policy does not adequately cover copyright issues, the organization may ask faculty to sign letters of agreement with specific language that spells out all rights and responsibilities for authoring simulations.

Organizations enter into contracts with vendors to purchase and lease simulation products. The administrators who sign must be fully aware of the obligations to which they are committing the organization. If a vendor does not deliver the goods and services that are promised, the administrator may consult with legal counsel to determine how to proceed against the vendor to seek relief.

According to Smith and Lammers (2014), ethical imperatives to maintain safety, avoid errors, and promote learning motivate simulation. If simulation teaches poor techniques, students may not be educated on how to deliver competent nursing care. This "failure to teach" can result in harm to patients and lead to legal liability. Faculty should follow the principles of evidence-based practice and teaching to ensure that their simulations reflect actual clinical situations.

Participating in simulation may lead to potential legal issues regarding students. Some ask students to sign a consent form that gives the organization wide latitude to record performance and use these recordings for evaluation. The form should make clear the intended purpose of the recording and how it may be used. Feedback about a student's performance may be revealed to classmates who are participating in a group simulation. Faculty need to be cognizant of accidentally sharing confidential information related to grading when discussing simulation performance in front of a group, such as during a debriefing session.

Third-party vendors may offer data collection and analytics as part of their product. However, these companies must institute safeguards that protect student information and collect data only for students who give informed consent to avoid violating the Family Educational Rights and Privacy Act (FERPA) federal privacy laws.

FACULTY ISSUES

The issues that faculty face depend on the roles that they are asked to assume when engaging in simulation. Faculty may be surrounded by a simulation team that frees them to concentrate on the pedagogical aspects of simulation. In smaller organizations, faculty may wear many hats and must take on the responsibilities of technology expertise, environment and avatar creation, user orientation, scheduling, and more. Each role comes with its own issues.

According to the FAST SIM©, faculty determine where and how simulation fits within the curriculum. A deep understanding of the factors that impact the curriculum is key to successful simulation integration. For example, curriculum decisions are influenced by rules and regulations from approving and accrediting bodies. Some state boards of nursing allow certain types of simulation to replace some portion of the mandatory clinical experience. Other state boards prohibit this. Faculty must judge the benefits and limitations of choosing care of patients in a **hardscape**

simulation center or of "real" patients in a clinical setting. Faculty may lack formal education in the pedagogical benefits of simulation and therefore make a poor case for its adoption and fumble its implementation (Hallmark, 2015). Training is critical to the successful integration of simulation into the curriculum.

Faculty need time to plan, design, develop, implement, and evaluate simulation. Issues include those related to workload and compensation for simulation-related efforts.

The FAST SIM© highlights the importance of technology in carrying out successful simulations. Faculty must have ready access to technology to participate in simulation either from an office on campus or an office at home. Budgets need to provide funds to equip the faculty with the hardware and software that is necessary to function at a high level. Organizations may offer to pay for better Internet service to ensure that online virtual simulation experiences run smoothly.

Policies related to the evaluation of faculty delineate what activities lead to a raise in salary, promotion, and tenure. The way in which simulation is viewed and valued by the organization can either encourage or discourage faculty from pursing this educational approach.

Verifying that faculty have the knowledge and understanding to manage a simulation-based learning environment can be difficult in an organization where the individual faculty member may have few or no peers. Administrators may ask faculty to show completion of courses, training programs, or workshops that pertain to virtual simulation. The SSH offers certification for healthcare simulation professionals called the Certified Healthcare Simulation Educator (CHSE; www.ssih.org/Certification/CHSE).

STUDENT ISSUES

Student issues related to simulation are affected by the type of simulation they encounter. Although virtual simulation may not necessitate students traveling to a physical simulation center, they may still be required to log in to a shared simulation experience on specific dates and times. These simulations may lead to scheduling conflicts with other priorities such as work.

Students who learn through virtual simulation face access challenges. Many online students have discovered that their courses allow them to upload, download, and interact with discussion boards for brief periods of time that require only minimal computer and Internet capabilities. They do not truly "learn" online but rather read books, study lessons, prepare posts, and write papers offline. It may be that when they are asked to connect to an online simulation that they need a computer that must meet higher standards and sustain an Internet connection throughout a lengthier session. Online programs and virtual simulation are especially attractive to students who live in remote, rural areas, but these are the very same students whose environments have the greatest problems achieving dependable Internet access. Purchasing new computer equipment that meets the minimum requirements for virtual simulation may be a financial burden, but it can be solved with money. Finding reliable access to the Internet in an area that does not provide this can be a barrier that can be overcome only by traveling to an area that does provide this level of service.

Virtual simulation requires technology to deliver it, so students require technical support to help them when they experience difficulties. If simulations can be taken independently, technical support may need to be offered 24/7 for students who choose to participate when not at work or caring for family.

The cost of education is always an issue for students. Unlike the faculty who may be given access to technology as a component of their job, students must usually pay for their own technology and, indirectly, the technology used by the faculty as well. The way in which simulation is financed by an organization may impact students who may be expected to pay additional fees for courses that include simulation. At times, students may receive financial aid that does not cover these additional fees, and they must pay the cost themselves. The organization needs to be aware of how students finance their education and make decisions about tuition and fees that give students the most affordable options.

FACULTY PREPARATION

Faculty preparation may be necessary at every step of the process of planning, implementing, and evaluating virtual simulation. Opportunities for training may be offered in a variety of ways.

One-on-one training may be done in settings where experienced users are available to mentor faculty. This is an excellent approach to sharing the perspective of how simulation is managed in the organization, but mentors are scarce resources, and may not be able to handle the demand of coaching several faculty.

Attending workshops pertaining to the faculty role in simulation can give the individual a wider perspective on the possible application of simulation and generate ideas on how to adapt it to one's own environment. Faculty may meet colleagues who share similar interests and engage in networking that continues beyond the event.

Much can be learned by taking advantage of educational courses online. The National League for Nursing operates the Simulation Innovation Resource Center (SIRC), which sells a course on developing faculty and others on curriculum integration, evaluating simulations, unfolding cases, debriefing, performing simulation research, and more (sirc.nln.org). The SIRC lists vendors that develop virtual simulation applications for the nursing education market.

Membership in professional organizations that focus on simulation provides faculty with many opportunities to learn about all aspects of simulation. The International Nursing Association for Clinical Simulation and Learning (INACSL) attracts members who are nurses teaching with simulation (www.inacsl.org). The SSH invites all healthcare professionals who have an interest in the use of simulation to join (www.ssih.org). Both associations provide its members with discounts on webinars and annual meetings, free access to their professional journals, networking opportunities, and the chance to become involved in efforts that can shape the future of simulation. SSH offers certification, including one for the CHSE and another for advanced educator (CHSE-A).

STUDENT PREPARATION

Students come to their educational experiences with a wide range of knowledge, skills, and attributes (KSAs). Some students quickly assimilate the KSAs necessary to be successful simulation learners. Others face struggles as they try to build competency not only in the use of the technology, but also in what may be a new type of learning for them.

Orientation to the simulation-based learning environment helps students become comfortable with what they encounter and lessens the impact of facing an unknown situation. Orientation may be done by creating a video of what to expect during a simulation, or a real-time tour of the simulation environment can be conducted to reduce anxiety and familiarize students with what to expect. Aspects of orientation may be documented in a guide or handbook that includes policies governing simulation activities, technical requirements, and technical support. Assigning a faculty mentor may also ease anxiety (Tiffany & Hoglund, 2014).

Some students may find it easy to suspend disbelief and quickly embrace the simulation-based learning environment. Others may face difficulty making the transition from "play acting" to experiencing a sense of realism. Preparing students for the virtual simulation may involve asking them to engage in learning that is not part of the simulation. For example, students may read background information related to case studies to familiarize themselves with what has happened before the visit in the simulated environment. Consider what other adjunct teaching materials can support student learning.

INFORMATION TECHNOLOGY/INFRASTRUCTURE AND SUPPORT

When preparing the instructional environment for simulation, **information technology (IT)** and infrastructure must be adequate to carry out the planned simulations. If these are lacking, the simulations may fail because they cannot be delivered or supported in a way that meets the needs of all students.

A major decision is whether to keep the IT and infrastructure in-house or contract for it. Large organizations may find it cost-effective to integrate the technology necessary to deliver simulation within their existing infrastructure. However, the need for knowledgeable technical staff must be considered as well. The technical expertise required for overseeing the organization's IT operations may not include the skills that are necessary to manage the IT that delivers simulation. In-house staff may undergo additional training, or the organization may decide to outsource technical management to another company.

The amount of bandwidth that simulation requires may be much higher than the organization can manage with its current infrastructure. This is another reason why outsourcing simulation may be a better decision than keeping it in-house.

Even if most of the simulation is being maintained and delivered externally, some level of in-house expertise is still necessary to communicate with the external company and to provide basic assistance to users, including faculty, students, and staff (see Appendix A).

KEY POINTS

- Comprehensive and well-planned preparation of the instructional environment is crucial to the success of virtual simulation integration.

- Faculty, administrators, students, and technology support staff, including designers and developers, all play pivotal roles in the success of virtual simulation and influence the integration of simulation into a curriculum.
- Challenges such as legal and financial issues, insufficient knowledge and understanding of simulation, lack of resources and support, role ambiguity, and work overload may jeopardize integration efforts.
- The advantages and benefits that come from learning through virtual simulation far exceed the obstacles of preparing the instructional environment to support integration.

SUMMARY

Preparing the instructional environment for simulation requires attention to the key components of the FAST SIM©. Faculty, administrators, students, and the technology all need careful consideration to create the momentum needed to carry out simulation-based learning experiences. All stakeholders need sufficient knowledge and understanding of simulation, appropriate to their role, to successfully learn with this educational approach. Legal and financial issues can shape the way in which the simulations are designed and delivered. Faculty time involved to prepare simulations is an often overlooked but important factor. Access issues to the Internet may impact faculty and students who participate in simulation from remote locations. The two exemplars that follow will help you assess and apply the content you learned in this chapter. Exemplar 1 (Box 8.2) explores how one college used a virtual health assessment pilot to improve assessment skills and Exemplar 2 (Box 8.3) solves a dilemma through a virtual community health practicum experience. Despite the challenges, the rewards that come from learning through virtual simulation make it well worth the resources devoted to preparing this instructional environment.

REFLECTIVE QUESTIONS

1. How well prepared is your institution to provide education in a virtual simulation environment? What limitations exist? What plans are in place to overcome them?
2. How well prepared are your faculty to teach in a virtual simulation environment? What opportunities exist for faculty to increase their KSAs with respect to teaching in a virtual learning environment (VLE)? What could be done to improve this situation?
3. How well prepared are your students to learn in a VLE? What barriers exist that prevent them from engaging fully in a simulation-based learning experience? What steps can the institution take to help students to minimize these barriers?

BOX 8.2 Exemplar 1—Virtual Health Assessment Pilot to Improve Assessment Skills

ABSTRACT

Teaching health assessment to online students can be challenging for both instructors and students. Students at one totally online RN-to-BSN program

(continued)

> **BOX 8.2 Exemplar 1—Virtual Health Assessment Pilot to Improve Assessment Skills** (*continued*)
>
> were asked to participate in a pilot study that compared the current practice of finding and assessing their own willing patients versus assessing a standardized virtual patient. Although the findings revealed advantages to using a virtual patient, the technological barriers faced by some students led to a decision not to adopt the virtual learning experience.
>
> ## INTRODUCTION
>
> A need exists to determine the nursing students' communication, examination, and documentation skills during a health assessment and their ability to synthesize the information gained from the patient encounter. Nursing students who practice interviewing patients in a virtual environment have shown that this is an effective approach to improving assessment skills (Sweigart, Burden, Carlton, & Fillwalk, 2014).
>
> Students in an online RN-to-BSN health assessment class were asked to find their own patients, who could meet their timeline and would be willing to share necessary, often sensitive, health information, to conduct a health assessment. The instructor had to grade the students without knowing the patients who were assessed. This made it difficult to discern the accuracy of the students' findings.
>
> The faculty learned about an online product that would let students log in to assess a virtual patient with various health conditions. These conditions would be known to the instructor but would need to be discovered by the learner. The student's activity would be tracked and analyzed to provide feedback to the instructor for evaluation purposes. The faculty predicted that this product could address the limitations with the current methods.
>
> The faculty approached a company that agreed to help the nursing program to conduct a pilot study that would compare both types of learning. The company reviewed the technical requirements for students and judged that the product would not exceed these and should be able to function properly.
>
> Any research studies involving human subjects must be submitted to the institutional review board (IRB) for approval prior to initiating the study and recruiting subjects. The IRB is designed for the protection of human subjects and evaluate each study in relation to the precautions in place in order not to harm the subjects and also in maintaining their privacy and confidentiality. The IRB ensures the safe, ethical treatment and well-being of human subjects involved in research. The IRB approved a proposal for an experimental design in which students in the treatment group would assess the virtual would assess the virtual patient. Training sessions for staff and faculty familiarized them with the product. Students who gave consent were assigned at random to class sections where they were provided access to the virtual patient or to sections where they completed the assignment by securing a person to assess. The assignments were almost identical.

(*continued*)

> **BOX 8.2 Exemplar 1—Virtual Health Assessment Pilot to Improve Assessment Skills** (*continued*)
>
> ## CHALLENGES
>
> Students completed an orientation to the product. The company handled tech-support calls and gathered information about the nature of problems reported. Immediately a small number of students could not meet the technical requirements for learning online. One was out of the country in a remote location with unreliable Internet access. Others lived in rural areas where their only access to the Internet was through satellite service. The students could connect for short periods of time, but the Internet service would repeatedly disconnect before students could complete their virtual health assessments. Still others had no access to Internet service in their homes. They would log on briefly at work or in a friend's home to quickly upload, download, and post but otherwise did not remain online for more than a few minutes at a time. One said she was "couch surfing" and had overstayed her welcome; therefore, she could not complete the assignment.
>
> The company reported that a significant number of students reporting issues used systems that did not meet the nursing program's minimum technical requirements. They had outdated operating systems, old browsers, and insufficient memory.
>
> ## RESOLUTIONS
>
> Students who were in the treatment group who faced technical issues dropped out of the pilot and completed the assignments using selected patients. Students were not penalized in any way for failure to complete the assessment with the virtual patient.
>
> ## SUMMARY
>
> Data were collected from those who did finish the health assessment with the virtual patient. The results revealed that conducting an online health assessment of a virtual patient did address most of the concerns with the current practice. However, the inability of a sizeable number of students to complete the assignment because of technical barriers led to a decision not to adopt the product.
>
> ## LESSONS LEARNED
>
> Many online students do not "learn online." Those with limited connectivity and older systems can be successful learners if the curriculum is designed in such a way that most of their learning can be accomplished offline with only brief periods of connectivity and modest memory and processing speed.

(*continued*)

> **BOX 8.2 Exemplar 1—Virtual Health Assessment Pilot to Improve Assessment Skills** (*continued*)
>
> The nursing program discussed enforcing the minimal technical requirements that would allow them to access and use the product. However, the faculty agreed that unless other aspects of the curriculum required this minimum level of technology, taking this stance could alienate a sizeable number of students who otherwise could take the program.
>
> The issue of older systems can be addressed with funding and the purchase of new hardware and software, but the inability to access reliable Internet service at any cost is a barrier that cannot be readily overcome. Students who live in rural, isolated areas without adequate Internet service are the same people who are geographically distant from campuses and in-class educational opportunities. Until more is done to reduce the connectivity gap, online programs that wish to enroll technologically-disadvantaged students will need to offer a curriculum that adapts to their environment.

> **BOX 8.3 Exemplar 2—Solving a Dilemma through a Virtual Community Health Practicum Experience**
>
> ## ABSTRACT
>
> Different state boards of nursing set different requirements for nurses to meet the standards to practice as public health nurses. An online RN-to-BSN program decided to offer a version of its community health nursing (CHN) course to incorporate learning experiences for students who reside in these states. This included taking a precepted practicum. When students in one state completed the CHN course without the practicum, the state allowed the nursing program to offer the students a practicum as a virtual learning experience.
>
> ## INTRODUCTION
>
> A small number of online RN-to-BSN students residing in a state with a requirement for a practicum in public health completed the version of the course without the practicum before these requirements were known. Communication with the state's board of nursing led to an agreement that the nursing program would offer the practicum to these students, who would take it in a virtual learning environment (VLE).
>
> The educational institution manages a very large and diverse VLE that could readily accommodate the needs for these students. Faculty teaching the course met with the VLE staff to discuss the scenarios that would meet the assignment criteria. The VLE staff identified potential sites, and the faculty explained what avatars would be needed for the students and patients.

(continued)

> **BOX 8.3 Exemplar 2—Solving a Dilemma through a Virtual Community Health Practicum Experience** (*continued*)
>
> The faculty and nursing staff coordinated their schedules with the students to set up three in-world experiences in which students would assume the roles of community health nurses, and the faculty and staff would play patients of varying ages, ethnicities, and socioeconomic levels. The VLE staff trained students. The faculty and nursing staff were already familiar with the VLE.
>
> The lead instructor created background information for the participants. Students received assignment guidelines and grading rubrics to inform them of what was expected to be successful during the encounters. Those playing patients obtained histories and suggested topics to mention during interactions, but they could also improvise their responses.
>
> ### CHALLENGES
>
> A major issue was finding days and times when all could meet. The program is totally asynchronous, so there is no need for everyone to interact in real-time. Students may be invited to webinars to interact with faculty, but these meetings were recorded and could be watched later, when it was convenient. The use of a virtual practicum learning experience was a unique situation, but if this was to be an on-going expectation, numerous options for days and times would need to be offered to accommodate the schedules of students, faculty, and staff.
>
> At first, the students had the usual questions about how to connect and how to manage their avatars, but these were quickly answered. The VLE coordinator minimized the need for students to learn how to navigate by putting the avatars in the proper meeting location prior to their logging in. The VLE coordinator also teleported people to the next meeting location as needed.
>
> One student was quiet throughout most of the initial experience. The nursing staff, in the role of the patient, prompted her to engage in conversation. Later, she explained she was unsure how to use the technology to speak up, but this improved through some trial and error. She also expressed difficulty suspending disbelief and remarked how new it all was to her. As time progressed, she became more comfortable with the virtual environment and could assume her role as the CHN when conversing with other avatars.
>
> ### RESOLUTION
>
> Despite the difficulties with scheduling, the students all agreed that this was a much better solution for them than attempting to secure a practicum setting and preceptor. Debriefing sessions were held after each scenario was completed, and it was clear that they were able to assume the role of the CHN and could assess the problems the patients and clients presented. They submitted assignments that met the grading rubric criteria and all successfully completed the practicum.

(continued)

> **BOX 8.3 Exemplar 2—Solving a Dilemma through a Virtual Community Health Practicum Experience** (*continued*)
>
> ### SUMMARY
>
> In this case, students needed a practicum experience to help them satisfy a state requirement that was previously unknown to them. The nursing program worked with the state's board of nursing to devise a plan that could be accomplished by leveraging the educational institution's exceptional VLE resources.
>
> ### LESSONS LEARNED
>
> Some situations may require a solution that is outside the box. When all stakeholders such as the regulators, accreditors, administrators, faculty, students, and VLE experts collaborate, a successful outcome can be achieved.

REFERENCES

Conrad, M. A., Guhde, J., Brown, D., Chronister, C., & Ross-Alaolmolki, K. (2011). Transformational leadership: Instituting a nursing simulation program. *Clinical Simulation in Nursing, 7*(5), e189–e195. doi:10.1016/j.ecns.2010.02.007

Hallmark, B. (2015). Faculty development in simulation education. *Nursing Clinics of North America, 50*(2), 389–397. doi:10.1016/j.cnur.2015.03.002

Smith, A. B., & Lammers, S. E. (2014). The ethics of simulation. In J. C. Palaganas, J. C. Maxworthy, C. A. Epps, & M. E. Mancini (Eds.), *Defining excellence in simulation programs* (pp. 592–596). Philadelphia, PA: Wolters Kluwer.

Sweigart, L., Burden, M., Carlton, K. H., & Fillwalk, J. (2014). Virtual simulations across curriculum prepare nursing students for patient interviews. *Clinical Simulation in Nursing, 10*(3), e139–e145. doi:10.1016/j.ecns.2013.10.003

Tiffany, J., & Hoglund, B. A. (2014). Teaching/learning in Second Life: Perspectives of future nurse-educators. *Clinical Simulation in Nursing, 10*(1), e19–e24. doi:10.1016/j.ecns.2013.06.006

CHAPTER 9

Nexus of Game Development: Curricular Integration and Faculty Development

ERIC B. BAUMAN, PENNY RALSTON-BERG, AND GREGORY E. GILBERT

LEARNING OBJECTIVES

Upon completion of this chapter, the reader will be able to:
- Briefly reflect on the experiential and contemporary pedagogy that supports game-based learning, mobile learning, and other emerging digital multimedia.
- Evaluate the processes related to game design and the integration of game-based and innovative digital solutions into the curriculum.
- Discuss the importance of evidence-based best practices and outcome measures in relation to integration of game-based learning and curriculum.

KEY TERMS

Anytime–anywhere learning
Burstiness
Created spaces
Designed experiences
Educational design
Educational games
Environments
Evidence-based education practices
Fit
Games
Game-based learning

Game-based teaching
Game designers
Game mechanics
Just-in-time (JIT) information
Just-in-time (JIT) learning
PICO (population, intervention, comparison group, outcome)
Psychometrics
Scaffolds
Simulations
Video games

This chapter addresses how and why faculty and staff should integrate and leverage game-based technology for their curricula. The chapter also advocates anytime—anywhere learning as the corollary for mobile learning facilitated through smart technology devices and mobile applications as it relates to video games, mobile app–based games, and simulation-based learning. It discusses the process of educational game development specific to clinical education and provides an approach for integration of such technology into the curricula, as well as introduces readers to the pedagogy supporting such technology. Definitions provided in this chapter and terms defined in the glossary are crafted through the lens of **educational design** to assist and inform teachers or faculty members wishing to integrate game-based learning solutions into their curricula. Readers should note that these definitions provide a conceptual introduction to the language of game design so that interested teachers can begin to understand the innovation process required to integrate existing games and mobile applications or develop new and novel games for integration into curricula. The chapter also provides a discussion on the merits of faculty support and professional development needed to promote successful integration of game-based mobile technology into the curriculum. Last, processes for outcome evaluation are discussed from both teaching and learning perspectives.

RELATION TO THE FAST SIM©

Faculty and administrators are increasingly inundated with recommendations for the integration of new and novel educational technology into the curricula. The integration of such technology without careful forethought, product vetting, and stakeholder buy-in often leaves faculty, administrators, and students frustrated. This said, students, often younger and more experieced with technology than faculty, come to academic and clinical learning settings with specific expectations related to the use of technology to meet their educational goals and professional aspirations. Faculty, however, are often ill-prepared to meet these expectations.

Although processes for integrating innovative educational technology into the nursing curriculum may not always be intuitive from the faculty and administrators' perspectives, the best and brightest students choose to attend institutions successfully integrating technology such as game-based applications into the curriculum in an effective and efficient manner (Bauman, 2010, 2012, 2016). The Faculty Administrators Students Technology Strategic Integration Model© (FAST SIM) framework supports **game-based teaching** and **game-based learning** from several perspectives. Faculty, administrators, and students are all stakeholders within the technology integration paradigm.

Games, particularly mobile games, are agnostic—games do not care who is learning from them or the player's level of academic expertise or clinical discipline. They need not be linear and are not sensitive to time and place. Well-designed games are learning machines promoting competence and mastery (Deterding, 2015). Games situate course content and curricular objectives through **designed experiences** (Squire, 2006) in **created spaces** (Bauman, 2007, 2010). Games are designed experiences leveraging faculty subject matter expertise so that players (i.e., the learners in the case of **educational games**) are guided through lessons by performance with measurable outcomes. Within the context of game development for nursing education, game performance should take place in **environments** (digital or otherwise) congruent with course objectives in meaningful ways that are directed toward eventual clinical practice settings and have meaningful and salient consequences. All gameplay activities in some manner exist in the real world or were conceived in the context of the designers' real-world experience. From this perspective gameplay takes place within the situated context of a game environment based on lessons drawn from real-world experience. Thus, to play an educational game requires players to immerse themselves in real-world experiences (Salen & Zimmerman, 2006). This is particularly true for well-designed educational games attending to the Ecology of Culturally Competent Design (Bauman & Games, 2011; Games & Bauman, 2011). When designed experiences are effectively leveraged with the created spaces associated with games, in this case digital games, it is possible to attend to the expectations of faculty, administrators, and students (Bauman, 2010, 2016; Bauman & Ralston-Berg, 2014a, 2014b).

GAME-BASED TEACHING AND LEARNING, AND MOTIVATION

Games, whether they are traditional games or **video games**, are most effective as teaching tools when they are integrated into a curriculum in meaningful ways, rather than used as supplemental content that students are free to leverage as an optional exercise. Consequently, faculty and instructional staff must take care to avoid requiring digital content simply because it is available. Administrators should avoid mandates pushing digital content onto faculty and into curricula before it is carefully evaluated and determined to be a good fit, promoting course objectives and curricular outcomes (Bauman & Ralston-Berg, 2014a, 2014b).

By *fit*, we mean administrators and faculty must be diligent when evaluating digital tools such as games and simulation activities. These tools must be relevant to intended outcomes, matching gameplay activities to overarching course and curricular objectives, as well as providing an alignment of objectives and activities with outcome assessments. It is important for learners to understand why an activity is necessary and how it relates to academic success. If games and simulation activities have a poor fit, learners may perceive them as busywork not directly related to their academic success and therefore not worth investment of their time or full attention. A clear fit in alignment with curricular objectives ties games and simulation activities to the curriculum in a clear and purposeful way (Ralston-Berg & Lara, 2013). A proper fit provides meaning to learners and raises learner engagement through intrinsic motivation.

Well-designed educational games support intrinsic motivation and learning. Within the context of game-based learning; shifting mechanics from extrinsic motivation to intrinsic motivation promotes engagement (Habgood & Ainsworth, 2011). In turn, learning activities should support intrinsic motivation to promote mastery over tangible and often disconnected rewards. Activities found within game narratives should be intrinsically motivating and progress in an intuitive manner. They should be apparent and immediate so that they support a sense of worth or value from the perspective of the player or learner. Games as intrinsically motivating educational tools reinforce behaviors to which learners are already committed to or hope to engage in in the future. They provide a sense of learner agency, such that playing and mastering the game prepares them for clinical practices in ways that are consistent with entry to postlicensure practice expectations and professional acculturation (Bauman & Games, 2011; Deterding, 2015; Games & Bauman, 2011). Shifting the teaching and learning paradigm from extrinsically motivating cues such as task-oriented hierarchical skill and drill exercises to intrinsically motivating opportunities designed to promote learner agency and mastery represent a higher order active learning resulting in deeper understanding (Bauman, 2007).

Digital games and simulation activities support mastery in learning (Gee, 2003; Klopfer, Osterweil, & Salen, 2009), but they should not be a replacement for other traditional forms of learning, including online learning supported by learning management systems. Blended learning has the potential to improve academic performance of learners (Hill, Chidambaram, & Summers, 2017) and is perhaps most effective when motivated learners are provided evaluation of and feedback about their performance. Blended learning provides students with the opportunity to adjust or modify behaviors (Swan, 2002). Integrating games and simulation activities, which provides formative and summative feedback, into the curriculum provides learners with support, instilling important learning principles, such as pattern recognition, into educational practice (Gee, 2003).

Educational game-based activities are most powerful when they support other forms of learning and serve as cognitive aids (Gee, 2007). The most utilitarian and powerful games and digital simulation activities act as tools supporting the continuum of the educational process. Well-designed and integrated games do not aspire to replace other modes of the educational process. Rather, innovative educational technologies such as digital games and simulation activities should strive to provide bridges between traditional teaching modalities and provide cognitive support throughout the formal curriculum and beyond into clinical practice. This is Bauman's Layered Learning Theory (see Figure 9.1; Bauman et al., 2014).

Although it is imperative that games selected for integration into the curriculum meet course and curricular objectives and goals, they need not be fun to be effective. To be effective, educational games must appeal to learners. Many puzzles and games in which people engage in are exceedingly difficult, yet people willingly engage in these puzzles and play these games. Why? Doing so provides a sense of mastery and often comes with social or professional rewards that individuals find intrinsically satisfying. Effective games provide challenges at the edge of learners' competence, yet provide achievable benchmarks encouraging mastery (Gee, 2005; Sharp, 2012). Games facilitating behavior change or mastery of learning improve performance or promote processes supporting continued patterns of behavioral change that drive performance.

Educators are cautioned to carefully select or build candidly purposeful games and digital simulation activities for integration into the curriculum. Students must see games as valuable to achieving their academic goals. Assigning a game as a required course activity can be fraught with peril. Selection and design of game-based learning activities, solving problems, adhering to best practices, which are

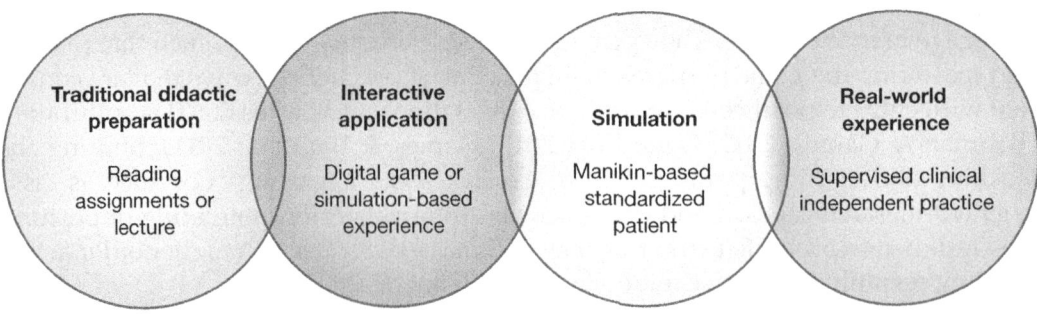

FIGURE 9.1 Bauman's Layered Learning Theory.

intrinsically motivating is imperative to successful implementation. In short, faculty and instructional staff must integrate games that students want to play!

ANYTIME–ANYWHERE AND JUST-IN-TIME LEARNING

Game-based mobile applications designed for tablets and smartphones, provide anytime–anywhere learning. Interactive or active learning activities are not limited to the constraints of classrooms and learning laboratories such as simulation centers. In addition, games are agnostic; they do not care who is learning from them or what expertise the player has because whoever engages in the game is free to learn from that experience.

Gee (2005) posited that games provide **just-in-time (JIT) information** in an on-demand way that is contextually relevant and situated within authentic contexts, which help learners project how lessons gleaned from gameplay informs future practice in actual clinical contexts. **Just-in-time (JIT) learning** allows students to acquire knowledge as they need it to support a continuum of learning in situated and contextually relevant paradigms.

Good video games leverage JIT learning to facilitate meaning-making and understanding among players to find or create solutions to in-game challenges that may also apply to real-world practice environments (S. S. Adams, 2009). In-game challenges should relate to both discrete and overarching gameplay and academic goals. In this way, the game provides ongoing cues and pearls to support proficiency and competency first and mastery later (Bauman & Ralston-Berg, 2014a). JIT cues and learning opportunities found throughout gameplay make relevant information easily accessible so that it need not be recalled from a distant and disjointed previous experience (Gee, 2003).

Prensky (2012) postulated that the amount of information relevant and available to educational processes is growing exponentially and that it is no longer efficient or even possible for experts, let alone students, to commit all relevant discipline-specific information to memory. From this perspective, teachers (or experts) should dedicate part of their practice to helping students learn where to find reliable and vetted information supporting and leveraging anytime–anywhere and JIT information to support clinical and professional practice. Knowing *how* to access and leverage information quickly is a salient point for nursing education and practice and all healthcare disciplines. Facilitating best practices and promoting positive patient outcomes is distributive by nature. Therefore, it is imperative that contemporary nursing students be taught and engage in informatics processes as part of their prelicensure training.

Video games leveraging informatics literacy by way of JIT access to information and anytime–anywhere learning opportunities not only increase player engagement and support player success but also situate a level of digital literacy for future practice (Bauman, 2012; Gee, 2003; Prensky, 2005; Squire, 2006). Learners practice making JIT decisions regarding required information and places where they can efficiently find it. Rather than mimicking a predetermined path or process, games and simulation activities encourage independent thought and decision-making based on the situation at hand (Aldrich, 2009). In games, rote memory is far less useful than students' ability to read and interpret the environment and mobilize the needed information (Oblinger, 2004). JIT learning mirrors real world clinical practice.

In practice, nurses and other clinicians do not have all the necessary information about any given patient prior to a clinical encounter. In other words, all practitioners face ill-structured or ambiguous problems. In clinical settings, known patient information in the form of a shift report or medical record is not always immediately or even readily accessible. Yet, traditional problem-based learning presents students with an "if/then" style of paradigm detached from actual practice. Nursing students often prepare for clinical encounters 12 to 24 hours before taking care of patients. The information gleaned in preparation is often irrelevant by the time they care for their patient. Modern video game design supports a model of information availability more accurately suited to clinical practice. In game design, information is presented through immersion in the environment, authentic interaction, and situational feedback. In **simulations**, learners make decisions and can self-correct based on immediate situational feedback from the results of their decisions. Over time, learners may achieve mastery through practice that is achieved through reflection and self-correction (Aldrich, 2009).

PROCESS OF EDUCATIONAL GAMES DEVELOPMENT

From a teaching and learning perspective, most successful game-design processes begin with identifying a problem. Faculty and teaching staff should identify an educational challenge solvable through game-based learning, such as developing pattern recognition skills needed to differentiate between various disordered breathing presentations. Educators should keep in mind that not all challenges are amenable to game-based solutions. A topic being difficult to teach or learn does not necessarily mean a game-based learning solution is the best solution. Faculty familiar with manikin-based simulation understand it is not a silver bullet for all aspects of nursing education. Understanding and evaluating a challenge within the curriculum and creating a new game or integration of an existing game to solve that challenge is a nuanced matter of *fit*.

Rote memorization is a boring and dreaded task. More intrinsic motivation and interest can be integrated into the experience by creating timed, low-fidelity games that support learning through memorization. Low-fidelity text and graphic-based simulations challenge learners' knowledge of process and procedure, as well as noncritical decision-making skills. High-fidelity decision-making simulations immerse learners in a situated environment testing performance under added stress and time constraints. Fully interactive, virtual team simulations and multiplayer games challenge decision-making ability, as well as communication, leadership, and teamwork skills.

As the complexity of the game or simulation increases, the costs and resources necessary to create and support it continue to grow. After identifying a problem and evaluating the potential fit for a game-based solution, it is important to subject such solutions to a cost–benefit analysis. When evaluating the cost–benefit of a game-based solution, consider investment time, cost, and complexity.

One consideration in designing game-based solutions is how soon a game or simulation must be ready for learners relative to the expected lead times of different solutions. If time is short, a lower-fidelity or modular version of the solution may be necessary. The solution may need to be scaled up over time rather than fully deploying a poorly designed initial solution.

Costs are also a major consideration. One must consider the costs of not only creating the solution, but also maintaining the game, troubleshooting bugs found in the game, providing rudimentary technical support, and updating the game: Will there be ongoing costs? Will there be a cost for students to license the game each semester? Faculty are unlikely to maintain a simulation activity or a video game developed from within the institution without ongoing support. Consider the technical aspects of a given solution's sustainability: "Will staff be available to support hardware and software associated with the video game or simulation activity? Will there be continued institutional support for these staff? Will staff be available to support faculty beyond initial visioning, development, and solution integration? Other questions to consider: How complex is the required solution? Can it be scaled up to accommodate more learners? Are other content areas or uses within its scope, or are its capabilities highly specific to one learning objective? If it is not scalable or is narrow in scope, is the proposed solution a one-time solution, specific to one use and not likely to be repurposed? For high expense solutions, consider a solution developed in a modular format that can be populated with content for different purposes. Think to the future and solve potential challenges at the onset of game or simulation proposal. At some point, the solution will need to be updated. Consider who will update the game or simulation activity. Are local staff capable of making content and software revisions to the solution, or will it be necessary to hire external consultants or develop collaborations among industry partners? When planning your game or simulation activity, you must consider all of these issues. Time spent meticulously planning your proposed game-based solution are time and money saved in the future.

Once you have identified a problem and selected a gamed-based solution, the next step is to vet the game-based solution for *fit*. This involves completing a cost–benefit analysis to support or reject your game for integration into the curriculum. If leveraging an existing game or creating a new game to address a problem or challenge survives fit testing, vetting, and the cost–benefit analysis, integration is a matter of determining how and where the game best **scaffolds** and supports course content and the curriculum. Integrating an existing game or digital simulation into the curriculum is much easier than developing a new digital solution from scratch. Very few faculty have the time or expertise to handcraft their own educational video game. Building a game from scratch often requires collaboration with third-party vendors and industry experts.

CONTEMPORARY PEDAGOGY SUPPORTING THE DIGITAL PARADIGM

Much of the pedagogical discussion supporting simulation, particularly manikin-based simulation, focuses on simulation as a technique supported by experiential learning theory. Kolb's experiential learning theory focuses on a continuous approach to learning through experience, in which new information or knowledge attained by learners is tested through active experimentation to form concrete experiences that drive reflective observations and abstract conceptualization (D. Kolb, 1984; A. Y. Kolb, Kolb, Passarelli, & Sharma, 2014). Simulation-based learning environments provide a chance for students to test newly acquired knowledge prior to imparting it in a clinical environment (Bauman, 2007; Euliano, 2001; Issenberg, McGaghie, Pertrusa, Lee Gordon, & Scalese, 2005; Tanner, 2006). Benner's experiential learning model (1984) supports thinking-in-action whereby previous experiences influence the quality of ongoing clinical decision-making. Schön's discussion (1983) of how professionals think-in- and on-action is also frequently cited in the simulation literature. Schön's discussion is salient because it emphasizes that there is substantial difference among those inexperienced learners who are only capable of reflecting on-action after the fact and those more experienced learners who are able to think and reflect in-action while an activity or experience is unfolding. D. Kolb, A. Y. Kolb, Benner, and Schön could not have known how their educational models and theories might be applied to game-based and simulation learning 30 years after their seminal work. These experiential learning models set the stage for contemporary models borne out of the integration of game-based and simulation activities that have emerged throughout nursing education and other clinical sciences education.

The Ecology of Culturally Competent Design (Bauman & Games, 2011; Games & Bauman, 2011) was developed to guide game-based learning and educational experiences taking place in virtual environments that attempt to address complex relationships among culture, identity, and learning. This design theory focuses on four key elements: activities, contexts, narratives, and characters. Games and Bauman (2011) suggested that these elements are crucial for nursing education, as well as other professions where acculturation and readiness for practice are essential. The Ecology of Culturally Competent Design draws from Squire's (2006) discussion of the designed experience specific to game-based learning whereby educators carefully craft in-game experiences to facilitate learning as performance to drive students towards anticipated academic goals and outcomes. Because clinical professions exist within a social paradigm, the Ecology of Culturally Competent Design also draws from Gee's (2003) theory of socially situated cognition.

Learning theories and technology supporting video games and simulation activities must be viewed from a contemporary perspective because traditional pedagogy alone may not be able to account for all of the variables associated with rapidly evolving technology. We are not advocating abandonment of traditional learning exercises. Rather, the most successful learning environments strive to engage learners on multiple levels and contemporary methodology. Using video games and digital simulation activities can serve as an adjunct to traditional teaching and learning methods. Leveraging multiple educational techniques to facilitate the transfer of knowledge and behavioral change among learners is more successful than limiting educational interventions to one technique.

Bauman's Layered Learning Theory (Bauman et al., 2014), displayed in a two-dimension linear illustration, should be conceptualized in three-dimensions like a multilevel tiered chessboard (see Figure 9.1). The analogy of the three-dimensional multilevel chessboard conveys nonlinear strategy and complexity associated with the multivariant educational process.

IMPORTANCE OF SOUND OUTCOME MEASURES

In **psychometrics**—the study of test measurement and test qualities—there are two chief concerns: reliability and validity. Reliability is consistency: Does a test provide consistent results with repeated administrations? The second issue, validity, refers to whether a test measures the concepts it purports to measure. For example, when testing students in a class on introduction to medical/surgical nursing, does the test adequately cover the concepts presented in the course? If the answer is yes, this would make the test valid. If questions on the examination dealt with advanced cardiac life support and other concepts not covered in the introductory course, the test would not demonstrate validity. The concept of validity relates to game-based learning and simulation activities. The correct outcomes must be measured. Without a valid game-based or simulation activity that maps back to the course goals and outcomes, educators may go to the trouble and expense of creating a learning activity that does not accurately reflect course learning objectives. In other words, games and digital solutions must be reliable such that outcomes are consistent over time. In addition, content must be valid such that the content being conveyed during gameplay or through immersion in the simulation or digital experience is in fact accurate and assessed through the **game mechanics** intended to assess performance.

Several quantitative methods for assessing content validity—the validity of the information included in the game or simulation activity—are beyond the scope of this text. For specific methodology for assessing content validity consult Lawshe (1975); Lynn (1986); Rutherford-Hemming (2015); and Wilson, Pan, and Schumsky (2012). Finally, Gilbert and Prion (2016) concisely describe how to carry out a validity study.

EVIDENCE-BASED EDUCATION PRACTICE

Making decisions based on evidence has come to the forefront of nursing and other healthcare disciplines. When implementing a novel teaching methodology or curriculum, we still want to make a sound evidence-based decision. Slavin (2008) concluded that new educational practices should be supported by evidence from rigorous experiments. Using **evidence-based education practices** protects students from ineffective curricular innovations. When a new game or simulation activity is developed, it is imperative to include an active research component. By deliberately including a psychometrician, statistician, or quantitative educational researcher on the development team, **game designers** are better positioned to ensure that important variables supporting educational outcomes are included throughout the design process and can be accurately measured through gameplay. Likewise, this process should include subject matter experts supporting game or simulation content so that they can collaborate with the statisticians to accurately frame salient research questions with measurable outcomes. Without integrating evidence-based practice into the game-design process, instructors, faculty, and administrators will not know whether a new game or innovative activity is valid and/or reliable.

One framework for formulating research questions is the **population, intervention, comparison group, and outcome (PICO)** framework (da Costa Santos, de Mattos Pimenta, & Nobre, 2007; Durbin, 2004; Richardson, Wilson, Nishikawa, & Hayward, 1995). Most well-operationalized research questions have all these components. Some may not have a comparison group, but when proposing a novel curriculum or an adjunct such as a game or digital simulation activity, an instructor would always be comparing the group of students who use the simulation activity or game to those who are not using it. An example of a good research question is: In a population of BSN students (P), do nursing students who practice two hours a week on a mobile application learning intervention to insert a peripherally inserted central catheter (PICC) line (I), have a higher first-time passage rate when tested on a placement of a PICC line (O) compared with nursing students practicing two hours a week inserting a PICC line in the simulation laboratory (C)?" Note that the research question does not have to be phrased in the P-I-C-O order.

An important component to consider when studying educational games is how "students" use them. If only time is recorded as a global variable, the nuances of time on task, time-in-state, or repeated measures as it relates to a given learning activity or task may be lost. Time as a global measure fails to illustrate the circumstances of gameplay as an educational intervention. If a student spends 16 hours over the course of a semester playing a game, we have failed only to understand how that gameplay unfolded. Did the student engage in the game 16 hours in a week, an hour a week over the 16-week term, or some other combination? How the game is played is pedagogically relevant and can and should be captured for further analysis by a construct called **burstiness**. Although it is beyond the scope of this text to examine burstiness in detail, the authors would refer you to Alves, Assunção, and Vaz de Melo (2016), Barabási (2005), Colman and Vukadinović Greetham (2015), and Goh and Barabási (2008).

KEY POINTS

- Game-based learning opportunities are most effective as teaching tools when they are integrated into a curriculum in meaningful ways, rather than used as supplemental content that students are free to leverage as optional exercises.
- As purposeful learning experiences, games must motivate and guide learners through lessons with the goal of achieving measurable outcomes.
- Educational game–based activities are most powerful when they augment other forms of learning modalities, such as online learning supported by learning management systems, and serve as cognitive aids.
- Effective game-based learning activities leverage the concepts of JIT and anytime–anywhere learning and fit to facilitate understanding among learners to create solutions to in-game challenges that may also be applicable to real-world environments.
- The development a game-based or simulation activity and the subsequent integration strategy must be underpinned by ongoing evidence-based research.

SUMMARY

This chapter has provided the reader with definitions to help frame processes related to game design and the integration of game-based and innovative digital solutions into the curriculum. Concepts of fit, JIT, and anytime–anywhere learning were discussed within the context of the educational digital paradigm. Furthermore, the chapter also presented a brief historical discussion of experiential pedagogy as the basis to introduce readers to contemporary pedagogy that supports game-based learning, mobile learning, and other emerging digital multimedia. In addition, the importance of evidence-based best practices and outcome measures were emphasized as part of a necessary evaluation process that should be integral to the design and integration of any new or novel educational intervention.

REFLECTIVE QUESTIONS

1. In this chapter, the authors propose that pedagogies, game-based learning design, and other virtual simulation platforms must be critically appraised to foster successful virtual simulation integration into nursing curriculum. Pedagogical issues are significant issues to consider because simulation itself is not sufficient to ensure effective learning. What are your thoughts on this?
2. The integration of game-based and innovative digital solutions into a curriculum requires a stepwise approach. Consider your institution and academic needs. What might be the first step in the integration process?
3. It is necessary to incorporate evidence-based best practices and outcome measures in relation to the integration of game-based learning into a curriculum. At what point in the integration process should best practices and outcome measures be considered? Why?

REFERENCES

Adams, S. S. (2009). What games have to offer: Information behavior and meaning-making in virtual play spaces. *Library Trends*, 57(4), 676–693. doi:10.1353/lib.0.0058

Aldrich, C. (2009). *Learning online with games, simulations, and virtual worlds: Strategies for online instruction.* San Francisco, CA: Jossey-Bass.

Alves, R. A. S., Assunção, R., & Vaz de Melo, P. O. S. (2016). *Burstiness scale: A highly parsimonious model for characterizing random series of events.* Proceedings from KDD '16: The 22nd ACM SIGKDD International Conference on Knowledge Discovery and Data Mining, San Francisco, CA. New York, NY: Association for Computing Machinery. doi:10.1145/2939672.2939852

Barabási, A. -L. (2005). The origin of bursts and heavy tails in human dynamics. *Nature*, 435(7039), 207–211. doi:10.1038/nature03459

Bauman, E. B. (2007). *High fidelity simulation in healthcare* (Doctoral dissertation). Retrieved from ProQuest Dissertations database. (UMI No. 3294196)

Bauman, E. B. (2010). Virtual reality and game-based clinical education. In K. B. Gaberson & M. H. Oermann (Eds.), *Clinical teaching strategies in nursing education* (3rd ed.). New York, NY: Springer Publishing.

Bauman, E. B. (2012). *Game-based teaching and simulation in nursing and healthcare.* New York, NY: Springer Publishing.

Bauman, E. B. (2016). Games, virtual environments, mobile applications and a futurist's crystal ball. *Clinical Simulation in Nursing*, 12(14), 109–114. doi:10.1016/j.ecns.2016.02.002

Bauman, E. B., Adams, R. A., Pederson, D., Vaughan, G., Klompmaker, D., Weins, A., . . . Squire, K. (2014). *Building a better donkey: A game-based layered learning approach to veterinary medical education* (pp. 372–375). Proceedings from GLS '10, Madison, WI. Pittsburgh, PA: Carnegie Mellon University ETC Press. ISSN 2164-6651 (print), ISSN 2164-666X (online).

Bauman, E. B., & Games, I. A. (2011). Contemporary theory for immersive worlds: Addressing engagement, culture, and diversity. In A. Cheney & R. Sanders (Eds.), *Teaching and learning in 3D immersive worlds: Pedagogical models and constructivist approaches.* IGI Global. doi:10.4018/978-1-60960-517-9.ch014

Bauman, E. B., & Ralston-Berg, P. (2014a). Serious gaming using simulations. In P. Jeffries (Ed.), *Clinical simulations in nursing: Advanced concepts, trends, and opportunities* (pp. 71–89). Philadelphia, PA: Wolters Kluwer—Lippincott Williams & Wilkins.

Bauman, E. B., & Ralston-Berg, P. (2014b). Virtual simulation. In J. Palaganas, J. Maxworthy, C. Epps, & M. E. Mancini (Eds.), *Defining excellence in simulation.* Philadelphia, PA: Wolters Kluwer—Lippincott Williams & Wilkins.

Benner, P. (1984). *From novice to expert: Excellence and power in clinical nursing practice.* Menlo Park, CA: Addison-Wesley.

Colman, E. R., & Vukadinović Greetham, D. (2015). Memory and burstiness in dynamic networks. *Physical Review E*, 92(1), 012817. doi:10.1103/PhysRevE.92.012817 da Costa Santos, C. M., de Mattos Pimenta, C. A., & Nobre, M. R. C. (2007). The PICO strategy for the research question construction and evidence search. *Revista Latino-Americana de Enfermagem, 15*(3), 508–511. doi:10.1590/S0104-11692007000300023

Deterding, S. (2015). The lens of intrinsic skill atoms: A method for gameful design. *Human–Computer Interaction, 30*(3–4), 294–335. doi:10.1080/07370024.2014.993471

Durbin, C. G. (2004). How to come up with a good research question: Framing the hypothesis. *Respiratory Care, 49*(10), 1195–1198. Retrieved from http://rc.rcjournal.com/content/respcare/49/10/1195.full.pdf

Euliano, T. Y. (2001). Small group teaching: Clinical correlation with a human patient simulator. *Advances in Physiology Education, 25*(1–4), 36–43. doi.org/10.1152/advances.2001.25.1.36

Games, I. A., & Bauman, E. B. (2011). Virtual worlds: An environment for cultural sensitivity education in the health sciences. *International Journal of Web Based Communities, 7*(2), 189–205. doi:10.1504/IJWBC.2011.039510

Gee, J. P. (2003). *What video games have to teach us about learning and literacy.* New York, NY: Palgrave-McMillan.

Gee, J. P. (2005). Good video games and good learning. *Phi Kappa Phi Forum, 85*(2), 33–37. Retrieved from http://norcalwp.org/pdf/Gee--Learning_Principles_Articles.pdf

Gee, J. P. (2007). *Good video games + good learning: Collected essays on video games, learning, and literacy.* New York, NY: Peter Lang.

Gilbert, G. E., & Prion, S. K. (2016). Making sense of methods and measurement: Lawshe's Content Validity Index. *Clinical Simulation in Nursing, 12*(12), 530–531. doi:10.1016/j.ecns.2016.08.002

Goh, K. -I., & Barabási, A. -L. (2008). Burstiness and memory in complex systems. *EPL, 81*(4), 48002. doi:10.1209/0295-5075/81/48002

Habgood, M. J., & Ainsworth, S. E. (2011). Motivating children to learn effectively: Exploring the value of intrinsic integration in educational games. *The Journal of the Learning Sciences, 20*(2), 169–206. doi:10.1080/10508406.2010.508029

Hill, T., Chidambaram, L., & Summers, J. D. (2017). Playing 'catch up' with blended learning: performance impacts of augmenting classroom instruction with online learning. *Behaviour & Information Technology, 36*(1), 54–62. doi:10.1080/0144929X.2016.1189964

Issenberg, S. B., McGaghie, W. C., Petrusa, E. R., Lee Gordon, D. L., & Scalese, R. J. (2005). Features and uses of high-fidelity medical simulations that lead to effective learning: A BEME systematic review. *Medical Teacher, 27*(1), 10–28. doi:10.1080/01421590500046924

Klopfer, E., Osterweil, S., & Salen, K. (2009). *Moving learning games forward: Obstacles, opportunities, & openness.* Cambridge, MA: The Education Arcade.

Kolb, D. (1984). *Experiential learning: Experience as the source of learning and development.* Upper Saddle River, NJ: Prentice Hall.

Kolb, A. Y., Kolb, D. A., Passarelli, A., & Sharma, G. (2014). On becoming an experiential educator: The educator role profile. *Simulation & Gaming, 45*(2), 204–234.

Lawshe, C. H. (1975). A quantitative approach to content validity. *Personnel Psychology, 28*(4), 563–575. doi:10.1111/j.1744-6570.1975.tb01393.x

Lynn, M. R. (1986). Determination and quantification of content validity. *Nursing Research, 35*(6), 382–385. doi:10.1097/00006199-198611000-00017

Oblinger, D. (2004). The next generation of educational engagement. *Journal of Interactive Media in Education.* Retrieved from https://www-jime.open.ac.uk/articles/10.5334/2004-8-oblinger

Prensky, M. (2005). Listen to the natives. *Educational Leadership, 63*(4), 8–13. Retrieved from http://www.ascd.org/portal/site/ascd/template.MAXIMIZE/menuitem.459d..._EL&javax.portlet.begCacheTok=token&javax.portlet.endCacheTok=token

Prensky, M. (2012). *Brain gain: Technology and the quest for digital wisdom.* New York, NY: Macmillan.

Ralston-Berg, P., & Lara, M. (2013). Fitting virtual reality and game-based learning into an existing curriculum. In E. Bauman (Ed.), *Game-based teaching and simulation in nursing and health care.* New York, NY: Springer Publishing. ISBN 9780826109699

Richardson, W. S., Wilson, M. C., Nishikawa, J., & Hayward, R. S. (1995). The well-built clinical question: A key to evidence-based decisions. *ACP Journal Club, 123*(3), A12–A13. doi:10.7326/ACPJC-1995-123-3-A12

Rutherford-Hemming, T. (2015). Determining content validity and reporting a content validity index for simulation scenarios. *Nursing Education Perspectives, 36*(6), 389–393. doi:10.5480/15-1640

Salen, K., & Zimmerman, E. (Eds.). (2006). *The game design reader: A rules of play anthology*. Cambridge, MA: MIT Press.

Schön, D. A. (1983). *The reflective practitioner: How professionals think in action*. New York, NY: Basic Books.

Sharp, L. A. (2012). Stealth learning: Unexpected learning opportunities through games. *Journal of Instructional Research, 1*, 42–48.

Slavin, R. E. (2008). Cooperative learning, success for all, and evidence-based reform in education. *Éducation et Didactique, 2*(2), 149–157. Retrieved from https://journals.openedition.org/educationdidactique/334

Squire, K. (2006). From content to context: Video games as designed experience. *Educational Researcher, 35*(8), 19–29. doi:10.3102/0013189X035008019

Swan, K. (2002). Building learning communities in online courses: The importance of interaction. *Education, Communication & Information, 2*(1), 23–49. doi:10.1080/1463631022000005016

Tanner, C. A. (2006). Changing times, evolving issues: The faculty shortage, accelerated programs, and simulation. *Journal of Nursing Education, 45*(3), 99–100.

Wilson, F. R., Pan, W., & Schumsky, D. A. (2012). Recalculation of the critical values for Lawshe's Content Validity Ratio. *Measurement and Evaluation in Counseling and Development, 45*(3), 197–210. doi:10.1177/0748175612440286

CHAPTER 10

Design and Creation of Virtual Gaming Simulations in Nursing Education

JENNIFER L. LAPUM, MARGARET ANNE VERKUYL, MICHELLE HUGHES, OONA ST-AMANT, DARIA ROMANIUK, LORRAINE BETTS, AND PAULA MASTRILLI

LEARNING OBJECTIVES

Upon completion of this chapter, the reader will be able to:
- Identify the process for designing and creating virtual gaming simulations in nursing education.
- Assess key decision points associated with game designs.
- Compare and contrast different forms of virtual environments and tools that inform game design.

KEY TERMS

Serious games
Virtual simulations
Virtual gaming simulation (VGS)

In virtual simulation, learners are immersed in simulated scenarios, engage in diagnostic reasoning, and experience the consequences of their clinical decisions (Duff, Miller, & Bruce, 2016; Koivisto, Niemi, Multisilta, & Eriksson, 2017). However, these consequences do not have a real-life impact, making it a safe learning environment for students and clients (Nelson, 2016; Verkuyl, Hughes, et al., 2017). **Virtual gaming simulation (VGS)** is a novel pedagogical tool and a type of virtual simulation that combines gaming features in a simulated learning experience (Verkuyl, Hughes, et al., 2017). These types of virtual gaming pedagogies provide deep-rooted learning in which the primary goal is education (Lynch-Sauer et al., 211; Verkuyl, Atack, Mastrilli, & Romaniuk, 2016).

In this chapter, an overview is provided of virtual learning environments and tools, followed by a discussion of two VGS exemplars related to a mental health assessment and prescription the of controlled substances. The former is focused on baccalaureate students, whereas the latter is focused on advanced practice nurses. These exemplars examine challenges encountered, resolutions considered, and lessons learned in VGS design. The team's reflections on design decisions and lessons learned are informed by the Faculty Administrators Students Technology Strategic Integration Model© (FAST SIM).

RELATION TO THE FAST SIM©

The authorship team did not directly apply the FAST SIM© in the design, creation, and implementation of the VGSs detailed herein. However, the FAST SIM© resonates with the team in terms of the key components to consider in game design, expected challenges, and possible resolutions. The iterative relationship between faculty, computer programmers, administrators, and students is vital to consider when integrating technological platforms into curricula so that key stakeholders are engaged in, and influence, the processes. In this chapter, the FAST SIM© model is applied as a method to reflect on and critique the groups' processes for making design decisions and to frame a discussion of the lessons learned in the process.

BACKGROUND

Experiential Nature and Learning Outcomes of Virtual Simulations and Games

Virtual simulations and **serious games** provide opportunities for experiential learning that expose learners to scenarios that simulate real life (Irwin & Coutts, 2015; Johnsen, Fossum, Vivekananda-Schmidt, Fruhling, & Slettebø, 2016). This pedagogical approach is commonly used to complement or partially replace in-person simulation and/or clinical practice. Recent research indicates that VGS has comparable learning outcomes to in-person simulation, specifically related to self-efficacy, knowledge gains, and student satisfaction (Verkuyl, Romaniuk, Atack, & Mastrilli, 2017). Integration of VGS into nursing education involves standardization in which all learners encounter the same experience (Verkuyl, Hughes, et al., 2017). The integration of technological platforms in nursing education also aligns with today's students, for whom technology has been embedded in everyday life from an early age (Miller & Jensen, 2014).

The experiential nature of virtual simulations and serious gaming gives rise to a host of learning outcomes. These modalities have the capacity to produce immersive learning experiences (De Gagne, Oh, Kang, Vorderstrasse, & Johnson, 2013; Ulrich, Farra, Smith, & Hodgson, 2014) that actively engage the learner's many senses (Foran, 2013; Saunder & Berridge, 2015). VGS and serious games, with the client portrayed in the simulation, have been shown to trigger emotional connections for the learner (Johnsen et al., 2016; Whyte, Smythe, & Scherf, 2015) and promote engagement with the topic (Duff et al., 2016; Irwin & Coutts, 2015; Ulrich et al., 2014). During these simulated experiences, learners are provided opportunities to integrate current knowledge while making clinical decisions based on client data and the surrounding environment (De Gagne et al., 2013). This strategy allows learners to practice problem solving and fortify clinical reasoning (Duff et al., 2016) while learning from their mistakes in safe environments (Nicolaidou et al., 2015; Saunder & Berridge, 2015; Ulrich et al., 2014) with no real consequences for clients (Verkuyl, Hughes, et al., 2017). Ultimately, the experiential nature of VGS helps learners prepare for expectations and skills required in clinical practice (Johnsen et al., 2016).

VIRTUAL LEARNING ENVIRONMENTS AND TOOLS

In the last decade, various virtual learning environments, such as The Neighborhood, Second Life®, Stilwell, Mirror Lake, Virtual Clinics, and others, have emerged

(Carlson-Sabelli, Giddens, Fogg, & Fiedler, 2011; Curran, Elfrink, & Mays, 2009; Giddens, 2007; Giddens, Fogg, & Carlson-Sabelli, 2010; Palumbo, De Gagne, & Murphy, 2016). These environments have gaming features that offer fictional web-based characters, communities, and scenarios focused on health care issues. The platforms create a space for teaching-learning to occur in multiple contexts, using multiple modes of communication (beyond words), and are adaptive to both high- and low-context learners (Carlson-Sabelli et al., 2011). Each virtual learning environment has varying levels of immersion, interaction, and fidelity contingent on the chosen platforms and tools.

Common types of virtual learning environments have been expanded since the emergence of Web 2.0 (Ghanbarzadeh, Ghapanchi, Blumenstein, & Talaei-Khoei, 2014), which involves a shift to more dynamic web applications and enhanced opportunity for user interaction and collaboration. The Neighborhood, for example, is a virtual community that features over 40 character stories brought to life through video clips, medical records, photos, and breaking news alerts (Giddens et al., 2010). This resource has been shown to augment learning by requiring higher-order thinking that is more imitative of real-life experiences, such as making sense of storylines and visual/audio/textual information compared to reading a textbook, which tends to be one-dimensional (Giddens et al., 2010). Other virtual environments incorporate film clips of actors (Cant & Cooper, 2014; Verkuyl, Hughes, et al., 2017) or animated characters such as avatars (Irwin & Coutts, 2015; Palumbo et al., 2016) playing patients in scenarios. Use of film clips provide experiences that allow learners to observe simulated scenarios, make clinical decisions, and influence the game's path (Verkuyl, Hughes, et al., 2017). Conversely, Second Life allows learners to participate in a virtual world through student-controlled avatars or virtual persons and to navigate clinical scenarios (Giddens et al., 2010).

Virtual learning tools are used in virtual simulation and serious games to immerse learners in interactive and dynamic storylines (Petit dit Dariel, Raby, Ravaut, & Rothan-Tondeur, 2013; Whyte et al., 2015). Game design aesthetics is used to create tension for the player and fortify the storyline (Breuer & Bente, 2010; Johnsen et al., 2016). *Game design aesthetics* refers to the tangible story and characters, as well as sensory phenomena, such as visual and aural elements, that dramatize encounters within the game (Clochesy, Buchner, Hickman, Pinto, & Znamenak, 2015; DeSmet et al., 2016; Johnsen et al., 2016; Saunder & Berridge, 2015; Whyte et al., 2015). Game scenarios and storylines can be enhanced by modifying environments, lighting, characters' vocal intonation, and facial expressions. In conjunction with aesthetics, the games' flow (including immersion, emotional reactions, and challenges, which the player encounters as while interacting and moving through a game) is important to gamification (Kapp, 2012). The concept of flow, which includes engagement, attentiveness, and pleasure in learning (Csikszentmihalyi, 1990; Shernoff, Csikszentmihalyi, Schneider, & Shernoff, 2014), has been applied to game design to enhance immersion (Faiola, Newlon, Pfaff, & Smyslova, 2013). Game flow and optimal user experiences are determined by interactive tools that provide a sense of agency and control for the user, offer challenging cognitive activities, create options to progress to the game's next level, and present immediate feedback (Clochesy et al., 2015; Faiola et al., 2013; Petit dit Dariel et al., 2013; Whyte et al., 2015). While culminating in a rich learning experience (Clochesy et al., 2015; Petit dit Dariel et al., 2013), the interactive environments associated with gamification facilitate the game's flow, learners' concentration on tasks, motivation to acquire skills, and learning opportunities (Breuer & Bente, 2010; Faiola et al., 2013; Johnsen et al., 2016). When VGSs are designed, consideration of the interactivity of the learning tools is essential for the enhancement of the game's aesthetics and flow to ensure balance between entertainment and learning (Breuer & Bente, 2010, Johnsen et al., 2016).

REQUIREMENTS AND COSTS

Virtual simulation and serious gaming requirements are multifold and require significant planning and preparation. Simulation design and creation is best achieved with interdisciplinary collaboration from clinical experts, educational specialists, administrators, instructional designers, application developers, computer programmers, multimedia production editors, and engineers (Botezatu, Hult, Kassaye Tessma, & Fors, 2010; Guise, Chambers, & Välimäki, 2012; Pittiglio, Harris, & Mili, 2011). In addition, nursing faculty members, with expertise in simulation and scenario development, are essential to the process (Kilmon, Brown, Ghosh, & Mikitiuk, 2010). It is beneficial to consider the integration of the cultural and multilingual context into VGS (Giddens et al., 2010; Guise et al., 2012) so that there is expansive uptake and relevance for application.

Costs are contingent on the project scope and complexity of the technological platform and learning tools (Foran, 2013), as well as the team's programming capacity and access to key stakeholders and resources. Although there are high costs at inception (Botezatu et al., 2010), experts indicate that virtual simulation is an economical alternative to in-person simulation (Anderson, Page, & Wendorf, 2013; Verkuyl, Romaniuk, et al., 2017); once produced, these simulations have the potential to be used by an unlimited number of learners. Most virtual simulation design and production costs range between $10,000 and $50,000 (Botezatu et al., 2010) with minimal maintenance fees (Verkuyl, Romaniuk, et al., 2017). However, there could be significant costs involved in modifying a VGS as new best practices emerge or with technological changes. To promote longevity, developers should design scenarios reflective of established best practices that are relevant and applicable across nursing programs. In comparison, in-person simulation is monetarily costly and labor intensive because of the need for laboratory space, high-fidelity manikin purchase and maintenance, and human resource facilitation of small student groups. Simulation laboratory costs can range from $100,000 to millions for state-of-the-art laboratories (Hanberg, Brown, Hoadley, Smith, & Courtney, 2007). Alternatively, students can access VGS from an electronic device such as a computer or cell phone at their convenience, which is advantageous compared with in-person simulation in which access to manikins is limited. Although some computers may lack the capacity to operate technologically sophisticated programs (Miller & Jensen, 2014; Pittiglio et al., 2011), most have sufficient power to support these platforms (Lynch-Sauer et al., 2011).

Although the literature has highlighted the many opportunities and challenges of integrating VGS into the nursing curriculum, educators are often left to navigate the nuances of this work. In this chapter, we offer two exemplars of successful implementation to better attend to some of the intricacies embedded in the process of this work.

KEY POINTS

- VGS is a novel type of virtual simulation that provides opportunities for experiential learning exposing learners to scenarios that are safe and resemble real life.
- Virtual game–based simulation fortifies the learner's capacity for problem solving and enhances clinical reasoning skills.
- Nurse educators should critically consider the combination of best practices for both gaming and nursing simulation to create meaningful educational experiences.
- The rapidly changing landscape of nursing education provides an opportune time for VGS research because of the equally rapid expansion of technology and virtual simulation.
- The integration of VGS into nursing education is a complex process that requires careful deliberation and attention. This process entails developing strategies to enhance game fidelity while weighing the significant costs involved in its technical development (Verkuyl et al., 2016).
- Because of its relative newness to nursing education, few standards specific to VGS, including best practices, have been established. The lack of standards of best practices for VGS in nursing education impedes its widespread development and implementation. Educators need to consider the combination of serious gaming best practices (Catalano, Luccini, & Mortara, 2014) with nursing simulation best practices (International Nursing Association for Clinical Simulation and Learning, 2016; Jeffries, 2005) to enhance educational value. The development of standards of best practices also needs to be considered within the context of rigorous educational theories so that meaningful VGS learning experiences are created.

SUMMARY

VGS is a novel pedagogical approach that combines virtual simulation and serious gaming. Learners are immersed in safe, interactive, and simulated experiences that resemble real life to enrich and deepen learning. In this chapter, an overview of virtual learning environments and tools was provided; following this summary you will review a discussion of two VGS exemplars, including challenges encountered in design, resolution considerations, and lessons learned. Nurse educators should critically consider the combination of best practices for both gaming and nursing simulation to create meaningful educational experiences. It is an opportune time for research because of the rapid expansion of virtual simulation and the advent of VGS. Empirical work helps establish best practice guidelines and standards for the use of this novel educational strategy.

Nursing education is changing to meet the learning needs of dynamic and technology-savvy students. The literature suggests that virtual simulation, combined with serious gaming, has the potential to be an effective teaching strategy and to address the shortage of clinical practice placements. This teaching strategy actively engages students in safe learning experiences that promote skills traditionally taught in clinical practice, such as problem solving, decision making, and critical thinking. Because of the rapid expansion of VGS in nursing education, it is an opportune time for further research so that the state of science is clear about its benefits, ways to best support learners, and ways to best guide and support educators in the effective design and implementation of this teaching modality into nursing curricula.

REFLECTIVE QUESTIONS

1. What gaming features could heighten learning for the undergraduate level nursing student?
2. How can the interactivity and fidelity of a VGS be enhanced?
3. What clinical situations would be suitable for a VGS? Describe in detail how one of the clinical situations you have identified could become a VGS.
4. How should VGS content and game experts collaborate with external partners when designing and creating games for nursing education?
5. How can VGS designers create film scripts to enhance the fidelity of the scene?
6. What is the best way to provide formative feedback at the end of the VGS?

VGS EXEMPLARS

Authors of this book chapter were involved in the design, creation, implementation, and evaluation of multiple VGSs, two of which are highlighted in this chapter (refer to Boxes 10.1 and 10.2). The design process, framed by Kolb's Experiential Learning Model (2015), assumes that knowledge is developed through a transformative experience. It is a model in which learners reflect on concrete experiences and assimilate them into concepts for revised action; the new concepts serve to create new experiences (Kolb, 2015). In the VGS, there are frequent opportunities for reflection and the application of nursing concepts, as well as for the learner to redo experiences within the game and reconsider decisions.

BOX 10.1 Exemplar 1—Mental Health Virtual Gaming Simulation

ABSTRACT

Exemplar 1 discusses a virtual gaming simulation (VGS) developed for undergraduate level nursing students. Faculty members from the Ryerson, Centennial, George Brown Collaborative Nursing Degree Program and digital education experts from the G. Raymond Chang School of Continuing Education at Ryerson University collaborated to produce the online, open-access resource, Therapeutic Communication and Mental Health Assessment: Knowledge and Practice, which includes learning modules and a VGS. The resource was designed as an interactive and experiential opportunity for learners to practice and develop skills as a community health nurse while conducting a mental health and interpersonal violence assessment in a simulated, virtual environment.

INTRODUCTION

The inception of the VGS emerged from nursing faculty who established a collaboration with an interdisciplinary team, including instructional designers, web developers, multimedia production editors, accessibility specialists,

(continued)

> **BOX 10.1 Exemplar 1—Mental Health Virtual Gaming Simulation (*continued*)**
>
> interactive design and audio recording specialists, standardized patients, and support staff. Project funding was secured through a grant from the Ontario Ministry of Training, Colleges and Universities. Administrative and operational support was provided by the director of e-learning at Ryerson University, who helped the team successfully apply for and receive these provincial funds. The funding to produce the modules and the VGS with approximately 13 decision points was $37,000 (CAD). However, significant time on the part of the nursing faculty members was provided primarily in-kind.
>
> The project goal was to produce a realistic portrayal of a nurse completing a mental health and interpersonal violence assessment while doing a home visit. These topics were chosen because mental health concerns and violence are pervasive issues that stretch across clinical settings, making the acquisition of assessment skills important for all nursing students. Furthermore, these issues tend to be overlooked in some settings and are often an underassessed domain of care. The VGS learning outcomes are based on foundational skills that are transferrable to all clinical settings and applicable to all nurses, allowing for broad uptake.
>
> The game design uses film clips of individuals acting out a scene. The filming was completed from the nurse's visual perspective; this means that within the VGS, the learner interacts in the role of nurse and sees the scene, played out by standardized patients, through the nurse's eyes. In this game, the learner (i.e., the nurse) must make a series of clinical decisions through the course of the scenario. The decision points are based on specific learning outcomes and topics contained in the online learning modules (i.e., therapeutic communication, mental status assessment depression, suicide risk, interpersonal violence).
>
> The opening scene involves the nurse knocking on the client's, Irina's, door. Immediately, the learner has to make a decision about how to respond when the client says "Who is it? What do you want?" These clinical decision points happen throughout the game. At each decision point, learners are offered three or four options to choose from, and their decision determines their experiences and results in a video depiction of the consequences of each choice made as they progress through the game. Another decision point example is when the nurse enters the client's apartment and Irina says, "Would you like to sit down?" The nurse scans the room and then is offered four options to choose from: remain standing, offer to sit down at the table, ask where to sit, or offer to sit down on the couch. In this case, the learner's decision should be based on personal safety.
>
> The team used three response choices at each decision point, including *correct, not the best, and incorrect*. Each scene flows into the next decision point when the learner chooses the correct response. If the learner chooses not the best or the incorrect response, the scene plays out depicting the nurse's action and client reaction for that particular response. Then, a window pops up to provide

(continued)

> **BOX 10.1 Exemplar 1—Mental Health Virtual Gaming Simulation (*continued*)**
>
> feedback, rationales, and a reflection question related to the learner's decision for not the best or incorrect response. At the end of the VGS, summary lists each decision point, the choices the student made, and links to content in the learning modules that pertain to the decisions.
>
> ## CHALLENGES AND RESOLUTIONS
>
> Funding is important because development of virtual simulations requires expertise and is time and labor intensive (Kilmon et al., 2010). Fortunately, online learning for postsecondary education is a component of the current provincial government's platform; thus, securing external funding with the administrative support from the university was not problematic for this specific VGS. However, it was difficult to estimate costs related to human resources in the grant proposal as the team was not familiar with the extensive time required for VGS development, and ultimately, a significant portion of the nursing faculty's time was not compensated. Although it depends on each game's complexity, it is advantageous to draw on the expertise of team members who have gone through the process of VGS development because they can provide reasonable estimates of the time commitment.
>
> Fundamental to design decisions is the fidelity of the VGS experience because it impacts learner engagement. Research has indicated that animated characters, such as avatars, do not look like a human and thus can lack realism (Kidd, Kinsley, & Morgan, 2012). Other virtual environments aim to heighten the reality with pictures of faces, textual information, and video clips (Giddens et al., 2010). On another project, a mix of nursing instructors and standardized patients acted out film scenes. The instructors experienced challenges acting out the incorrect responses, making it at times obvious to learners when responses were not correct. In addition, the instructor's lack of experience in acting resulted in multiple retakes. In this exemplar, the acting was performed completely by actors. As a result, the film clips were more realistic, enhancing the VGS fidelity. It was also cost-effective because the video-shooting time and retakes were significantly decreased.
>
> Game developers were aware that technological challenges can impact the VGS experience, including learning to navigate a virtual environment and sophisticated software programs that affect learners' experiences. These potential challenges provided an impetus for the development team to conduct a usability study before implementing the VGS into the nursing curriculum. The usability study was informed by two factors that affect technology acceptance: ease of use and perceived usefulness (Davis, 1989). The study sample included 12 nursing instructors and students. As a result of the study, changes were made (such as preliminary instructions on how to play the game) to enhance ease of use and increase VGS uptake (Verkuyl, Romaniuk, & Mastrilli, in press).

(continued)

> **BOX 10.1 Exemplar 1—Mental Health Virtual Gaming Simulation (*continued*)**
>
> Effective marketing to and support from stakeholders is crucial to enhancing integration into curricula. The literature has indicated that faculty members who are not enthusiastic and supportive of virtual simulations have been reported to negatively impact students' perceptions of these learning experiences (Carlson-Sabelli et al., 2011). Like all innovations, early adopters are important so that acceptance and integration into the curricula is smooth. As noted elsewhere in two separate usability studies (one related specifically to this VGS), support was gained for adopting this pedagogical strategy when nursing instructors were given opportunities to play the game and provide feedback so that refinements could be made during the development process (Verkuyl et al., 2016; Verkuyl et al., in press). In addition, one of the game's developers taught a health assessment course with similar learning objectives and sought feedback from the course instructors. The team decided to pilot the VGS within the course, and over 1000 students have played the game. A focus group study was conducted to explore students' experiences, which found positive outcomes related to satisfaction, high levels of engagement, and enhanced knowledge and self-efficacy (Verkuyl, Hughes, et al., 2017). The overall response from the course instructors and the students who have played the game has been overwhelmingly positive. Several colleges and universities from across Canada and elsewhere are now using this VGS in their programs as a result of the team's networking and dissemination at conferences.
>
> The challenge of how to debrief following a VGS became apparent as a result of the focus group's study of students' experiences (Verkuyl, Hughes, et al., 2017). Debriefing is pivotal following simulation (Van Heukelom, Begaz, & Treat, 2010) to facilitate students' reflection, critical thinking, learning, and future performance (Center for Medical Simulation, 2016; Decker, 2007; Dreifuerst, 2009; Rudolph, Simon, Raemer, & Eppich, 2008). The focus group study suggested that the game's self-debrief (facilitated through the feedback provided to learners) may not have been sufficient; the study participants used the focus group as a way to debrief their experiences (Verkuyl, Hughes, et al., 2017). There is a significant gap in the literature on how to debrief following a VGS. Future research is needed to explore alternative debriefing methods in virtual simulations so that what the International Nursing Association for Clinical Simulation and Learning (INACSL) (2016) refers to as "a heightened learning" is preserved. Even though INACSL's *Standards of Best Practice: Simulation* were developed to support effective simulation and learning by incorporating these standards in simulation design and development, they have not been fully conceptualized to address virtual simulation.
>
> ## LESSONS LEARNED AND SUMMARIZATION
>
> The team's involvement in game development and implementation of this VGS has led to a number of lessons learned and key takeaways to consider as other
>
> *(continued)*

> **BOX 10.1 Exemplar 1—Mental Health Virtual Gaming Simulation (*continued*)**
>
> nursing faculty members begin thinking about getting involved in developing and implementing VGSs into curricula. It is important to clearly identify the purpose and expected learning outcomes that the VGS is being designed to achieve. This step provides direction when writing decision points and guidance when aligning the VGS with curricula learning outcomes. The team members are strong proponents of film clips as the technological platform for VGS. This platform appears to enhance the simulation fidelity because learners watch and interact with real people. The enhanced fidelity increased learner engagement and connection to the characters because their intellect was activated on cognitive, emotional, and visceral levels (Verkuyl, Hughes, et al., 2017).
>
> VGS design and creation are complex initiatives that require interdisciplinary teams so that expertise can be capitalized as needed. It is important for web developers to create a user-friendly, customizable software platform that can be easily adopted and used by faculty and students. In addition, content experts and nursing faculty support are crucial for advocating uptake into nursing curricula. Technological expertise related to platforms and gaming also reduce the risks for technical glitches and enhance learning outcomes. When the VGS is used as a learning strategy, adequate technical support for both students and faculty members help decrease episodes of frustration with the new learning modality. The chapter authors note the value of including, from the inception of game development, a comprehensive plan for both formative and summative evaluations that can benefit future developers and researchers in this field.
>
> ### PAUSE AND REFLECT
>
> As the team pauses and reflects, they are left to consider how to enhance the technological sophistication of future VGSs. Students who have played the VGS voiced interest in having increased gaming features. There is limited research on what VGS features motivate engagement, increase tension, and enhance the learning experience.
>
> *Source:* Ryerson University. (n.d.-b). Therapeutic communication and mental health assessment. Retrieved from https://de.ryerson.ca/games/nursing/mental-health

> **BOX 10.2 Exemplar 2—Pediatrics: Prescribing Controlled Substances**
>
> ### ABSTRACT
>
> Exemplar 2 discusses a VGS developed for advanced practice nurses. In this VGS, the learner assumes the role of a nurse practitioner (NP) assessing an adolescent client in a primary care clinic to determine the appropriateness of prescribing a controlled substance. The client's reason for seeking care is "difficulty focusing at school." The simulation goal is for learners to assess,

(continued)

BOX 10.2 Exemplar 2—Pediatrics: Prescribing Controlled Substances (*continued*)

diagnose, and ultimately determine treatment based on best practices related to controlled substances. At each decision point, learners choose from three or four options. When learners successfully select the correct answer, they move on to the next scenario. Learners are prompted to critically reflect on their responses, then are asked another question and provided with two options if they do not select the correct answer.

INTRODUCTION

Following a conference presentation, staff from the Canadian Association of Schools of Nursing (CASN) approached faculty members associated with the VGS detailed in Exemplar 1 and voiced interest in this learning strategy. The CASN staff inquired whether a VGS could be developed as part of a current online learning project for NP-Resource Prescribing Controlled Drugs and Substances. At the time of the request, the online learning project was partially complete, and there was a tight deadline to develop the VGS to meet CASN's deadline.

To meet the five-month deadline, it was decided to follow a similar design akin to the film clips described in Exemplar 1. The subject experts were nursing faculty who began by making decisions on the game design and flow. Later in game development, other team members (i.e., instructional designer, videographer, web developer) became involved in the process. It was difficult to use an identical design because the modules were not embedded within this VGS because CASN developed these separate from the game. In addition, the comprehensive documents (i.e., consultation notes, assessment notes, documentation, prescriptions) involved a long script that could not be directly embedded in the VGS; thus, these documents opened in another window when playing the VGS. Also, the label "incorrect response" was not used because it did not lend itself best to the topic. Rather, the label "not the best" was used for responses that were identified as not the correct response. In this VGS, there was provision of feedback for all responses, and leading questions were provided to help direct the learner to the right answer. At the end of the VGS, a summary page provided all the questions the learner answered, with the correct answers highlighted in different colors from answers that were not the best responses. This VGS did not include hyperlinks to the modules for each decision point. At the end of the VGS, the learner is provided with the number of questions it took them to complete the game with the shortest route being 13 questions/responses.

This VGS begins with 14-year-old Owen sitting in a clinic room focused on his digital music player. The NP enters and greets the client and his mother, who states that the school requested that Owen sees a healthcare professional because he is having trouble focusing and needs medication to help him pay attention. The learner (i.e., the NP) is presented with three options on how

(*continued*)

> **BOX 10.2 Exemplar 2—Pediatrics: Prescribing Controlled Substances** (*continued*)
>
> to respond (i.e., address lack of focus, discuss medication, or address school experience). The scenario continues to the next scene and decision point if the learner chooses "address school experience" (i.e., the correct response). Otherwise, the scenario continues based on the response that was not the best and provides feedback. The learner is then given the option of choosing from two or three responses until the correct response is chosen. As the VGS continues and the learner chooses the correct responses, the client begins to open up about his situation, and the learner is able to complete a comprehensive assessment to determine Owen's need for a controlled substance.
>
> ### CHALLENGES AND RESOLUTIONS
>
> The development team made the decision to insert the comprehensive notes in a PDF document that opened in a new window to be viewed. This formatting was required because the subject experts felt it was important for the NP in the scenario to read these notes while playing the VGS to make specific clinical decisions. Although the web designer felt opening a document in a new window took away from the basics of gaming design, it was an essential solution based on the substantive content required in this context. CASN staff and the NPs who have played the VGS have anecdotally responded positively to the format and content.
>
> Because of the tight timeline for creation, the actors were not provided film scripts in a timely manner so memorization of lines was not achievable. This challenge specifically affected the NP who had the most lines. Fortunately, the film's point of view was from the NP's perspective because the learner plays the game as the NP. Thus, the actor playing the NP was not visually filmed and was able to read directly from the script. Despite this resolution, there appears to be less natural speech when someone reads from a script, so the NP's lines were audio-recorded separate from the filming. These audio-recordings were used in areas where the tone/words sounded scripted. In future game development, the film scenes should be acted out a few weeks before recording and lines adjusted for a final script.
>
> At the end of the VGS, as the Exemplar 1 noted, learners received a report with feedback for each decision made and an autogenerated indication of the level of their ability. However, some questions within the VGS are more important to ask than others, but this was not factored into the assigned level of ability. Therefore, the learner could have a false sense of their assessment ability. At the end of the VGS in Exemplar 2, the learner received a list of the number of specific decisions made with feedback and the number of responses that took them out of a perfect score of 13. There was no autogenerated judgement regarding the learner's skill, decreasing the risk of potentially making a faulty assessment of their ability.

(continued)

> **BOX 10.2 Exemplar 2—Pediatrics: Prescribing Controlled Substances (*continued*)**
>
> ### LESSONS LEARNED/SUMMARIZATION
>
> The team's involvement in game development and implementation of this VGS has led to several lessons learned. Game design and creation is a complex and lengthy process. It is important to include the whole team as early as possible in the process with an estimated 4- to 12-month timeline contingent on the game's complexity and the team members' time commitment. Involvement and consultation of the full team from the beginning of game development would have prevented some of the challenges that occurred. In future filming for VGS, the team would advance some of the preparatory work. For example, it is helpful to role-play the scenarios with the actors a few weeks before the filming so that script issues can be identified early. This strategy would allow for the script to be finalized ahead of time, giving actors the opportunity to fully memorize it.
>
> ### PAUSE AND REFLECT
>
> As the team pauses and reflects, they are left to consider how to best approach VGS development with external partners. They must address how they would plan for script design and feedback.
>
> *Source:* Ryerson University. (n.d.-a). Pediatrics: Prescribing controlled substances. Retrieved from https://de.ryerson.ca/games/nursing/treatment-plans/#

REFERENCES

Anderson, J., Page, A., & Wendorf, D. (2013). Avatar-assisted case studies. *Nurse Educator, 38*(3), 106–109. doi:10.1097/NNE.0b013e31828dc260

Botezatu, M., Hult, H., Kassaye Tessma, M., & Fors, U. (2010). As time goes by: Stakeholder opinions on the implementation and use of a virtual patient simulation system. *Medical Teacher, 32*(11), e509–e516. doi:10.3109/0142159X.2010.519066

Breuer, J., & Bente, G. (2010). Why so serious? On the relation of serious games and learning. *Journal for Computer Game Culture, 4*(1), 7–24. Retrieved from http://www.eludamos.org/eludamos/index.php/eludamos/article/view/vol4no1-2/146

Cant, R., & Cooper, S. (2014). Simulation in the Internet age: The place of Web-based simulation in nursing education. An integrative review. *Nursing Education Today, 34*(12), 1435–1442. doi:10.1016/j.nedt.2014.08.001

Carlson-Sabelli, L., Giddens, J., Fogg, L., & Fiedler, R (2011). Challenges and benefits of using a virtual community to explore nursing concepts among baccalaureate nursing students. *International Journal of Nursing Education Scholarship, 8*(1). doi:10.2202/1548-923X.2136

Catalano, C., Luccini, A., & Mortara, M. (2014). Guidelines for an effective design of serious games. *International Journal of Serious Games, 1*(1), 1–13. doi.org/10.17083/ijsg.v1i1.8

Center for Medical Simulation. (2016). Debriefing as defined by CMS. Retrieved from https://harvardmedsim.org/resources-other.php

Clochesy, J., Buchner, M., Hickman, J., Pinto, M., & Znamenak, K. (2015). Creating a serious game for health. *Journal of Health & Human Services Administration, 38*(2), 162–173. Retrieved from http://www.jstor.org/stable/24463889

Csikszentmihalyi, M. (1990). *The psychology of optimal experience.* New York, NY: Harpers & Row.

Curran, C., Elfrink, V., & Mays, B. (2009). Building a virtual community for nursing education: The town of Mirror Lake. *Journal of Nursing Education, 48*(1), 30–35. doi:10.3928/01484834-20090101-03

Davis, F. (1989). Perceived usefulness, perceived ease of use, and user acceptance of information technology. *MIS Quarterly*, *13*(3), 319–340. doi:10.2307/249008

Decker, S. (2007). Integrating guided reflection into simulated learning experiences. In P. Jeffries (Ed.), *Simulation in nursing: From conceptualization to evaluation* (pp. 73–85). New York, NY: National League for Nursing.

De Gagne, J., Oh, J., Kang, J., Vorderstrasse, A., & Johnson, C. (2013). Virtual worlds in nursing education: A synthesis of the literature. *Journal of Nursing Education*, *52*(7), 391–396. doi:10.3928/01484834-20130610-03

DeSmet, A., Thompson, D., Baranowski, T., Palmeira, A., Verloigne, M., & De Bourdeaudhuij, I. (2016). Is participatory design associated with the effectiveness of serious digital games for healthy lifestyle promotion? A meta-analysis. *Journal of Medical Internet Research*, *18*(4), e94. doi:10.2196/jmir.4444

Dreifuerst, K. (2009). The essentials of debriefing in simulation learning: A concept analysis. *Nursing Education Perspectives*, *30*(2), 109–114.

Duff, E., Miller, L., & Bruce, J. (2016). Online virtual simulation and diagnostic reasoning: A scoping review. *Clinical Simulation in Nursing*, *12*(9), 377–384. doi:10.1016/j.ecns.2016.04.001

Faiola, A., Newlon, C., Pfaff, M., & Smyslova, O. (2013). Correlating the effects of flow and telepresence in virtual worlds: Enhancing our understanding of user behavior in game-based learning. *Computers in Human Behaviour*, *29*(3), 1113–1121. doi:10.1016/j.chb.2012.10.003

Foran, A. (2013). Learning from experience: Shared constructs in virtual reality and occupational therapy. *International Journal of Therapy & Rehabilitation*, *18*(7), 362–369. doi:10.12968/ijtr.2011.18.7.362

Ghanbarzadeh, R., Ghapanchi, A., Blumenstein, M., & Talaei-Khoei, A. (2014). A decade of research on the use of three-dimensional virtual worlds in health care: A systematic literature review. *Journal of Medical Internet Research*, *16*(2), e47. doi:10.2196/jmir.3097

Giddens, J. (2007). The Neighborhood: A web-based platform to support conceptual teaching and learning. *Nursing Education Perspectives*, *28*(5), 251–256.

Giddens, J., Fogg, L., & Carlson-Sabelli, L. (2010). Learning and engagement with a virtual community by undergraduate nursing students. *Nursing Outlook*, *58*(5), 261–267. doi:10.1016/j.outlook.2010.08.001

Guise, V., Chambers, M., & Välimäki, M. (2012). What can virtual patient simulation offer mental health nursing education? *Journal of Psychiatric & Mental Health Nursing*, *19*(5), 410–418. doi:10.1111/j.1365-2850.2011.01797.x

Hanberg, A., Brown, S., Hoadley, T., Smith, S., & Courtney, B. (2007). Finding funding: The nurses' guide to simulation success. *Clinical Simulation in Nursing*, *3*(1), e5–e9. doi:10.1016/j.ecns.2009.05.032

International Nursing Association for Clinical Simulation and Learning. (2016). Standards of best practice: Simulation. *Clinical Simulation in Nursing*, *12*, S48–S50. doi:10.1016/j.ecns.2013.06.005

Irwin, P., & Coutts, R. (2015). A systematic review of the experience of using Second Life® in the education of undergraduate nurses. *Journal of Nursing Education*, *54*(10), 572–577. doi:10.3928/01484834-20150916-05

Jeffries, P. (2005). A framework for designing, implementing, and evaluating simulations used as teaching strategies in nursing. *Nursing Education Perspectives*, *26*(2), 96–103.

Johnsen, H., Fossum, M., Vivekananda-Schmidt, P., Fruhling, A., & Slettebø, Å (2016). Teaching clinical reasoning and decision-making skills to nursing students: Design, development, and usability evaluation of a serious game. *International Journal of Medical Informatics*, *94*, 39–48. doi:10.1016/j.ijmedinf.2016.06.014

Kapp, K. (2012). *The gamification of learning and instruction: Game-based methods and strategies for training and education*. San Francisco, CA: Pfeifer.

Kidd, L., Kinsley, S., & Morgan, K. (2012). Effectiveness of a Second Life® simulation as a teaching strategy for undergraduate mental health nursing students. *Journal of Psychosocial Nursing & Mental Health Services*, *50*(7), 28–37. doi:10.3928/02793695-20120605-04

Kilmon, C. A., Brown, L., Ghosh, S., & Mikitiuk, A. (2010). Immersive virtual reality simulations in nursing education. *Nursing Education Perspectives*, *31*(5), 314–317.

Koivisto, J., Niemi, H., Multisilta, J., & Eriksson, E. (2017). Nursing students' experiential learning processes using an online 3D simulation game. *Education and Information Technologies*, *22*(1), 383–398. doi:10.1007/s10639-015-9453-x

Kolb, D. (2015). *Experiential learning: Experience as the source of learning and development* (2nd ed.). Upper Saddle River, NJ: Pearson.

Lynch-Sauer, J., Vandenbosch, T., Kron, F., Gjerde, C., Arato, N., Sen, A., & Fetters, M. D. (2011). Nursing students' attitudes toward video games and related new media technologies. *Journal of Nursing Education, 50*(9), 513–523. doi:10.3928/01484834-20110531-04

Miller, M., & Jensen, R. (2014). Avatars in nursing: An integrative review. *Nurse Educator, 39*(1), 38–41. doi:10.1097/01.NNE.0000437367.03842.63

Nelson, R. (2016). Replicating real life: Simulation in nursing education and practice. Providing learners the experiences without the risks. *American Journal of Nursing, 116*(5), 20–21. doi:10.1097/01.NNE.0000437367.03842.63

Nicolaidou, I., Antoniades, A., Constantinou, R., Marangos, C., Kyriacou, E., Bamidis, P., . . . Pattichis, C. S. (2015). A virtual emergency telemedicine serious game in medical training: A quantitative, professional feedback-informed evaluation study. *Journal of Medical Internet Research, 17*(6), e150. doi:10.2196/jmir.3667

Palumbo, M., De Gagne, J., & Murphy, G. (2016). Interprofessional care of elders: Utilizing the virtual learning environment. *Journal of American Association of Nursing Practitioners, 28*(9), 465–470. doi:10.1002/2327-6924.1236

Petit dit Dariel, O., Raby, T., Ravaut, F., & Rothan-Tondeur, M. (2013). Developing the serious games potential in nursing education. *Nurse Education Today, 33*(12), 1569–1575. doi:10.1016/j.nedt.2012.12.014

Pittiglio, L., Harris, M., & Mili, F. (2011). Development and evaluation of a three-dimensional virtual hospital unit: VI-MED. *Computers, Informatics, Nursing, 29*(5), 267–271. doi:10.1097/NCN.0b013e318222ef46

Rudolph, J., Simon, R., Raemer, D., & Eppich, W. (2008). Debriefing as formative assessment: Closing performance gaps in medical education. *Academic Emergency Medicine, 15*(11), 1010–1016. doi:10.1111/j.1553-2712.2008.00248.x

Ryerson University. (n.d.-a). Pediatrics: Prescribing controlled substances. Retrieved from https://de.ryerson.ca/games/nursing/treatment-plans/#

Ryerson University. (n.d.-b). Therapeutic communication and mental health assessment. Retrieved from https://de.ryerson.ca/games/nursing/mental-health

Saunder, L., & Berridge, E. (2015). Immersive simulated reality scenarios for enhancing students' experience of people with learning disabilities across all fields of nurse education. *Nurse Education in Practice, 15*(6), 397–402. doi:10.1016/j.nepr.2015.04.007

Shernoff, D., Csikszentmihalyi, M., Schneider, B., & Shernoff, E. (2014). Student engagement in high school classrooms from the perspective of flow theory. In *Applications of Flow in Human Development and Education* (pp. 475–494). Netherlands: Springer. doi:10.1007/978-94-017-9094-9_24

Ulrich, D., Farra, S., Smith, S., & Hodgson, E. (2014). The student experience using virtual reality simulation to teach decontamination. *Clinical Simulation in Nursing, 10*(11), 546–553. doi:10.1016/j.ecns.2014.08.003

Van Heukelom, J., Begaz, T., & Treat, R. (2010). Comparison of postsimulation debriefing versus in-simulation debriefing in medical simulation. *Simulation in Healthcare, 5*(2), 91–97. doi:10.1097/SIH.0b013e3181be0d17

Verkuyl, M., Atack, L., Mastrilli, P., & Romaniuk, D. (2016). Virtual gaming to develop students' pediatric nursing skills: A usability test. *Nursing Education Today, 46*, 81–85. doi:10.1016/j.nedt.2016.08.024

Verkuyl, M., Hughes., M., Tsui, J., Betts, L., St-Amant, O., & Lapum, J. (2017). Virtual gaming simulation in nursing education: A focus group study. *Journal of Nursing Education, 56*(5), 274–280. doi:10.3928/01484834-20170421-04

Verkuyl, M., Romaniuk, D., Atack, L., & Mastrilli, P. (2017). Virtual gaming simulation for nursing education: An experiment. *Clinical Simulation in Nursing, 13*(5), 238–244. doi:10.1016/j.ecns.2017.02.004

Verkuyl, M., Romaniuk, D., & Mastrilli, P. (in press). Virtual gaming simulation of a mental health assessment: A usability study.

Whyte, E., Smyth, J., & Scherf, K. (2015). Designing serious game interventions for individuals with autism. *Journal of Autism & Developmental Disorders, 45*(12), 3820–3831. doi:10.1007/s10803-014-2333-1

CHAPTER 11

Virtual Gaming in Nursing Education

NATÁLIA DEL ANGELO AREDES, SUZANNE HETZEL CAMPBELL, AND LUCIANA MARA MONTI FONSECA

LEARNING OBJECTIVES

Upon completion of this chapter, the reader will be able to do:
- Explore the use of serious games as a viable method for educating nurses.
- Assess present resources that use serious games for education in the health professions.
- Explain the steps to consider when developing serious games.
- Appreciate the challenges and opportunities for the use of virtual gaming in nursing education.

KEY TERMS

Active learning
Active video games (AVGs)
Debriefing
Emotional design
Engagement
Gameability
Game dynamic
Game mechanics
Games for learning
Gamification
Heuristic
Human-computer interaction (HCI)
Prebriefing
Prototyping
Serious games (SGs)
Target users

It is important that we explore ways to provide associations between recreation and education. **Serious games (SGs)** offer the opportunity to have fun playing a game while learning. As we learn how to harness the power of instructional technologies and associate positive emotional experiences such as having fun with learning, we can transform education and begin to achieve a learner-centered paradigm.

RELATION TO THE FAST SIM©

This chapter relates to the faculty aspect of the Faculty Administrators Students Technology Strategic Integration Model© (FAST SIM). Faculty must be able to assume the beginner role of technology user, move to the experienced roles of designer/developer and innovator, and then move into the expert roles of researcher and pedagogy synthesizer. Faculty influence the use of SGs and ways to merge pedagogy, content, and technology to facilitate learning, and they help the model's cog keep moving and advancing understanding of and capabilities in relation to moving to a learner-centered paradigm.

TEACHING–LEARNING THROUGH VIRTUAL (SERIOUS) GAMING

In the past, games have been used for education to create a climate of fun and excitement, encouraging students' sense of competitiveness and curiosity. Today, with advanced technology and various devices becoming popular even in developing countries, SGs are an upcoming trend. An updated systematic review of the literature combined outcome information related to SGs or **games for learning** (the terms are used interchangeably) and found that, of the articles fitting inclusion criteria, game genres included simulations (14), simulation games (10), and role-playing games (Boyle et al., 2016). Games in this review addressed topics such as exercise (Pichierri, Murer, & de Bruin, 2012), rehabilitation (Hurkmans, Ribbers, Streur-Kranenburg, Stam, & Van Den Berg-Emons, 2011), quality of life (Chen, Hsieh, Wei, & Kao, 2011), and advanced life support training (Boyle et al., 2016; Cook, McAloon, O'Neill, & Beggs, 2012). Researchers using virtual games recognize that player characteristics, game features, and the context of play variables all have an influence on game outcomes and require further study (Boyle et al., 2016). In addition, studies examining skill acquisition outcomes were more common with higher-quality randomized controlled trials (RCTs) in health, and three notable ones looked at triage skill performance (Knight et al., 2010), knowledge retention and proficiency in CPR team training (Creutzfeldt, Hedman, & Fellander-Tsai, 2012), and advanced cardiac life support or advanced cardiovascular life support (ACLS) performance in India (Delasobera et al., 2010).

As identified in the **NMC Horizons Report** (Johnson, Adams Becker, Estrada, & Freeman, 2014), SG use is predicted as a short-term goal for adoption in education. SGs are educational games that use *fun* to engage students while incorporating entertainment components, such as animated and motivating resources, to support the learning experience. Once created, SGs can be reused and students can make mistakes in a safe environment and repeat the game until they reach their goals (or mastery). SGs can be projected in many formats, including simulating real situations (De Freitas & Neumann, 2009). This feature has been very successful among health educators who perceive SGs as an interesting opportunity to provide meaningful learning experiences through entertainment, capture students' curiosity, and motivate them to be active learners.

Thus, in the context of active methods for learning, technology innovation and **gamification** can strengthen nursing faculty strategies to engage students in the teaching–learning process. It is important to emphasize that the technology does not do it by itself and that the use of virtual games in education requires developing SGs that connect to learning objectives and expected competencies while being mindful of users' interests.

More and more health courses in higher education, including nursing, have increased their use of educational technologies as a way to prepare students prior to practical experiences in clinical environments with live patients and problems requiring teamwork and quick decision making. Students recognize the potential of SGs as resources that offer fulfillment and motivation to learn. In addition, SGs have the potential to enhance clinical reasoning and decision making and skills' training in cognitive, procedural, and behavioral areas.

Despite the focus on virtual games use in a simulation format, many SGs have been developed with varying themes and **gameability** heuristics. It is interesting for faculty and students to know what resources are available and to use them to suit course purposes. Some SGs are freely available, and others are not; it is important to mention that gamification in learning has increased interest in private companies, building most likely on the concept of the billion-dollar entertainment gaming industry. Given this, educators must be vigilant to the quality of resources and the accuracy of evidence-based research and clinical protocols used to develop the games for nursing education. Also, there is still a language barrier for some games because many countries have been creating them for their own use; therefore, partnerships between faculty at universities to translate and validate the SGs for domestic use is an exciting opportunity.

There are resources available on the Internet, including SG in pharmacology, aiming to provide a memory exercise for drug groups and their function (Foronda & Bauman, 2014; Lancaster, 2013), and Second Life®, technology through an innovative interface for clinical case solving through the use of avatars so that students can interact with previously created avatars representing patients or health team members and respond with interventions through their own avatars, defining responses and describing conduct by recording their voices (Anderson, Page, & Wendorf, 2013; Foronda & Bauman, 2014). Other research examining the use of games in healthcare include a systematic review of **active video games (AVGs)** to increase physical activity (Peng, Crouse, & Lin, 2012), another systematic review of the use of games for health-related outcomes, including health education of practitioners and patients (Primack et al., 2012), and the cognitive and motivational effects of playing games (Wouters, van Nimwegen, van Oostendorp, & van der Spek, 2013). Specifically in nursing, SGs have been used to teach pharmacology (Lancaster, 2013), safety training for home health care workers (Darragh et al., 2016), life-support training (Cook et al., 2012), neonatal nursing care with preterm newborns (Fonseca et al., 2015), health education for children (Dias et al., 2016), and empathetic responses and attitudes about older adults with an aging game (Henry, Ozier, & Johnson, 2011). Some see virtual gaming simulation as an experiment (Verkuyl, Romaniuk, Atack, & Mastrilli, 2017), but there is no question that much research is needed in this area.

Following the success of clinical simulation as an **active learning** strategy for nursing and other health professions, virtual simulation using SGs is gaining widespread focus and has demonstrated positive results in learning, providing a student-centered approach and triggering curiosity in the process of researching responses and rationale to support actions. From a patient safety perspective, SGs using virtual simulation represent an opportunity for students to experience "thinking and acting like a nurse" in a virtual and safe scenario that represents reality and allows students to respond, knowing that if they make an error virtually, real patients will not be affected. When mistakes happen in a virtual world, it is possible, and necessary, for students to try again and again until they feel safe about the skill or knowledge they are developing.

In nursing, many SGs cover complicated themes such as trauma, cardiorespiratory resuscitation (Boada et al., 2015), clinical evaluation, and care interventions for maternal health, pediatrics, and adults in general (Aredes, 2016; Fonseca et al., 2015).

Considering the lifelong learning and professional development inherent for nurses, SGs can also provide a way for nurses to keep up to date, learn about evidence-based practice, and build capacity with knowledge translation of new research. In addition, SGs can help nurses educate their communities, providing information about relevant health promotion or chronic disease management through entertainment. In Brazil, our research group has created a SG called *e-Baby Family* to help parents identify respiratory problems in newborns, both in the hospital and at home, with scenarios on how to manage situations such as visitors with the flu, outside trips with a newborn, and choking (at home).

Creating SGs with virtual simulation requires following steps carefully to ensure the quality of the final product and alignment of the game to learning objectives. This is discussed in detail later in the chapter. In addition, it is crucial to have a strong relationship and clear communication with the information technology (IT) team to translate the health information accurately to animations and gameability.

ENACTING SCENARIOS/ACTIVITIES

Developing the virtual setting

To develop an SG with virtual simulation, some authors have suggested good practices to accommodate its main features (Marfisi-Schottman, George, & Tarpin-Bernard, 2010; Preece, Rogers, & Sharp, 2007). Based on our experience and literature review, we have developed the following schema (refer to Figure 11.1).

In the scope definition, the authors choose a theme based on students' learning needs, faculty needs in specific areas, alignment with clinical practice demand (health and social context), and/or literature trends based on epidemiology, representing a broad impact on communities in the present or future. In all cases, it is important to consider the relevance and impact of the SGs, matching the cost and effort to the broad reach that it will have and the multiple areas it will serve.

For game format and functionality, it is recommended to play games already available online and use these existing games to approximate desirability, **target users**, learning goals, and resources. It is also important to know gameability heuristics before SGs development, and this content is usually discussed in validation studies.

A detailed description of the game based on the authors' intention and plan helps inform decisions and is connected with script definition. This description

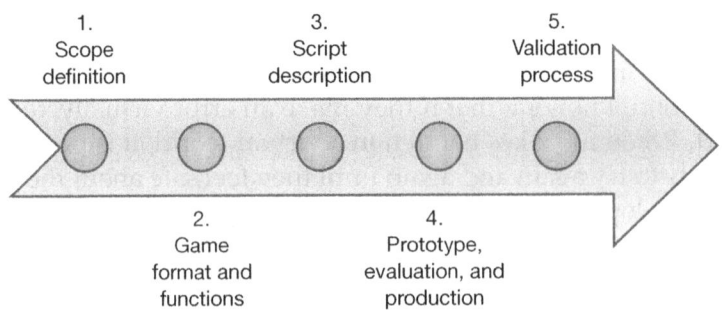

FIGURE 11.1 Virtual simulation game development process.

helps the creator decide on the appropriate bottoms, colors, texts (i.e., fonts, styles), **game dynamic**, SG major format, and goals and specific features in the game (e.g., rewards, phases, tips, retry, reset and pause, save). As the presented SGs is a virtual simulation, the script acts as a storyboard describing the objectives, scene/context within which the situation to be solved arises, expected actions from users, feedback on actions (e.g., correct or incorrect, redirection of user if necessary), outcome in the simulation showing users what happened after their intervention (Farra et al., 2016).

Then **prototyping** is crucial for providing author feedback on what is possible or feasible according to the script. IT experts on game development provide valuable contributions regarding **game mechanics**, gameability, and other related **heuristics** such as interface, educational elements, content, and multimedia. However, mixing health and IT professionals requires a clear understanding of previously defined goals, technological reach, and capture intended by the authors, translation between knowledge areas, and most important, detailed scripts for communication.

Given our experience, this step is most critical and has the potential for greatest friction between educators and IT, representing an opportunity for authors to be vigilant, attentive, and flexible. Strategies for success include revisiting the first draft (script) of the game multiple times and tracking changes throughout the process, ensuring that the learning goals previously defined are represented, and evaluating the robustness of the SG. Prototyping does not need to use time-consuming technology to be evaluated by both the authors and the IT team. To save costs, looking for other resources that provide a vision for future products is encouraged.

After production, a validation process is a good practice for ensuring quality and determining how accurately the final version of the game aligns to the scripted game's heuristics. There are some instruments for validating SG, such as Playability Heuristic Evaluation for Educational Computer Games (PHEG; Mohamed & Jafaar, 2012), Heuristic Evaluation for Digital Educational Games (HEDEG; Valle, Vilela, Parriera Junior, & Inocencio, 2013), and EGameFlow (Fu, Su, & Yu, 2009). See Table 11.1.

Other instruments help in this process even though they were not specifically developed for SG—digital content in general; these include software for different purposes and virtual environments of learning, based on heuristics of usability, accessibility, and inclusion.

TABLE 11.1 SG Validation Instruments

Instrument	Key Features
PHEG	Validation with experts in heuristics: Interface, content, multimedia, educational aspects, gameability

HEDEG	Validation with experts or users:
	  Interface, content, multimedia, educational aspects, gameability
	  HEDEG is adapted from PHEG and contains additional and modified items in the described heuristics.

EGameFlow	Validation with users: Concentration, goal clarity, feedback, challenge, autonomy, immersion, social Interaction, knowledge improvement

Heuristics of usability, accessibility, and inclusion have been studied in computer design to adapt software to users' needs, helping developers worldwide to format their digital content to provide engaging and quality digital navigation. This is a very important component for the validation process and requires the definition of a theoretical framework, use of a validated questionnaire, and contribution from experts in performing this type of evaluation.

Nevertheless, considering that SGs incorporate educational aspects, it is crucial to assess the pedagogical approach taken in the development of the games, its relevance for learning, and students' satisfaction in using SGs when learning. The instruments mentioned earlier can be helpful when considering the gap in the research in this area and the increasing use of digital educational games.

Validation can be performed by multiple groups, including experts in games and technology, nurses as clinical experts, and students, professionals, or consumers in the target population of users. Each group offers suggestions relevant to the quality and impact of the SGs, and their input provides an external review of the match between the created SG and its goals, as well as assists in making modifications to improve the technology and learning experience.

Other differential aspects to consider during SG development are the concepts of **human-computer interaction (HCI)** and **emotional design**. HCI is the discipline that studies how people interact with computers, analyzing the connection between design and computation from a humanistic and ergonomic perspective, considering the experience of use and users' preferences (Xavier, Garcia, & Neris, 2012). Adopting HCI knowledge to SG creation certainly aggregates quality by aiming to provide the best experience possible to the final user, which is especially important in the educational field when motivation and satisfaction in use are determinants of the learning process and meaningful use of technology as support.

Another component we highlight is emotional design as the area that studies emotions evoked by technologies or products' use, which can occur during the use of a SG (Norman, 2008). SG must go beyond realism, it has to incorporate advanced knowledge of design aiming to generate positive emotions from users, thus motivating access and learning experiences (Fonseca et al., 2014).

IMPORTANCE OF PREBRIEFING AND DEBRIEFING

More than playing an SG, students must reflect on challenges faced or problems presented in the game that lead to the clinical reasoning and decisions that they have made in phases. This reflection can occur during **debriefing**, which is commonly used in laboratory simulation. Debriefing is a wide field of knowledge in education that is guided by different referential branches. The key difference with debriefing in the context of SG is the timing: Should **prebriefing** with an introduction to the SG come first and at what point should debriefing occur? Given that one of the advantages of computational games is that there is no need for laboratory use or faculty support in real time, is there a different approach that can be recommended for debriefing after SGs?

These authors concur that it is relevant to offer after-gaming encounters in person in which students and facilitators can discuss the experience following typical simulation debriefing techniques (International Nursing Association for Clinical Simulation and Learning [INACSL] Standards Committee, 2016). We encourage, when possible, arranging for all members of the team (i.e., educators, IT, staff, and students) to come together to discuss the students' learning experiences during the virtual game. This will provide an opportunity for free discussion and reflection, and conclusions can be drawn from the collective input that could lead to several outcomes, including enhancing the student's knowledge and understanding of the content and making necessary alterations to the game, approach, and evaluation.

In other contexts, when located in a hybrid or exclusively online perspective, other strategies for debriefing, such as forums in virtual environments mediated by faculty, can be identified. In the current INACSL *Standards of Best Practice: Simulation Debriefing*, criterion 3 was amended from the previous version. The criterion formerly recommended that "debriefing be facilitated by a person(s) who observed the simulated experience" (Decker et al., 2013, p. S28). The revised criterion recommends that debriefing be, "facilitated by a person(s) who can devote enough concentrated attention during the simulation to effectively debrief the simulation-based experience" (INACSL Standards Committee, 2016, pp. S22). Modification to the language for this criterion allows for adherence to the standards with regard to debriefing simulation which occurs in virtual learning environments. Box 11.1 provides suggestions for debriefing virtual simulation using an online conferencing platform based on the INACSL standards. Debriefing using an online platform can also be used for prebriefing, including file exchange, discussions on the theme by participants in virtual chats or forums itself, access to relevant videos in the interest area, and other multimedia resources available on virtual environments.

We believe the success of prebriefing and debriefing is more a result of the facilitator's knowledge of its assumptions and strategies for operational aspects in different contexts than of the way it is performed. In spite of this, we encourage moments of face-to-face interaction to strengthen faculty analysis of students' needs in learning, deep comprehension of difficulties and potentialities, and the relational context and exchange of experiences and conversations beyond verbal or written communications.

One strategy for total virtual debriefing already exists in SG; it indicates errors and hits at the end of the game, so that students can identify errors and retry. We also believe that it is plausible and pedagogically relevant to offer further readings and additional materials for remediation, including scientific literature that helps students understand their errors or hits, providing evidenced-based practice, research studies, and suggested intervention/protocols on the theme so that they are adequately supported to retry.

Regarding prebriefing for the area of neonatal care within baccalaureate and licensure nursing courses, we have been using other materials developed by our research group (Adolescent and Childs' Health Nursing Research Group—GPECCA) and already in use by the University of São Paulo; these include booklets, software containing multimedia, e-books, and other games complementing conventional classes.

ASSESSMENT

SGs can be used to assess students' learning. Considering several types of SGs with different goals and actions exist, each one must establish a plan for measuring learning and recording scores through errors and hits in the game's progress. It is possible to

> **BOX 11.1 Debriefing Virtual Simulation Using a Web-Based Conferencing Platform: Lessons Learned**
>
> - When scheduling debriefing sessions, limit the number of participants to a maximum of 10 students per session. More than 10 students inhibited participation and made conversation difficult when multiple students attempted to contribute at once to the discussion. High participant engagement is a hallmark of strong debriefings because it leads to deeper levels of learning and increases the likelihood of transfer to the clinical setting. Conversely, too few students in a session diminished the depth of the conversation.
> - Schedule multiple debriefing sessions per week and allow students to self-select and register for the day and time that best suits their schedule. This strategy improved attendance and allowed for flexible scheduling if a student was unable to attend a debriefing.
> - Schedule debriefing sessions to occur within the shortest amount of time after completion of the learning activities. Ideally, debriefing should occur immediately following the simulation activity.
> - Incorporate a best-practice meeting with all course faculty on a regular basis and attend at least one debriefing session facilitated by another faculty member. Collaborative meetings and observation of other faculty-preceptor sessions are strategies for promoting quality and consistency among course sections.
> - Select tools designed to assist in evaluating and developing debriefing skills, as well as allow for assessing debriefings from a variety of disciplines and courses, varying numbers of participants, a wide range of educational objectives, and various physical and time constraints. Examples are the Debriefing Assessment for Simulation in Healthcare© (DASH) Score Sheet and the Debriefing Assessment for Simulation in Healthcare© (DASH) Instructor Version (Simon, Raemer, & Rudolph, 2010, 2012).

record a log to be used by teachers later during debriefing, highlighting the moments when the student made mistakes and clarifying the content and expected actions.

In addition, more than recording the action sequences performed by the user assessing it, SG technology can provide immediate or fast feedback for students, indicating when and why errors were made. Providing explanations of why the action is wrong is a very important feature because it integrates a crucial component in pedagogical approach, guiding students to understand the subject better, reasons that their choice of action is incorrect, and possible other solutions to the problem, ultimately allowing success with another chance.

Even when a second chance is given, scores can register grades/status considering only the first action outcome; that is, even if the game offers students a second chance after they did something wrong, their assessment identifies the error for further debriefing and as a measure for comparison in next attempts.

Scores for assessment status during games can assume many versions of graphic representation, such as numbers, percentages, symbols of rewards (i.e., stars, coins), or colored bars marking progress of success and failure. This assessment is key to the gamification perspective, motivating and engaging the user in seeking better results in further attempts, regardless of a competitive or collaborative approach in games.

Other assessments can be done during a game experience for learning; these include number of clicks and main objects clicked (demonstrating users' interest and focus), satisfaction, and emotional impact. All perspectives are relevant because they represent heuristics of interaction between the human and the computer, aiming to improve quality and outcomes derived from this relation (see human–computer interaction definition and details in the following sections of this chapter).

A current challenge is to assess the impact on students' learning. Identifying data demonstrating student learning would allow testing of the feasibility of SG use as a tool for better learning results. The challenge in measuring learning is because of its complex nature as a multifaceted phenomenon that includes different domains, such as cognitive, behavioral, and procedural knowledge. In addition, different learning theories and correlated matters are exemplified by learning styles and individual timing for processing information, making it difficult to prove technology and digital games as supportive for better learning. This challenge is faced by all educators because there is no formula or recognized gold standard assessment.

In researching learning in nursing students, we focused on the cognitive branch, capturing learning by the use of close-ended questions that allowing for objectivity, reduced bias, and quantitative methods of calculating outcomes. In spite of using this method of assessment, we adopt constructivism in education and recognize the importance of assessing learning through games in a broader perspective. It is more than close-ended questions, using for example measurement techniques to assess the impact on students' behavior in the health team. We also need to assess their behavior with patient and family during procedures common to practice and decision-making in clinical setting or solving clinical cases.

Therefore, this is a key area for future research in nursing education; it represents an opportunity for evaluation of new SGs and other educational tools and strategies.

EVALUATING THE VIRTUAL LEARNING EXPERIENCE

SGs aim to concretize formal learning through ludic and entertainment; therefore, investigations in satisfaction and motivation for learning are necessary but are not limited to these variables. Other important research objectives are the role of SGs in self-regulated learning assuming autonomy for active methods in education (Hacker, 2016).

Considering this emergent need for research, it is necessary to make progress in metacognitive understanding of SGs by interpreting the process of learning and the way that knowledge is built, supported by learning theories and the educational psychology field (Hacker, 2016). That is why SGs must follow theoretical references in pedagogy as problematization, projects pedagogy, and problem-based learning (e.g., incorporating learning goals before its development and in the phases on *Developing Virtual Setting*).

We encourage adoption of a progressionist pedagogical approach from the point of view of the teaching–learning process, valuing students' active role and previous experiences as a starting point for future learning, faculty as facilitators and not unique holders of knowledge, and the use of clinical and social contexts to create learning experiences that are potentially meaningful and prepare professionals for real challenges and demands of the healthcare system (Ausubel, 2000; Freire, 2016).

We highlight the importance of not only developing educational tools, but also testing them. There is interest in understanding how SGs can improve understanding, **engagement**, satisfaction, motivation, curiosity, and clinical impact through critical thinking and decision making. Regarding impact analysis, the literature provides scarce publications to determine technology benefits on higher education because of limitations on research methods such as bias control, sample size, and focus only on satisfaction (Diehl, Souza, & Gordan, 2014).

Researchers indicate high levels of students' satisfaction by using SGs for learning (Anderson, Page, & Wendorf, 2013; Aredes, 2016), not differences on critical thinking comparing with and without avatars technology for clinical case resolution (Morey, 2012), not differences on cognitive impact (Fonseca, Aredes et al., 2015). On the other hand, researchers (Anderson et al, 2013; Day-Black, Merrill, Konzelman, Williams, & Hart, 2015; Hara et al., 2016; Lumsden, Edwards, Lawrence, Coyle, & Munafo, 2016) believe in games and other technologies for learning, considering their resources and processes to facilitate students with their knowledge building. It is crucial to analyze investigation methods that are applicable to education to represent the impact on evidence.

LESSON LEARNED: SGs FOR NEONATAL AND PEDIATRIC NURSING LEARNING IN BRAZIL

As discussed earlier in this chapter, we believe in the importance of active methods of learning and the use of clinical and social context plus epidemiology to support scopes on games. Within a discipline of neonatal care for nursing students, we developed a SG named e-Baby, initiated in 2010 with a partnership among faculty members from University of São Paulo, Brazil, and Higher School of Nursing of Coimbra, Portugal.

It is a sequence of games using the same format of virtual simulation with validated heuristic and emotional design with students and experts from both technology and clinical nursing areas. The games are organized by basic human needs (Wanda Horta nursing theory, based on Maslow human needs theory), and the series are Oxygenation, Circulation, Thermoregulation, Skin integrity, and Nutrition (Horta, 1979).

The scope inside each sequence was defined by a literature review and multiple meetings with clinical staff of a neonatal unit. Prematurity is a main concern in many countries and is the main cause of neonatal mortality in the world (15.4%), according to a recent report (Liu et al., 2015). The causes are intrapartum complications (10.5%) and neonatal sepsis (6.7%), and neonatal mortality represents 44% of infant deaths globally.

Aiming to improve learning for neonatal nurses on premature newborns' care, and mindful of the local and global demand for this information given the global healthcare context, e-Baby offers students the opportunity to perform clinical evaluation and interventions in a preterm baby in a virtual Isolette. The clinical case was developed by researchers using results from the literature review and nurses' opinion about what is more relevant for students to know before coming to clinical practice in the hospital. The game provides the necessary tools to subsidize clinical evaluation and gives feedback on hits and errors, adding detailed comments on errors that explain why the action was not correct based on scientific evidence.

The images (refer to Figure 11.2) show some of the screenshots from the game, which can be accessed freely through the university website at the following URLs:

http://www2.eerp.usp.br/site/grupos/gpecca/objetos/ebaby
http://gruposdepesquisa.eerp.usp.br/gpecca/ebaby2

Research on e-Baby has demonstrated that it is relevant to clinical practice, validated on heuristics for games, results in a high level of satisfaction among

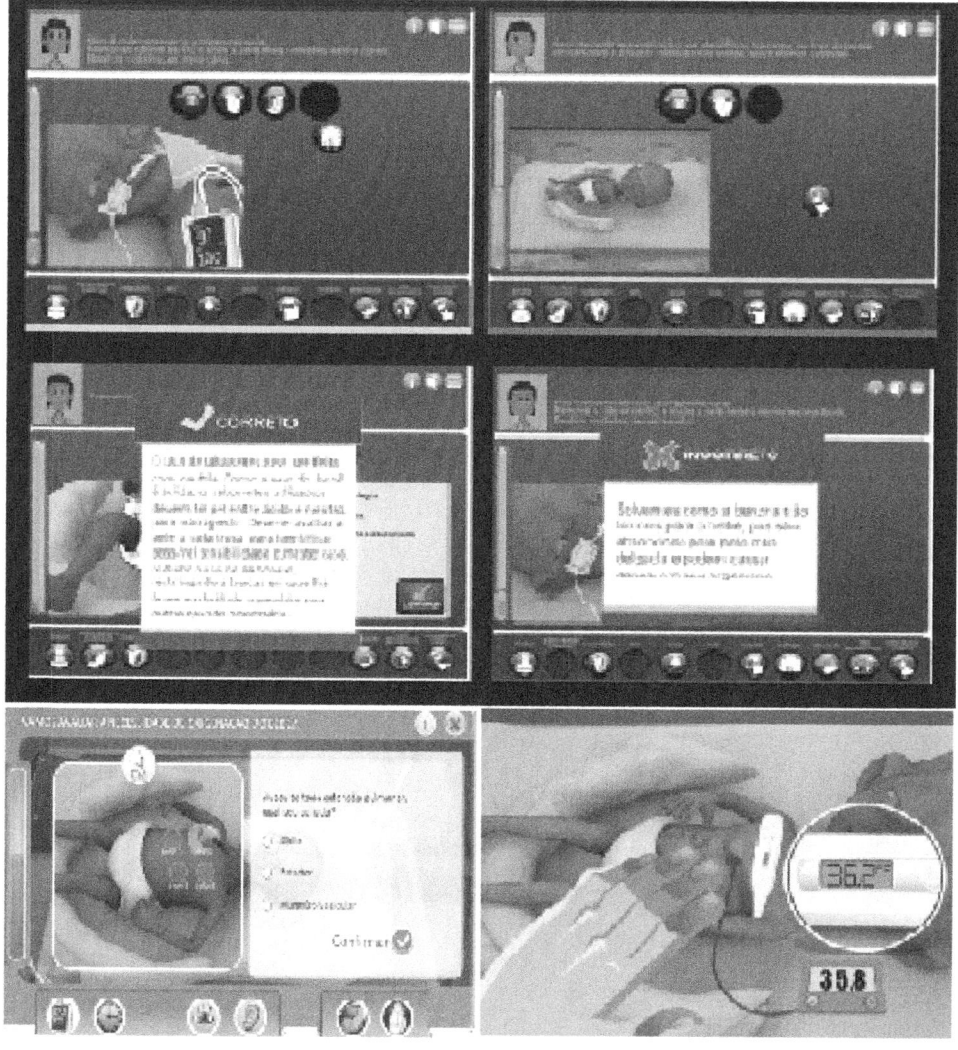

FIGURE 11.2 Screenshots of e-Baby serious game.

students, improves learning over time when associated with lectures and practicums, but is similar to conventional approaches when comparing control and experimental groups (Aredes, 2016; Fonseca et al., 2014, 2015).

A version of e-Baby had been created to support health education as mentioned before in this chapter. The SG e-Baby Family can be accessed freely by all Internet users as a product developed by the public university with financial support from government and research foundations to strengthen trustworthy information in health regarding child care (gruposdepesquisa.eerp.usp.br/gpecca2/?page_id=181). It uses avatars as caregivers, offers a game experience based on two different contexts (hospital and home), and teaches users how to identify trouble breathing by interpreting oxygen saturation, cardiac rate, and other signs such as cyanosis and intercostal retractions (refer to Figure 11.3). In addition, explanations about how to react in situations of infants' choking and other challenges with the baby are included in the SG.

Other SGs were developed to support the teaching–learning process in neonatal care and focus on preterm infants; these include breastfeeding (Ferecini, Goes, Fonseca, Leite, & Scochi, 2012) and environmental control of noise and luminosity in hospital units (Fonseca et al., 2013).

For the pediatric area, our research group in partnership with other researchers developed an SG for children so that they can understand obesity and ways to prevent or manage it with entertainment (Dias et al., 2016).

DigesTower is a SG developed collaboratively by graduate students and faculty members from the schools of nursing and computer science at two different universities in Brazil, and its aim is to provide a game for children to learn about healthy food and obesity prevention and management. The user plays the human body role

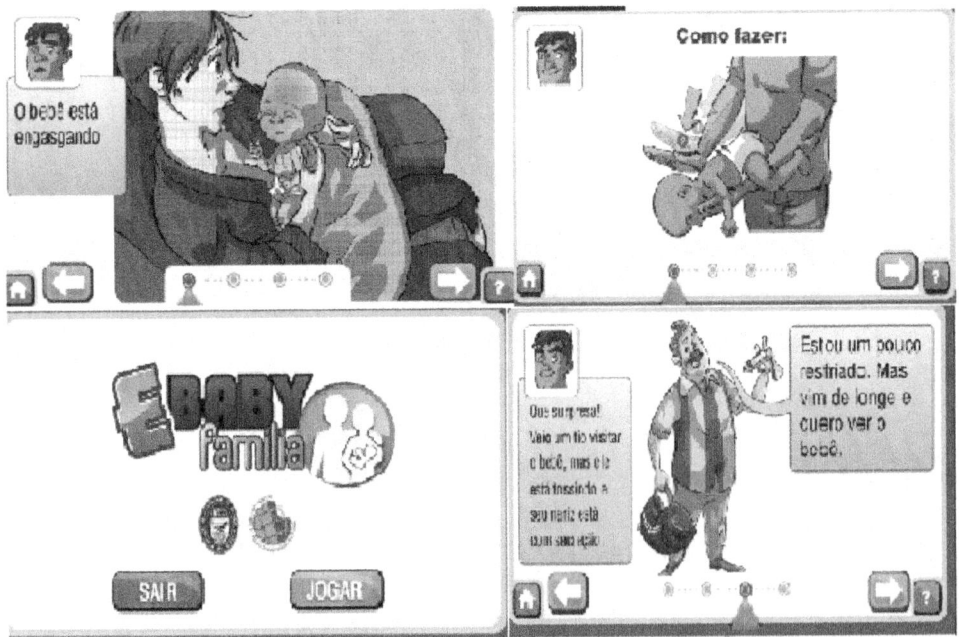

FIGURE 11.3 Screenshots of e-Baby Family.

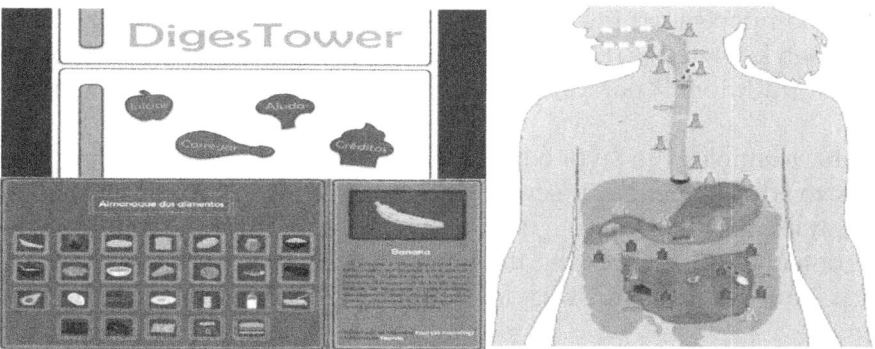

FIGURE 11.4 Screenshots of DigesTower.

by selecting foods and digesting them by using mastication and proper enzymes for different components (carbohydrates, proteins, fat, and vitamins). By selecting the desired food, children consult an almanac to understand better what basic components are in their foods and the level required to digest the food chosen (refer to Figure 11.4). Depending on the choices they make, they have more or less difficulty maintaining a healthy weight during the game and start understanding obesity prevention and management. The game also incorporates information about physiology, which is relevant for health education.

We believe SGs are a strong tool for engaging students in learning. Students gain better knowledge and understanding not only by being motivated to study and learn in a fun way but also by being given a powerful source of information and interaction that is relevant to their lives. SGs provide a different perspective, more aligned with Y-generation interests and social behavior, compared with traditional education (e.g., reading books, rote memorization of material that may have little relevance).

KEY POINTS

- When planning before developing, you should use a theoretical approach contemplating steps similar to those described in this chapter.
- You must exercise special care with communication between IT teams and creators, aiming to facilitate comprehension through a different knowledge field.
- Pay attention to learning objectives and pedagogical approaches to define the student's role in the game.
- It is important to focus on data and actions based on scientific evidence and contextual relevance.
- Partnerships and articulations between health professionals and academics are necessary to strengthen research quality and exchange of knowledge from both perspectives.

SUMMARY

SGs offer users the opportunity to learn and are connected to fun (e.g., "playing a game"), creating an association between education and recreation. Considering that emotion impacts learning processes and that positive emotions while learning can strengthen knowledge (Daniels et al., 2009), gamification is an ally for changing education's traditional paradigm into a more playful and student-centered approach.

Using this technology to favor education is imperative when analyzing worldwide challenges to educate people at several levels, especially considering the contemporaneous context of mobile device use and web access. It can help in understanding difficult content and in processing the tons of information we have available on the Internet in a fun way, as long as its development follows reliable data from scientific literature.

REFLECTIVE QUESTIONS

1. Consider the term *serious game* and describe what it means from a faculty perspective and from a student perspective.
2. SGs aim to concretize formal learning. How would you research their role in self-regulated learning? Describe the research questions or hypotheses you would propose and the results you would expect.
3. Discuss the importance of using active methods of learning with clinical and social context plus epidemiology to support the scope of games. Describe in detail the active learning methods you would use to develop the clinical and social context while including epidemiological concepts.

REFERENCES

Anderson, J. K., Page, A. M., & Wendorf, D. M. (2013). Avatar-assisted case studies. *Nurse Educator, 38*(3), 106–109. doi:10.1097/NNE.0b013e31828dc260

Aredes, N. D. A. (2016). *Technology and education in nursing: An experimental study towards gameability, student's autonomy and learning styles* (Thesis doctorate). Nursing School of Ribeirão Preto, University of São Paulo, Ribeirao Preto, Brazil.

Ausubel, D. (2000). *Aquisição e retenção de conhecimentos: uma perspectiva cognitiva*. Lisboa, Portugal: Plátano Edições Técnicas.

Boada, I., Rodriguez-Benitez, A., Garcia-Gonzalez, J. M., Olivet, J., Carreras, V., & Sbert, M. (2015). Using a serious game to complement CPR instruction in a nurse faculty. *Computer Methods and Programs in Biomedicine, 22*, 282–291. doi:10.1016/j.cmpb.2015.08.006

Boyle, E. A., Hainey, T., Connolly, T. M., Gray, G., Earp, J., Ott, M., . . . Pereira, J. (2016). An update to the systematic literature review of empirical evidence of the impacts and outcomes of computer games and serious games. *Computers & Education, 94*, 178–192. doi:10.1016/j.compedu.2015.11.003

Chen, P. Y., Hsieh, W. I., Wei, S. H., & Kao, C. L. (2011). Interactive Wiimote gaze stabilization exercise training system for patients with vestibular hypofunction. *Journal of NeuroEngineering and Rehabilitation, 9*(1), 1–19. doi:10.1186/1743-0003-9-77

Cook, N. F., McAloon, T., O'Neill, P., & Beggs, R. (2012). Impact of a web based interactive simulation game (PULSE) on nursing students' experience and performance in life support training—A pilot study. *Nurse Education Today, 32*(6), 714–720. doi:10.1016/j.nedt.2011.09.013

Creutzfeldt, J., Hedman, L., & Fellander-Tsai, L. (2012). Effects of pre-training using serious games technology on CPR performance—An exploratory quasi-experimental transfer study. *Scandinavian Journal of Trauma, Resuscitation, and Emergency Medicine, 20*(79), 1–9. doi:10.1186/1757-7241-20-79

Daniels, L., Stupnisky, R., Pekrun, R., Haynes, T., Perry, R., & Newall, N. (2009). A Longitudinal analysis of achievement goals: From affective antecedents to emotional effects and achievement outcomes. *Journal of Educational Psychology, 101*, 948–963. doi:10.1037/a0016096

Darragh, A. R., Lavender, S., Polivka, B., Sommerich, C. M., Wills, C. E., Hittle, B. A., . . . Stredney, D. L. (2016). Gaming simulation as health and safety training for home health care workers. *Clinical Simulation in Nursing, 12*(8), 328–335. doi:10.1016/j.ecns.2016.03.006

Day-Black, C., Merrill, E. B., Konzelman, L., Williams, T. T., & Hart, N. (2015). Gamification: An innovative teaching-learning strategy for the digital nursing students in a community health nursing course. *ABNF Journal, 26*(4), 90–95.

Decker, S., Fey, M., Sideras, S., Caballero, S., Rockstraw, L. (R.), Boese, T., . . . Borum, J. C. (2013, June). Standards of best practice: Simulation standard VI: The debriefing process. *Clinical Simulation in Nursing, 9*(6S), S27–S29. doi:10.1016/j.ecns.2013.04.008

De Freitas, S., & Neumann, T. (2009). Computers & education the use of "exploratory learning" for supporting immersive learning in virtual environments. *Computers & Education, 52*(2), 343–352. doi:10.1016/j.compedu.2008.09.010

Delasobera, B. E., Goodwin, T. L., Strehlow, M., Gilbert, G., D'Souza, P., Alok, A., . . . Mahadevan, S. V. (2010). Evaluating the efficacy of simulators and multimedia for refreshing ACLS skills in India. *Resuscitation, 81*(2), 217–223. doi:10.1016/j.resuscitation.2009.10.013

Dias, J. D., Mekaro, M. S., Lu, J. K. C., Otsuka, J. L., Fonseca, L. M. M., & Mascarenhas, S. H. Z. (2016). Serious game development as a strategy for health promotion and tackling childhood obesity. *Revista Latino-Americana de Enfermagem, 24*, e2759–e2768. doi:10.1590/1518-8345.1015.2759

Diehl, L. A., Souza, R. M., & Gordan, P. A. (2014). Gaming habits and opinions of Brazilian medical school faculty and students: What's next? *Games for Health Journal, 3*(2), 1–7. doi:10.1089/g4h.2013.0069

Farra, S., Miller, E. T., Hodgson, E., Cosgrove, E., Brady, W., Gneuhs, M., & Baute, B. (2016). Storyboard development for virtual reality simulation. *Clinical Simulation in Nursing, 12*(9), 392–399. doi:10.1016/j.ecns.2016.04.002

Ferecini, G. M., Goes, F. S. N., Fonseca, L. M. M., Leite, A. M., & Scochi, C. G. S. (2012). Avaliação de um website sobre o aleitamento materno do prematuro. *Cienc Cuid Saude, 11*(4), 642–649. doi:10.11606/T.22.2012.tde-28022012-142326

Fonseca, L. M. M., Aredes, N. D. A., Dias, D. M. V., Scochi, C.G.S., Martins, J. C. A., & Rodrigues, M. A. (2015). Serious game e-Baby: Nursing students' perception on learning about preterm newborn clinical assessment. *Revista Brasileira de Enfermagem, 68*(1), 13–19. doi:10.1590/0034-7167.2015680102

Fonseca, L. M. M., Dias, D. M. V., Goes, F. S. N., Seixas, C. A., Scochi, C. G. S., Martins, J. C., & Rodrigues, M. A. (2014). Development of the e-Baby serious game with regard to the evaluation of oxygenation in preterm babies: Contributions of the emotional design. *Computers, Informatics, Nursing, 32*(9), 428–436. doi:10.1097/CIN.0000000000000078

Fonseca, L. M. M., Goes, F. S. N., Medeiros, M. J., Castro, F. S. F., Zamberlan-Amorim, N. E., & Scochi, C. G. S. (2013). Development of a learning object for caring for the sensory environment in a neonatal unit: noise, light and handling. *Journal of Nursing Education and Practice, 3*, 11–18. doi:10.5430/jnep.v3n2p1

Foronda, C., & Bauman, E. B. (2014). Strategies to incorporate virtual simulation in nurse education. *Clinical Simulation in Nursing, 10*(8), 412–418. doi:10.1016/j.ecns.2014.03.005

Freire, P. (2016). *Pedagogia do oprimido* (62nd ed.). Rio de Janeiro, Brazil: Paz e Terra.

Fu, F. L., Su, R. C., & Yu, S. C. (2009). EGameFlow: A scale to measure learners' enjoyment of e-learning games. *Computers & Education, 52*, 101–112. doi:10.1016/j.compedu.2008.07.004

Hacker, D. J. (2016). The role of metacognition in learning via serious games. In R. Zheng & M. K. Gardner (Eds.), *Handbook of research on serious games for educational applications* (pp. 19–40). Hershey, PA: IGI Global.

Hara, C. Y. N., Aredes, N. D. A., Fonseca, L. M. M., Silveira, R. C. C. P., Camargo, R. A. A., & Goes, F. S. N. (2016). Clinical case in digital technology for nursing students' learning: an integrative review. *Nurse Education Today, 38*, 119–125. doi:10.1016/j.nedt.2015.12.002

Henry, B. W., Ozier, A. D., & Johnson, A. (2011). Empathetic responses and attitudes about older adults: How experience with the aging game measures up. *Educational Gerontology, 37*(10), 924–941. doi:10.1080/03601277.2010.495540

Horta, W. A. (1979). *Processo de enfermagem*. São Paulo Brazil: EPU.

Hurkmans, H. L., Ribbers, G. M., Streur-Kranenburg, M. F., Stam, H. J., & Van Den Berg-Emons, R. J. (2011). Energy expenditure in chronic stroke patients playing Wii Sports: A pilot study. *Journal of NeuroEngineering and Rehabilitation, 8*(38), 1–7. doi:10.1186/1743-0003-8-38

International Nursing Association for Clinical Simulation and Learning. (2016). INACSL Standards of best practice: Simulation debriefing. *Clinical Simulation in Nursing, 12,* S21–S25. doi:10.1016/j.ecns.2016.09.008

Johnson, L., Adams Becker, S., Estrada, V., & Freeman, A. (2014). *NMC horizon report: 2014 higher education edition.* Austin, TX: The New Media Consortium.

Knight, J. F., Carley, S., Tregunna, B., Jarvis, S., Smithies, R., de Freitas, S., . . . Mackway-Jones, K. (2010). Serious gaming technology in major incident triage training: A pragmatic controlled trial. *Resuscitation, 81*(9), 1175–1179. doi:10.1016/j.resuscitation.2010.03.042

Lancaster, R. J. (2013). Serious game simulation as a teaching strategy in pharmacology. *Clinical Simulation in Nursing, 10*(3), e129–e137. doi:10.1016/j.ecns.2013.10.005

Liu, L., Oza, S., Hogan, D., Perin, J., Rudan, I., Lawn, J. E., . . . Black, R. E. (2015). Global, regional, and national causes of child mortality in 2000–13, with projections to inform post-2015 priorities: An updated systematic analysis. *Lancet, 384,* 430–440. doi:10.1016/S0140-6736(14)61698-6

Lumsden, J., Edwards, E. A., Lawrence, N. S., Coyle, D., & Munafo, M. R. (2016). Gamification of cognitive assessment and cognitive training: A systematic review of applications and efficacy. *JMIR Serious Games, 4*(2), e11–e25. doi:10.2196/games.5888

Marfisi-Schottman, I., George, S., & Tarpin-Bernard, F. (2010). *Tools and methods for efficiently designing serious games.* The 4th European Conference on Games Based Learning ECGBL, Copenhagen, Denmark.

Mohamed, H., & Jaafar, A. (2012). *Analyzing critical usability problems in educational computer game (UsaECG).* Proceedings of the IASTED International Conference on Human-Computer Interaction, Chamonix, France.

More, D. J. (2012). Development and evaluation of web-based animated pedagogical agents for facilitating critical thinking in nursing. *Nursing Education Perspectives, 33*(2), 116–120.

Norman, D. (2008). *Emotional design: Why we love (or hate) everyday things.* New York, NY: Basic Books.

Peng, W., Crouse, J. C., & Lin, J. H. (2012). Using active video games for physical activity promotion: A systematic review of the current state of research. *Health Education & Behaviour, 40*(2), 171–192. doi:10.1177/1090198112444956

Pichierri, G., Murer, K., & de Bruin, E. D. (2012). A cognitive-motor intervention using a dance video game to enhance foot placement accuracy and gait under dual task conditions in older adults: A randomized controlled trial. *BMC Geriatrics, 12*(1), 74. doi:10.1186/1471-2318-12-74

Preece, J., Rogers, Y., & Sharp, H. (2007). *Interaction design: Beyond human computer interaction.* New York, NY: John Wiley & Sons.

Primack, B. A., Carroll, M. V., McNamara, M., Klem, M. L., King, B., Rich, M., . . . Nayak, S. (2012). Role of video games in improving health-related outcomes: A systematic review. *American Journal of Preventive Medicine, 42*(6), 630–638. doi:10.1016/j.amepre.2012.02.023

Simon, R., Raemer, D. B., & Rudolph, J. W. (2010). *Debriefing Assessment for Simulation in Healthcare (DASH)© student version.* Boston, MA: Center for Medical Simulation. Retrieved from https://harvardmedsim.org/wp-content/uploads/2017/01/DASH.SV.Short.2010.Final.pdf

Simon, R., Raemer, D. B., & Rudolph, J. W. (2012). *Debriefing Assessment for Simulation in Healthcare (DASH)© instructor version.* Boston, MA: Center for Medical Simulation. Retrieved from https://harvardmedsim.org/wp-content/uploads/2017/01/DASH.IV.ShortForm.2012.05.pdf

Valle, P. H. D., Vilela, R. F., Júnior, P. A. P., & Inocêncio, A. C. G. (2013). Hedeg-heurísticas para avaliação de jogos educacionais digitais. *Nuevas Ideas en Informática Educativa TISE.* XVIII Conferência Internacional sobre Informática na Educação, 9–11. Dezembro, 2013, Porto Alegre, Rio Grande do Sul, Brasil.

Verkuyl, M., Romaniuk, D., Atack, L., & Mastrilli, P. (2017). Virtual gaming simulation for nursing education: An experiment. *Clinical Simulation in Nursing, 13*(5), 238–244. doi:10.1016/j.ecns.2017.02.004

Wouters, P., van Nimwegen, C., van Oostendorp, H., & van der Spek, E. D. (2013). A meta-analysis of the cognitive and motivational effects of serious games. *Journal of Educational Psychology, 105*(2), 249.

Xavier, R. A. C., Garcia, F. E., & de Almeida Neris, V. P. (2012, November). Decisões de design de interfaces ruins e o impacto delas na interação: um estudo preliminar considerando o estado emocional de idosos. In *Proceedings of the 11th Brazilian Symposium on Human Factors in Computing Systems* (pp. 127–136). Brazilian Computer Society.

CHAPTER 12

Nursing Student Simulation Scenarios Within a Virtual Learning Environment

PAMELA L. GRANT

LEARNING OBJECTIVES

Upon completion of this chapter, the reader will be able to:
- Select student learning experiences in virtual environments.
- Develop learning experiences in virtual environments.
- Evaluate the student learning experience in virtual environments.

KEY TERMS

Avatars
Scenario
Simulation
Virtual

Some may argue that nursing has used **simulation** throughout the history of nursing education and continues to do so today whether it is with low- or high-fidelity manikins in rooms that look like hospital rooms with present day equipment or through role play in a classroom setting. Simulation has many advantages for nursing education, some of which include creating safe learning environments for students and reinforcing information learned in the classroom; it also has the advantage of being available in inclement weather as well as 24 hours a day for student access. Claman (2015) noted that it has been over a decade since the National League for Nursing (NLN) prioritized nursing education reform through innovative teaching methods. "The development of internet-based education platforms is providing more higher education opportunities for local, national, and international learning communities over long distances" (Claman, 2015, p. 13). Claman considered learning as being dependent on structured, intelligent interaction and communication to facilitate high levels of critical thinking: "The delivery of content in novel and dynamic ways takes on greater importance as curriculums that are partially or completely online become a larger part of nursing education" (p. 15). Faculty perception of computer-assisted learning is a variable that could impact the success of online education. "Faculty must advocate for sufficient training and ongoing administrative support including adequate resources such as hardware, maintenance, reliable connectivity, and ongoing training" (p. 15).

Technology has allowed nursing simulation to enter another realm that is the **virtual** learning environment. The virtual learning environment can be created to look similar to real communities, disaster areas, or homes, with avatars populating that environment. According to Lau and Lee (2015), "Avatars in immersive virtual reality are a crucial vehicle for various interactions and communications among participants" (p. 6). **Avatars** in the virtual environments can be created to simulate people, and nursing student avatars to interact with them. Avatars used by faculty are able to speak and can interact with student's avatars in real-time role play or be programed to behave in looped consistent patterns. Virtual learning environments have the advantage of being available for access around the clock, as well as around the world, by participants. This availability is the reason learning may occur under numerous circumstances and has limitless possibilities for collaboration. The World Health Organization (WHO, 2010) stated, "After almost 50 years of enquiry, the World Health Organization and its partners acknowledge that there is sufficient evidence to indicate that effective interprofessional education enables effective collaborative practice" (p. 7). The challenge was globally to all educators to create interprofessional collaboration as a necessary step in preparation to help make a practice-ready workforce to respond to local health needs.

The key objective to simulation is to give students an opportunity to experience possible future professional situations in which they must react. O'Connor (2015) suggested that instructors share their work experiences and their challenges and encourage students to explore and learn from their mistakes. "Instructors should speak from direct and personal experience within their field so, when using technologies as part of the learning environment, instructors should provide evidence of their own work in the area" (O'Connor, 2015, p. 166). To the extent possible, faculty will want to give students relatable information about the simulation by sharing professional experiences with them.

Frequently, students have more information about a given situation in a **scenario**; for example, they may know what type of disaster has occurred, they may have client names and health history, or they may know what role they have in the scenario. These are all pieces of information that they may not necessarily have in a lived experience as students or working professionals. Having some prior knowledge about what they are about to encounter helps the student navigate the experience. Another important aspect to being given prior information about the scenario is that students can better translate what took place during the scenario into lived experiences as a future healthcare professional. Debriefing after virtual learning experiences allows students to share thoughts on what went well and did not go well and ask the "what-if" questions for a real-life experience.

The advantage to using virtual reality, rather than a real-life experience, is that in real life, students could be immersed in an environment that could cause them harm. After all, it is perfectly acceptable to send student nurse avatars into a burning plane crash site at a chemical company to triage the injured. The other obvious advantage to using virtual learning environments is creating scenarios that would be otherwise impossible to provide for students in the real world. Another important factor noted by Tilton, Tiffany, and Hoglund (2015) is that "utilizing virtual simulation offered a consistent clinical learning experience for all students and decreased the challenge of securing an adequate number of quality clinical placements in the community" (p. 395).

RELATION TO THE FAST SIM©

This chapter relates to the model of Faculty Administrators Students Technology Strategic Integration Model© (FAST SIM) mainly through faculty and student perspectives. Administration must be on board for virtual learning environments to be created and to survive. When addressing virtual learning environments, Lee, Lee, Wong, Tsang, and Li (2010) stated, "This type of technology effectively simulates the experience of being immersed within a virtual world. Its application in nursing skills training, particularly in the mental nursing aspect, is noteworthy" (p. 362). Successful learning through simulation in a virtual world requires buy-in from administration, faculty, students, and technical support involved in the educational environment. Tokel and Isler (2015) stated, "Virtual worlds can focus on the productive use of a system to increase learning as well as the prolonged use to provide fun and enjoyment" (p. 262). Hernández, González, and Muñoz (2014) noted that online learning involved two levels and that topics were linked to curricular framework and, in the classroom, were linked to the faculty–student interaction. "The interrelations of all these factors inevitably condition the potential to teach and learn and, furthermore, that teaching and learning are possible through cooperation" (Hernández et al., 2014, p. 30). The combination of enjoyment and learning in a virtual learning environment facilitates student participation. For successful learning to occur within virtual learning environments, all stakeholders must be committed to facilitating strategic integration of learning for students.

A rather sweeping example of learning through simulation would be the U.S. government. Lau and Lee (2015) noted, "The Government of the United States has been using highly immersive simulators to teach solders to operate military helicopters, flights and tanks since the 1970s" (p. 7). Some of the same benefits for using computer simulation in the military apply to learning in nursing. Students are able to enter into unsafe environments and learn how to respond as professionals; computer simulations also provide consistent learning opportunities for students. "The advantage of using a virtual reality to enhance students' learning experiences is not only about creating computer simulations for them to tackle real-world situations, but also creating unusual environmental stimulation to motivate them to explore new ideas" (Lau & Lee, 2015, p. 15).

Selecting Student Learning Experiences in a Virtual Environment

One of the first things to consider when creating a learning experience in a virtual learning environment is the audience. In this case, the audience would be the students in the classroom or perhaps in a web-based classroom. All of the usual considerations for educators must take place—student level, course objectives, and student learning needs within the concepts or content, as determined by the educator. Some examples in community health might be disaster triage, community assessment, or assessment of a client's home environment, all of which can be created in a virtual learning environment.

Although three community-related options were mentioned, the home assessment for a client will be used as the selected example. Ideally, there would be a scenario that includes information about the client and why the student will be visiting the home. The American Association of Colleges of Nursing (2012) identified graduate-level Quality and Safety Education for Nurses (QSEN) competencies that require enough knowledge to analyze factors influencing safety and skills and including the use of existing resources to implement safety improvements. Essentially, students need to be able to assess the living arrangements of the client and determine if the home is safe. If the home is not safe, students must address what needs to happen to make the home safe enough, for example, for a client to return home after surgery. When the postoperative client returns home, perhaps the stairs are missing some spindles under the hand rail. Loose rugs, an empty pantry, or a space heater plugged into an extension cord might be a little less obvious. We want students to demonstrate the ability to identify safety issues within the home and then to address or find workable solutions to resolve issues so that the client may return home.

Virtual learning environments work well for this example; imagine having to explain what is needed in lecture format. In the virtual learning environment, students can look around, identify concerns, and then contemplate how best to address the issues identified. Faculty have to be familiar with what the students see and do during the scenario so that they can debrief students once the virtual learning experience comes to an end. The debriefing is an opportunity for students to critically think about the virtual learning simulation and self-reflect about their responses. Debriefing can be a fun and interesting experience because conversations tend to be translated to real-world situations.

Following the example of the home assessment, students may want to know:

- How much will it cost to make modifications to the home?
- Will the modifications have to be short or long term?
- What types of resources are available?
- What alternatives are there if the client cannot return home?

The possibilities are rather endless, depending on student interests and their ability to brainstorm ideas to resolve identified issues. Students may have had a similar family situation that they may share during debriefing as well.

Developing the Learning Experience in a Virtual Environment

Developing a learning experience in a virtual world environment may depend on what you have to work with in the beginning of the process. If there is something in place, it may be a matter of evaluating what the learning needs of the students are, or if it is possible to have input on creating the environment, there are some options. Knowing what is available is paramount to creating the learning opportunity (e.g., if there a virtual environment already developed, if there will be an opportunity to create the learning environment); each has its own challenge.

Working from the standpoint of having your virtual environment in place, the best option is to evaluate what is available in that environment. If possible, a learning experience should be created within that environment. Generally, it is a matter of determining how you are going to use the space and what is in it. The best situation is having an environment that supports the learning objectives for students. For example, if a learning objective is for students to understand the concept of triage, an environment with programed, injured avatars would be needed. Ideally, the avatars would represent a variety of injuries incurred at the disaster site. To triage, students would need to have information pertaining to a triage system such as simple triage and rapid treatment (START). Handouts for students might include a decision tree using START or a worksheet that accounts for all of the disaster victims and category choices for students to use for triage during the simulation.

There are several aspects to consider when deciding on the learning experience. Students need to be able to move through the virtual environment, and this can be accomplished by assigning avatars. Another approach in a classroom setting would be to display the virtual environment in front of the class and faculty move the avatar through the virtual leaning environment. Faculty should have time to gain experience operating the avatar during their demonstration.

With that in mind, several skills may be needed before students are able to successfully navigate the virtual world. If the learning experience can be accomplished in one location within the virtual environment, students will need to learn how to walk, run, and fly. If it requires moving to different locations within the virtual environment, students must learn to transport the avatars to various locations throughout the virtual world. For the sake of time, walking, running, and flying can be accomplished in the learning environment with some allotted time if the exercise is to be completed during class time. In fact, if class time is being used, dedicating the first five to ten minutes to learning to move will be time well spent; a show of hands can indicate mastering walking, running, and flying. Transporting avatars to different locations takes a bit more time to master. Once everyone in class has gained the skills needed to move, the exercise in the virtual environment may begin.

Creating the learning experience in a virtual world needs guidance by using specific instructions, finding certain objectives, or answering questions. Once again, a decision on in-class activity or independent student activity must be decided. Password protection for the virtual learning environment is desirable to maintain control over the number of people entering the site. It is also, desirable to prevent interlopers or unintended participants who may access the site.

Going back to the home assessment example, to be done in class, the home may have as many as 100 safety items of concern or 25 safety items students need to identify as issues. Having to list the concerns students identify helps them stay on task. Combining the number of issues to be identified within a time limit serves to avoid losing class time to distraction. Faculty want to keep in mind that avatars can be modified and transporting to other locations can happen. Students may have great fun if given the freedom to explore. A word to the wise: Keep students on task and busy to accomplish the learning exercise!

There are multiple ways of keeping students engaged in a virtual environment. Depending on the learning experience, a combination of the following may be useful:

- Answering open-ended questions in class or in the virtual learning environment or writing them for students to answer at a later time

- Locating items or faculty using an avatar in the virtual environment displayed in front of the class, where students may follow along and locate items
- Asking questions and creating conversation throughout the observation in class or in the virtual learning environment
- Creating a list for students to fill in as they follow along
- Developing a worksheet, perhaps with multiple-choice answers

There may be other options, depending on availability and the learning needs of the students. A list or a worksheet for students to fill in facilitate, participation and conversation related to the learning experience. The use of worksheets or packets directs the learning experience, gives the students some idea what faculty may be looking for, and ultimately helps faculty examine student participation. Discussion board questions are an option for online classrooms that may be posted for class participation after students have entered the virtual learning environment. The goal is to find the best way to make learning fun and interesting. With that in mind, any handouts should be evaluated with some criteria in mind:

- Is there enough information for the student to make sense of the assignment and not be too overwhelming?
- Are there sufficient questions, grids, and lists to fill in with needed information but not be too tedious?
- Most important, can the paperwork be filled out within the allotted time?

Evaluating the Student Learning Experience in a Virtual Environment

Evaluation is dependent on faculty needs—will a grade be given? Or will points for participation be given? Will the learning experience count toward clinical hours? Depending on what faculty wants to accomplish, evaluation may vary greatly. Another consideration may center on student satisfaction of the learning experience. Analyzing data from test scores for improvement may help determine whether progress is being made through the virtual learning experience. Understanding the specific needs of the faculty, students, and school helps determine the best form of evaluation.

Providing packets for the virtual learning experience helps students write down information as they go through the exercise. These can be collected after the experience, providing some data on student involvement and achievement. The packets may also guide faculty in making modifications to improve the learning experience, especially if an evaluation form is attached. Evaluation from students about the learning experience clarifies what faculty requires from students and provides useful information on what students like or dislike about their learning experience.

Nicely and Farra (2015) stated that "the blending of cooperative learning and learning-by-teaching theoretical frameworks provided an environment that enhanced knowledge acquisition and improved student' ability to effectively triage disaster victims" (p. 335). In this example, cooperative learning combined technology students and nursing students to create an experience in a virtual learning environment. Each group had their own expertise to bring to the table. However, learning in a virtual world can incorporate other disciplines in healthcare, as well as shared teaching and learning among students. For example, a student with work experience as a paramedic might have a real-life experience working during a disaster to share with fellow nursing students.

KEY POINTS

- As a teaching modality, simulation has been used in varying capacities throughout the history of nursing.
- With the modern advent of virtual simulation, the learning environment can be designed to mirror areas similar to real-world communities, clinical settings, or homes that have avatars representing actual people.
- The ability to modify and manipulate these environments, as well as incorporate components such as professionals from other disciplines, offers wide-reaching positive advantages to faculty, administrators, and students.
- When creating virtual simulation scenarios, students may need instructor guidance and specific user instructions to enhance success in the virtual learning environment.
- When developing simulation activities, it is recommended to include a variety of opportunities for students to access instructional information aimed at improving their performance in the virtual environment and achieving learning outcomes.
- Enhanced student engagement is well worth the time and effort of creating virtual learning experiences.
- Students can easily get sidetracked if given the opportunity.
- Adjustments can be made to the learning experience as needed.
- Virtual worlds offer students the possibility of going places that are impossible to reach in the real world.

SUMMARY

Simulation in nursing is one of many methods used for teaching students. Teaching and learning in a virtual learning environment has many advantages for administrators, faculty, and students. One of the advantages includes the use of other disciplines to help create or participate in a virtual world learning experience. Virtual worlds provide faculty with a way of presenting possible real-life scenarios without the risk of injury to participants. Karaman and Orban Özen (2016) noted that learners seek the benefit of, and obtain assistance to achieve, learning tasks, which allow them to apply and transfer what they learn in an online environment to the real world (refer to Boxes 12.1 and 12.2). Flexibility in creating learning experiences in a virtual world has the advantage of providing variation for students as well.

> **BOX 12.1 Exemplar 1—Disaster Triage**
>
> ### ABSTRACT
>
> The platforms used to create the learning disaster-triage experiences were within Second Life® (SL), a virtual world platform, and were already in place. The challenge was in using the created resources in SL for learning experiences for nursing students.
>
> ### INTRODUCTION
>
> The disaster sites had been previously created and were available for use in SL. One site was of a crashed airplane that was burning at a chemical factory. Police avatars blocked entry into the area, which added a slight element of apprehension because crossing such a line is not what would normally be done. The other site had a burning tanker truck on its side that had crashed through a fence outside a warehouse with stacked wooden crates. Prior to entering the virtual learning environment, students were exposed to community emergency response team (CERT), and the use of simple triage and rapid treatment (START) as a part of the disaster content covered in community health. Both sites had programed avatars moving around; when student avatars approached the avatars on site, pertinent information pertaining to each character appeared on the screen in drop-down boxes, such as their vital signs, name, and condition. During the exercise, students were asked to note the condition of the avatars, their surroundings, and ultimately triage the programmed avatars as red, yellow, green, or black.
>
> For the airplane crash site, a prebriefing packet was created for students to assist with learning and engagement. The packet included a triage decision tree; an explanation of the red, yellow, green, and black tag codes; instructions to maximize the total number of survivors; a sheet providing the background of the scenario (e.g., number of victims, smoke that is release chemicals into the air); and a documentation grid that allowed students to record the victim's vital signs, activity, complaint, and tag color. Students were asked to list chronic concerns for the primary and secondary (students) victims, comments about the disaster site, and the disaster that occurred. Many students wrote about needed resources at the site, organization of the site, and long-term effects for the people involved in the disaster. Claman (2015) stated, "In the development of curricular content and facilitation of delivery for an immersive experience, educators might consider allotting time at the beginning of class for structured social activities" (p. 16). An example of an activity that would allow students to socialize and become familiar with the environment might include encouraging them to share ideas from didactic content prior to the exercise in the virtual learning environment.
>
> Debriefing occurred immediately after the students completed the experience. Depending on the number of student participants, debriefing can be

(continued)

> **BOX 12.1 Exemplar 1—Disaster Triage (*continued*)**
>
> challenging, especially if more than 30 students participated. Thirty minutes was allotted for discussion after the experience; however, the time varied depending on class size and student involvement. Frequently, "what-if" questions came up during the debriefing; examples include: What if the person is almost dead? What should we tag them? Or how would you know as a first responder what chemicals were being released? How can you stay safe? Discussions frequently led to what happens after victims are transported, which allowed for a conversation about decontamination prior to hospital entry. A debriefing facilitator may wish to wrap up the session by asking students how the disaster might have been avoided or mitigated.
>
> ## CHALLENGES IDENTIFIED
>
> Some challenges identified for providing an opportunity for students to triage during a disaster simulation were:
>
> - Keeping students safe and yet providing great learning experiences
> - Giving students an opportunity to respond without fear of failure and answering the "what ifs" during debriefing
> - Evaluating options that may mitigate or prevent disasters
> - Keeping some students on a task or engaged in the simulation
> - Limiting the number of student participants in a virtual environment to provide a consistent learning experience while mitigating technical issues with avatar performance
>
> ## STAKEHOLDER PERSPECTIVES
>
> ### Administrative
>
> From an administrative perspective, there is a low risk of liability for student–faculty injury within the virtual world learning environment. There is potential to expand learning opportunities for all levels of students within a program. The cost is relatively low to implement and can be used by multiple students for an extended time.
>
> ### Faculty
>
> For faculty, the use of simulation in the virtual provides "hands-on" experience that reinforces didactic classroom instruction. The virtual world learning environment provides consistent learning opportunities. There is a relatively low liability risk to students and faculty who participate in disaster simulation in a virtual world.

(continued)

> **BOX 12.1 Exemplar 1—Disaster Triage (*continued*)**
>
> Student
>
> The ability to enter a virtual learning environment allows students to evaluate situations safely. Simulation provides students with an opportunity to ask "what-if" questions, which students frequently have about various disaster situations. Another benefit for students is perhaps a first-time exposure to potential real-life situations.
>
> Resolutions
>
> Students tend to be satisfied with learning experiences in virtual learning environments. The potential for student engagement is increased when they are given the opportunity to critically think and participate. There is flexibility with each learning group to accommodate student needs through debriefing after the virtual world learning experience.
>
> Frustration
>
> Frequently there is not enough buy-in from administration because of lack of understanding or bias. This lack of support makes using virtual learning environments extremely challenging. Keeping ahead of adventurous students in the virtual world can be challenging if students decide to experiment with the avatars or transport to different locations.
>
> Summarization
>
> In summary, using a virtual world for a triage learning experiences provides an opportunity to go into an unsafe environment, such as a disaster area, without risking harm. It is possibly the only way to create a disaster environment apart from recreating a disaster with real people and moulage. However, the virtual world remains intact once students are finished with the learning experience and is ready for the next group of students. Providing a consistent teaching–learning experience for each class of students avoids student complaints of inequality in learning experiences. The advantage of virtual learning environments enables the faculty to have consistent learning experiences with the ability to adjust elements within the learning experience.
>
> **LESSONS LEARNED**
>
> What worked?
>
> What worked well with virtual learning experiences would have to be student enthusiasm for new experiences in learning. From a student's perspective the opportunity to evaluate situations critically and then discuss strategies and observations, along with addressing the "what-if" questions related to the learning experience, can be powerful. In many ways the learning is more impactful because it seems to stay with students and may be a continued topic of conversation.

(continued)

> **BOX 12.1 Exemplar 1—Disaster Triage (*continued*)**

What did not work?

Challenges in a virtual world platform can be the technical glitches; too many student avatars in the same location can cause slow responses and lags in the responses of programed avatars. From this perspective, student frustration with being able to complete the assignment may cause problems. The easiest way to correct the situation is to alleviate congestion within the site if possible. Another work-around is to project the image in class with the faculty moving the avatar through the environment and allowing students to follow along. This approach works well if the class size is greater than 20.

What would you do the same in the future?

Creating worksheets to go with the virtual learning environment seems to assist students in staying on task. The worksheets can be as simple as creating a list, checking boxes on a grid, or answering multiple-choice questions. The more open-ended, thought-provoking questions should be saved for in-class discussion or could be worked on in groups to be turned in at the end of class.

What would you do differently in the future?

Some approaches to doing things differently in the future would entail collecting information on what students found uninteresting or what detracted from the learning experience. Decide on a method to keep students focused and take the exercise seriously. A combination of student feedback and observation should help faculty find a successful working method of keeping students on task.

What will you take away from this experience?

Some students are very serious and want to get everything they can from the learning opportunity, whereas others get sidetracked. Some of the ways that students get sidetracked are as follows: changing avatar appearances, traveling to other areas outside of the learning experience, or simply not participating by doing other things online. The ultimate challenge is keeping all students engaged; this can also be a matter of knowing your particular batch of students and minimizing their ability to stray.

What advice would you offer to others in the same situation?

Although it may seem incredibly challenging, using virtual learning environments provides opportunities to increase student involvement once they are engaged. The best recommendation would be to continue to look for ways to improve the learning experience in the virtual world. Get student feedback

(continued)

> **BOX 12.1 Exemplar 1—Disaster Triage (*continued*)**
>
> on what they think about the learning experience; students appreciate knowing you are interested. Implement suggestions where feasible; keep trying different approaches to keep things interesting.
>
> *Source:* Claman, F. (2015). The impact of multiuser virtual environments on student engagement. *Nursing Education in Practice, 15*, 13–16. doi:10.1016/j.nepr.2014.11006; Lau, K. W., & Lee, P. Y. (2015). The use of virtual reality for creating unusual environmental stimulation to motivate students to explore creative ideas. *Interactive Learning Environments, 23*(1), 3–18. doi:10.1080/10494820.2012.745426

> **BOX 12.2 Exemplar 2—Community Assessment and a Home Health Assessment**
>
> ## ABSTRACT
>
> This exemplar addressed students' ability to effectively assess a community and home setting within a virtual learning environment. Both learning activities provided an opportunity for active participation by students, but differed due to the limitations of the assessment environments.
>
> ## INTRODUCTION
>
> Students interacted in two separate environments during a community health course. The community assessment experience required the student to analyze a community environment setting, and the home setting required the student to assess living conditions for a person or family. The learning environments included similar learning objectives.
>
> Assessment of any community requires sufficient scale to encompass population-wide interventions that would entail measurable results. In a virtual learning environment, this can be accomplished through a simulated community setting in which students may make observations. The ability of students to interact in more than one type of setting is beneficial to learning. For example, creating an urban community and a suburban community offers students an opportunity to assess aspects of both environments. The communities may encompass common concerns such as safety. Available resources can be another aspect of evaluation in a virtual learning environment. Other concerns may include the presence of disease-carrying pests, pollution, and waste, as well as the resources that might be available to address these issues. The community assessment within a virtual learning environment may be less overwhelming to students than driving through an actual community but still demonstrate the principles of community assessment without the risk of physical harm. Karaman and Orban Özen (2016) noted that students are able to take a role actively, rather than passively, and that barriers between faculty and students were broken down in virtual learning environments.
>
> The same idea of active participation of students applies to the individual home assessment in a virtual learning environment. Although homes

(continued)

> **BOX 12.2 Exemplar 2—Community Assessment and a Home Health Assessment** (*continued*)

vary, some of the same concerns exist; for example, loose rugs, exposed wiring, lack of lighting or running water, and stairways or the number of steps—all relate back to the client. Depending on the home and client situation, this learning experience can facilitate student understanding of home evaluation and its relevance to health care. Home assessment also gives students some understanding of the concerns that need to be addressed before a client may be discharged from care.

CHALLENGES IDENTIFIED

Working with students who are performing assessments while immersed in a virtual environment can be fun; however, keeping them on task and engaged was challenging. A combination of worksheets, lists, and in-class discussions pertaining to potential risks and solutions can be very helpful for maintaining student engagement. Depending on faculty preference, the assessments in a virtual learning environment can be accomplished with or without faculty presence while students complete lists or worksheets in the virtual setting. Simulated community assessment in the virtual world can greatly assist student understanding of conducting similar tasks in an actual environment, which may be difficult for some students to comprehend without an example.

STAKEHOLDER PERSPECTIVES

Administrative

From an administrative perspective, there is no risk to students and faculty in entering unhealthy environments in the virtual world. Another positive aspect is the controlled learning experience, which translates to learning experience consistency among students. Once the virtual world or environment is created, it is relatively inexpensive to provide for large numbers of students.

Faculty

From a faculty perspective, some benefits are consistent learning experiences that may be adjusted to fit curricular and student learning needs. One drawback is the occasional time commitment to creating and implementing a simulated learning activity. However, some activities can be completed collaboratively or with students in groups, which can save time for faculty.

Student

From a student perspective, varying learning experiences from PowerPoint and lecture to active participation in applied learning can be a refreshing change of pace. Immersive virtual world learning experiences may challenge students to

(*continued*)

> **BOX 12.2 Exemplar 2—Community Assessment and a Home Health Assessment** (*continued*)

think and act in a manner consistent with their intended new role as a nurse. For some students, this opportunity can be new and exciting; for others, it may be out of their comfort zone.

Resolutions

One satisfaction with working in the virtual world is that changes can be made as needed to the learning experience to accommodate students. There is flexibility in adjusting the written assignments, as well as the presentation of content. The ability to make changes to enhance the learning experience is a plus; it is not necessary to start from the beginning.

Frustration

Conversely, the ability to make frequent changes within the learning experience may be time-consuming and frustrating for faculty. Student buy-in varies because some students like the use of a virtual learning environment but others do not. The technical aspects from frequent updates to platform changes can be another challenge.

Summarization

Overall, using a virtual learning environment for simulation is worth the time and effort. Students can be challenged without being put on the spot as they might be in a simulation laboratory. Using a virtual world for learning may facilitate some abstract concepts through controlled immersion into the virtual learning environment.

LESSONS LEARNED

What worked?

Aspects that worked well for teaching and learning in a virtual environment were that the experiences could be tailored to meet student learning needs. Much of the learning took place during debriefing after completion of the learning activity in the virtual world. Classroom conversations about community needs or the needs to be addressed in the home were great discussion topics. Students were able to use their own experiences to evaluate and critically think about resources and ways to mitigate future problems. Keeping track of student concerns and solutions enabled the faculty and developers the opportunity to modify and enhance the simulation experience.

What did not work?

Technical issues and students who struggled to overcome learning obstacles detracted from the benefits of the learning experience. Although the technical

(continued)

> **BOX 12.2 Exemplar 2—Community Assessment and a Home Health Assessment** (*continued*)

issues may or may not be avoidable, finding ways to minimize such distractions is critically important. The need to work with students who struggle will likely be a challenge regardless of the teaching method used. Keeping students engaged in the activity was also challenging. It is important to keep students busy but not overwhelm them with the virtual world.

What would you do the same in the future?

Some of the things worth repeating would be the use of virtual learning experiences for simulation. Creating worksheets, allowing students to work in pairs, and tracking student comments are worth continuing. The combination of virtual world simulation and postsimulation immersion conversations generates wonderful learning experiences for all involved.

What would you do differently in the future?

The challenges of teaching in the virtual world can be well worth the effort to create learning experiences and keep up with the technology. Faculty and developers must be creative when developing virtual learning experiences. Modifying the way the activity unfolds for students' gives faculty control of the experience. Unlike PowerPoint and lecture, virtual learning experiences require student participation. Through evaluation of student participation, faculty may make modifications and facilitate better results for the next learning opportunity.

What will you take away from this experience?

There may be several takeaways from using virtual worlds for teaching, but the biggest opportunity is the interaction between students and faculty. Having conversations in class after completing an exercise in a virtual learning environment can be enriching because students are forced to think critically. Regardless of the scenario, it was surprising to note the well-thought-out responses from students when they became more deeply immersed with virtual patients.

What advice would you offer to others in the same situation?

Some suggestions for using a virtual world platform for teaching would be to advocate for the student learning experience. Always strive to make the learning experience worthwhile and something memorable for students and thoroughly examine what did not go well with prior attempts to create such opportunities in the virtual world.

Source: Karaman, M. K., & Orban Özen, S. (2016). A survey of students' experiences on collaborative virtual learning activities based on five-stage model. *Educational Technology & Society, 19*(3), 247–259.

REFLECTIVE QUESTIONS

1. What kind of virtual world would allow you to take students where you want them to go? Describe a scenario that you could develop to guide student learning.
2. How can you best stimulate student learning? Discuss why your answer would stimulate learning.
3. If you were a student, would you want to participate in the learning experience? Provide a rationale for your answer.
4. Describe how you would know what students learned from the experience.

REFERENCES

American Association of Colleges of Nursing. (2012). QSEN education consortium: Graduate-level QSEN competencies knowledge, skills, and attitudes. Retrieved from http://www.aacnnursing.org/Portals/42/AcademicNursing/CurriculumGuidelines/Graduate-QSEN-Competencies.pdf

Claman, F. (2015). The impact of multiuser virtual environments on student engagement. *Nursing Education in Practice, 15,* 13–16. doi:10.1016/j.nepr.2014.11006

Hernández, N., González, M., & Muñoz, P. (2014). Planning collaborative learning in virtual environments. *Comunicar, 42,* 25–32. doi:10.3916/C42-2014-02

Karaman, M. K., & Orban Özen, S. (2016). A survey of students' experiences on collaborative virtual learning activities based on five-stage model. *Educational Technology & Society, 19*(3), 247–259.

Lau, K. W., & Lee, P. Y. (2015). The use of virtual reality for creating unusual environmental stimulation to motivate students to explore creative ideas. *Interactive Learning Environments, 23*(1), 3–18. doi:10.1080/10494820.2012.745426

Lee, L., Lee, J., Wong, K., Tsang, A., & Li, M. (2010). The establishment of an integrated skills training centre for undergraduate nursing education. *International Nursing Review, 57*(3), 359–364. doi:10.1111/j.1466-7657.2009.00796.x

Nicely, S., & Farra, S. (2015). Fostering learning through interprofessional virtual reality simulation development. *Nursing Education Perspective, 36*(5), 335–336. doi:10.5480/13-1240

O'Connor, E. A. (2015). Open source meets virtual reality: An instructor's journey unearths new opportunities for learning, community, and academia. *Journal of Educational Technology Systems, 44*(2), 153–170. doi:10.1177/004723951567158

Tilton, K. J., Tiffany, J., & Hoglund, B. A. (2015). Non-acute-care virtual simulation: Preparing students to provide chronic illness care. *Nursing Education Perspectives, 36*(6), 394–395. doi:10.5480/14-1532

Tokel, S. T., & Isler, V. (2015). Acceptance of virtual worlds as learning space. *Innovations in Education and Teaching International, 52*(3), 254–264. doi:10.1080/14703297.2013.820139

World Health Organization. (2010). Framework for action on interprofessional education and collaborative practice. Retrieved from http://www.who.int/hrh/resources/framework_action/en

CHAPTER 13

Enhancing the Rigor of Virtual Simulation

SIMON JR COOPER AND FIONA BOGOSSIAN

LEARNING OBJECTIVES

Upon completion of this chapter, the reader will be able to:
- Assess approaches to enhancing rigor in the development, implementation, and evaluation of virtual simulation.
- Examine the five recommended stages of development of a virtual simulation program.
- Appreciate the importance of and steps necessary to trialling a virtual simulation prior to full integration with an established curriculum.

KEY TERMS

Asynchronicity	Inter-rater reliability
Consequential validity	Nontechnical skills
Construct validity	Predictive validity
Content validity	Reliability
External validity	Rigor
Face validity	Stakeholders
Feasibility	Test–retest reliability
Internal consistency reliability	Validity
Internal validity	

Clinical simulation has changed significantly over the last three decades. The emergence of resuscitation manikins in the 1960s (Laerdal, n.d.) led to increasingly complex, high-fidelity equipment able to mirror aspects of the clinical world. However, scenarios and simulations need to integrate the myriad of complex and demanding aspects of a clinical setting, taking into account the technical and nontechnical aspects of healthcare. This is particularly difficult to do, even for an experienced instructor, and makes the consistent quality repetition and assessment of the same scenario difficult. This is of concern in assessing complex performances in which poor reliability and lack of consistency in standards (Bloxham, 2015) can result in inequitable assessment of learners. The introduction of virtual simulation programs enables safe repetition of practice in standardized scenarios that, if rigorously developed, can support validity and reliability. More important, this form of delivery is increasingly feasible with web-based access and may reduce face-to-face instructor time. The approach is also cost-effective overall, with reports suggesting that, although costly to design and develop, it becomes significantly cheaper than face-to-face approaches over time (Cooper et al., 2017).

In this chapter, we focus on enhancing rigor across the five stages of development of virtual simulation programs, drawing on our experience of developing a patient deterioration management program known as Feedback Incorporating Review and Simulation Techniques to Act on Clinical Trends (FIRST2ACTWeb™ [first2act-web.com]; see Box 13.1). The program includes background educational materials,

---

BOX 13.1 E-Simulation Spotlight

FIRST2ACT and FAST2ACTweb

PROBLEM

Research demonstrates that student nurses have good theoretical knowledge. Evidence demonstrates that the recognition and management of deteriorating hospital patients is a problem throughout the world and contributes to many adverse outcomes. Students often fail to respond appropriately, and as anxiety levels increase, student performance and awareness of the situation significantly decrease. Students frequently and erroneously fixated on a single issue.

RESEARCH

Research findings indicated that the educational experiences that incorporate simulation-based skills demonstration, reflection, and feedback had a significant impact on participants' reported learning. Further study supports that students grouped together in teams to review patient notes and conduct time series analyses produced a significant improvement in patient-management skills, which translates to better clinical outcomes in the actual healthcare setting.

SOLUTION

The best way to resolve this issue is to practice in simulated settings. The FIRST2ACT program includes assessment test, as well as simulation and feedback techniques, that are delivered face-to-face to individual participants by a team of four or five instructors over ½ to 2 hours. Based on the outcomes from FIRST2ACT, a web-based simulation program called FIRST2ACTweb was developed. FAST2ACTweb is a virtual simulation learning program that includes quizzes, presentations, and scenario-based interactive videos. The total time needed to complete the program is 1 to 2 hours. Participants may pause between pages and repeat scenarios as needed. FAST2ACTweb has been implemented in a variety of studies with nurses, midwives, and paramedics. The program was originally intended for Australian nursing students but is also applicable to international healthcare students and staff. Outcomes demonstrate that FIRST2ACT and FAST2ACTweb have positive impact on decision making in the clinical setting, on educational outcomes, and on teamwork.

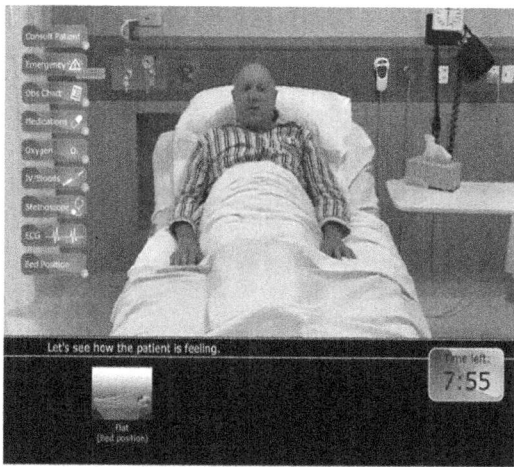

FIGURE 13.1 FIRST2ACTWeb screen shot.

precourse and postcourse knowledge tests, and three interactive management scenarios (acute myocardial infarction [AMI], hypovolemic shock, and chronic obstructive pulmonary disease). Each scenario is based on a video recording of a simulated patient experiencing sudden deterioration in a hospital setting and a range of interactive tasks (mouse clicks that generate pop-up videos) such as assessing vital signs and administering oxygen or cannulation (see Figure 13.1). Performance data are collated, enabling feedback. Further examples are drawn from a similar program called Rescuing a Patient in Deteriorating Situations (e-RAPIDS [www.youtube.com/watch?v=fRE9GVWhQhA]; Liaw et al., 2016) that also focuses on the management of patient deterioration but uses photographic elements as opposed to interactive video to simulate patients (see Figure 13.2).

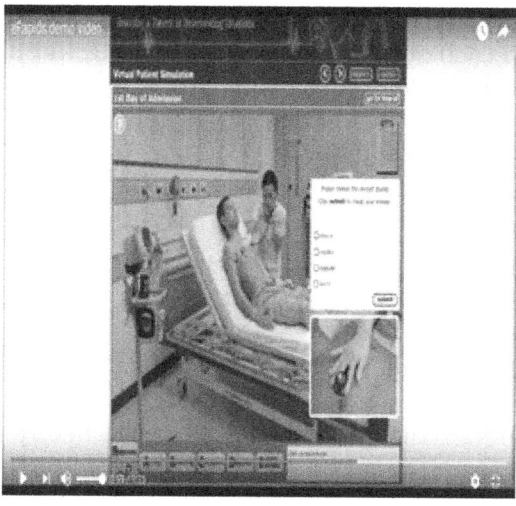

FIGURE 13.2 e-RAPIDS screen shot.
Source: Adapted from https://courseware.nus.edu.sg/RAPIDS/e-simulation/

RELATION TO THE FACULTY ADMINISTRATORS STUDENTS TECHNOLOGY STRATEGIC INTEGRATION MODEL© (FAST SIM)

Faculty members must be able to assume the experienced and expert levels dealing with the innovator and researcher roles; adding rigor to virtual simulation is paramount. Faculty must be able to conduct an appropriate needs assessment to determine appropriate solutions and pull **stakeholders** together to discuss integration strategies and research outcomes.

RIGOR AND VIRTUAL SIMULATION

Rigor is key to designing and building a high-quality virtual simulation education program and assessment. **Rigor** relates to the *scrupulous* and *meticulous* conduct of virtual simulation through structured and controlled planning of educational program design, coupled with a methodological commitment to careful, consistent, and diligent assessment. In reality, absolute rigor is rarely achievable. However, an intellectual approach that recognizes constraints, prejudices, biases, and important influences and that balances these with considerations of validity, reliability, and **feasibility**, should result in a robust and enduring virtual simulation program.

Validity is concerned with the *accuracy and credibility* of the program and assessment. Does the program or assessment truly represent the construct being taught or assessed? Validity addresses a number of elements; for example, responding to whether the "right" things being taught and assessed encompasses both **face validity** and **content validity**. Does the program encourage good learning techniques? This relates to **consequential validity**. Does educational success predict good future performance? This is relevant to **predictive validity**. Each of these elements should be considered in the design and assessment of virtual simulation.

Reliability, on the other hand, is concerned with the *stability and consistency* of the program and assessment. Can the program be uniformly repeated, and does the assessment dependably pass and fail the "right" learners? Reliability also addresses a number of elements; for example, responding to whether different assessors of the same thing agree with each other relates to **inter-rater reliability**. Would the learner obtain a similar result if retested without additional learning? This reflects *retest reliability*. Does the learner respond uniformly to different items that measure the same construct?' This examines *internal consistency*. Each of these elements warrants consideration in the design and assessment of virtual simulation. The key is to achieve maximal validity and reliability in both program design and assessment.

Fundamentally though, the design of any education program is likely to be subject to compromise, which may impact the rigor of the program and assessment. This is where feasibility must either be theoretically considered or pragmatically tested. There is debate in the literature around feasibility, with the terms and concepts used interchangeably and inconsistently (Eldridge et al., 2016). Feasibility can apply in virtual simulation design and assessment to determine the viability of an idea, to estimate important parameters, and to test methods, procedures, components, and uncertainties. Questions around feasibility should determine "whether something can be done, should we proceed with it, and if so, how" (Eldridge et al., 2016, p. 8).

In short, feasibility considers the practicality of the education program. Whether feasibility is determined through theoretical risk management or is formally tested using a trial, it has four common aspects that require deliberation: technical (physical and human resources), economic (cost/benefit analysis), operational (systems and settings), and schedule (time allocation and deadlines). For example, an educational program or assessment must be feasible to produce within the resources and time available and it must be feasible for learners to complete; that is, it must neither be too long nor too complex.

In summary validity, reliability, and feasibility contribute to the rigor of virtual simulation education programs and assessment methods (see Figure 13.3). So, with these issues in mind, where do you start if you want to build a virtual simulation?

DEVELOPING VIRTUAL SIMULATION

Designing and developing virtual simulation requires a staged approach, although in our experience, these stages are not necessarily undertaken in a linear fashion. Sometimes a creative insight occurs during a later stage, requiring revision of previous stages. It is important not only to be open to these flashes of inspiration, but also to deliberate their merits in the context of rigor. Many design meetings can be hijacked by creative ideas that lack validity, or reliability, feasibility or that merely detour the project.

Stage 1: Determining Aims and Objectives

First, to ensure the materials are valid, consider the program's focus, aims, and objectives. You may also like to reflect on what you want your program to change, including specific outcomes for learners related to knowledge, attitude, or skills or wider impacts of their behavior. For example, you may want to influence attitudes or change clinical practice or impact patient outcomes. The aims statement should include explicit reference to the target audience and population, the simulation type, and the intended outcomes because these help keep project activities focused.

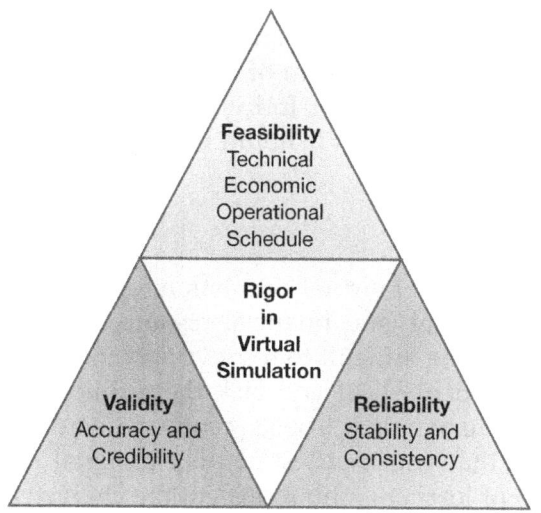

FIGURE 13.3 Rigor and virtual simulation.

In developing the FIRST2ACTWeb program, the project team explicitly listed the *aim* as a simulation-based learning program for healthcare students and professionals that aims to improve skills in recognizing and managing acutely deteriorating patients. Then in each section within the program and course manual, we listed the *objectives*, such as: To identify essential actions in the management of a deteriorating patient or to describe oxygen delivery devices. Note here that aims are general statements regarding the intentions of the program, whereas objectives are desired learning outcomes.

Stage 2: Designing Materials

Once the aims and objectives of your virtual simulation program are determined, the next challenge is to develop applicable education and assessment materials. The project team may adapt existing material or decide to develop their own. In either case, if the virtual simulation program has a clinical focus, consideration must be given to ensuring that contemporary, evidence-informed, best clinical practice underpins the development of program materials. Although there is unlikely to be a universal agreement on this principle, in practice linking evidence to design can be complicated, as there may be variance between national or international. To overcome this in the FIRST2ACTWeb program, we selected key guidance from the International Liaison Committee on Resuscitation (ILCOR), accepting that regional practices and guidelines may differ to some degree.

Once a set of materials have been drafted, checking *face validity* is important, with validation conducted by experts in the nominated setting. In the FIRST2ACTWeb program, we envisioned that the education program might have global uptake; as a result, face and content validity was completed by a panel of international experts who discussed and decided on the applicability of each element. *Content validity* is also a critical requirement if your program includes the development of an assessment tool. The validity of the content can then be measured to calculate the content validity index (CVI; Polit & Beck, 2006). For example, you may want to assess the **nonechnical skills** in a group of learners and therefore develop a rating scale/checklist measuring leadership, teamwork, and levels of situation awareness. In this case, team members would independently rate the relevance of each item using a five-point scale (1 = not at all relevant to 5 = most relevant). The CVI is calculated for each item and the sum of all items is based on the proportion of experts with a rating of three or more. Individual items with a CVI of greater than 0.78 are acceptable, and the total CVI should be greater than 0.90 (Cant & Cooper, 2014; Cooper et al., 2010).

Stage 3: "Real Life" Testing

The design and development of virtual simulation represents a considerable investment of intellectual, technical, and financial resources. Any errors in educational design and materials may be difficult to retrieve and correct once committed to the virtual environment, particularly if you lack the technological expertise or if the project budget has been expended. Consequently, when developing a virtual program, we recommend that you first test or pilot material in a face-to-face setting with a selected group of learners who represent the characteristics of the intended audience of the virtual simulation.

In the FIRST2ACTWeb education program, we produced a course manual, an audio slide lecture, and three patient deterioration scenarios. Assessment materials included preknowledge and postknowledge tests, self-assessment of confidence and competence, assessment of teamwork and situation awareness, and Objective Structures Clinical Examination (OSCE) performance rating forms. These included yes/no responses to performance checks: Was a nonrebreather mask selected? Was the blood pressure taken? Was an ECG performed? In testing, we used a live simulated patient in eight-minute scenarios with performance rating forms and tested these across a range of learners with varied characteristics and clinical experience.

After a sample group of learners have completed the program and relevant assessments, a number of checks relating to reliability can be performed. Returning to our example for the teamwork rating scale, we assessed how closely related the individual items were as a group using a statistical test known as Cronbach's alpha, which measures **internal consistency reliability**. Furthermore, for the FIRST2ACTWeb program, we were able to measure the *inter-rater reliability* of the OSCEs during face-to-face testing. Two instructors directly observed learners complete each scenario, and on completion, instructors immediately and independently rated the individual performance items. Once the documentation was complete, the two instructors discussed any discrepancies, confirming agreement via the video recording of the performance to make a fair and equitable judgment on performance. When a group of learners are assessed in this way, it is possible to formally test the inter-rater reliability using statistical tests such as Kappa and intraclass correlation coefficients. Likewise, the **test–retest reliability** can also be measured when a learner repeats the same test at a later date.

Stage 4: Adapting Materials for Virtual Simulation

The transition from "real life" to a virtual simulation environment requires specific technical skills to augment clinical, simulation, and educational expertise. The key to this stage is to have engaged a software programmer (or an educational designer, with appropriate technical capabilities) from the start of the project, as this person is likely to have insights into programming issues that may influence the pedagogy and use of the program. For example, programming in Adobe® Flash®, as opposed to HTML5, precludes video replay on portable (non-Flash compatible) devices. Stone (2016) identified how a teamwork approach to design learning, in which designers and academics collaborate, is important for compatibility and accessibility of curriculum, content, and delivery.

Consider if there are any technological outcomes of the project that should be monitored and reported, because these may require additional process planning and specific data collection. A number of models of technological utility can be used to guide thinking about this aspect of the project. Venkatesh, Morris, Davis, and Davis (2003) proposed a model that incorporates user experiences, user behavior, performance expectancy, effort expectancy, and social influence. We used this model previously in testing video capture technology and found it useful for assessing user acceptance and use of technology (Strand, Fox-Young, Long, & Bogossian, 2013), aspects fundamental to successful virtual simulation.

There are additional considerations regarding users. At this stage, you need to consider writing disclaimers in relation to the educational content if, as mentioned, international guidelines differ. Online presentation and the format of material require thought and programming for feedback mechanisms. For example, consider if and how you provide results of performance to users, whether onscreen or sent directly to learners' email accounts.

Significant work is required in the development of the virtual simulation components whether filming simulated patients or, in the case of e-RAPIDS, gathering photographic elements. Writing a storyboard is a central component of good design, as are the authenticity and psychological fidelity (believability) of the scenarios. Although the use of photographed stills or even computer-generated patients (avatars) can be economical in terms of technical production, these may come at the price of authenticity and psychological fidelity. However, if mistakes are made in the development of the scenarios or if practices or guidelines change, it may be possible to reprogram the avatar relatively easily.

In the FIRST2ACTWeb program, we took a unique approach and video-recorded trained actors for various components of each eight-minute scenario. This included gradual deterioration in the first four minutes, with increasing signs and urgency of more acute deterioration for the final four. Many virtual responses in the form of "pop up" clinical actions were also necessary, and where possible, the action and responses (e.g., assessment of tympanic temperature, auscultation of the chest) were recorded using the same actor. Actors could not be expected to have their veins cannulated, so filming of intravenous cannulation was performed using a close-up of a staff member's arm with some consequent reduction in fidelity in scenarios. Yet this overall approach ensured that each scenario was of high fidelity with acute deterioration demanding and challenging action from learners. Once filmed, however, each video sequence was locked, limiting the programmers' ability to change a scenario at a later date. Developers should also consider the resource-intensive nature of such approaches because the filming and editing of scenarios takes considerable time and resources.

Rating performance in scenarios in virtual simulation is critical for both formative feedback and summative assessment purposes. In FIRST2ACTWeb, we designed a scoring system based on the nominal "yes/no" OSCE assessment tested in the face-to-face development stage. Over time, this developed into a weighted system reflecting the refinement of our thinking, where it became increasingly apparent to us that learners needed to not only "do the right thing," but also do it at the right time. For example, in the AMI scenario, a score of 2 was awarded when glyceryl trinitrate was given, with an additional score of 1 if the drug was given in the first four minutes of the scenario. In comparison, a score of 1 was allocated where the patent was positioned semi-upright compared with a score of 2 + 1 when the patient was positioned upright in the first four minutes of the scenario.

As in face-to-face development, the scoring system was checked for *face validity* by a panel of international clinical experts. This included intense discussion around the equity of the scoring of various tasks, which in the relatively simple scoring system we devised was not completely resolved. Gaining consensus on the applicable performance tasks and their timing is difficult especially when virtual simulation inevitably limits the learner to one task at a time compared with the clinical setting in which a team performs multiple tasks simultaneously.

Feedback and debriefing mechanisms are critical to any simulation programs (Cant & Cooper, 2011). E-learning approaches, in general, lack the capacity for learner–teacher engagement (Al-Shorbaji, Atun, Car, Majeed, & Wheeler, 2015), and in virtual systems, this may be emphasized because of **asynchronicity** and one-way communication in which detailed two-way communication through question-and-answer sessions is not possible. In the initial development of FIRST2ACTWeb, we provided learners with general feedback statements about what they "should do" after each scenario. However, in later versions, we tailored more detailed feedback to their performance score, such as "you did this, but don't forget to do that next time." Feedback relating to postsimulation knowledge tests was also possible by presenting learners with detailed responses about the questions they answered correctly and the answers to those they did not.

Further considerations when developing virtual simulation programs relate to the tacit dimensions of assessment. Is the program oriented and designed to be instructional and educative without the additional pressures of assessment? Does the program include formative assessment elements (i.e., assessment *for* learning) and/or summative assessment approaches (i.e., assessment *of* learning)? Are criteria designed to make the processes of judgement about performance transparent? What is the purpose of the judgement of performance, and is passing performance required or not?

We know that assessment does drive learning, and assessment may therefore be one motivator (among others) for learners to complete a program. In the case of health care professionals, there are also employment and professional licensure issues to consider. The essential conditions are that the assessment approach is rigorous, valid, and reliable and that it "passes" the right learner. If you decide to set criteria for a passing performance then the Angoff technique is a useful approach (Ricker, 2006). An example is detailed in Table 13.1. To set the "pass-mark" in FIRST2ACT, OSCEs complete the procedure with a group of approximately five expert clinicians/educators. It is useful to record the relevant characteristics and experience of each assessor.

Stage 5: Trialling, Implementing, and Evaluating a Virtual Simulation Program

After the development and adaption of materials from the real-life setting, extensive trials for implementation in a virtual simulation environment are necessary. Trialling is critical to determine whether you have done "enough piloting and feasibility work to be confident that the intervention—in this case the virtual simulation—can be implemented as intended" (Lancaster, 2015, p. 2). Although pilot and feasibility studies are sometimes viewed as synonymous, it is important to distinguish the purpose and therefore the design of each in the context of virtual simulation.

A pilot study involves a small preliminary trial run of the virtual simulation program and assessment and evaluation methods to test whether the components work together and to make any improvements (Lancaster, 2015; Thabane et al., 2010) before the virtual simulation is implemented on a larger scale. An internal or "within organization" pilot test should be conducted to identify and correct program issues prior to testing across a wider population. Inevitably, there will be issues, and using an adaptive trial design allows modifications to be made either prospectively, concurrently, or retrospectively (Thabane et al., 2010).

TABLE 13.1 Modified Angoff Pass-Mark Setting (A Worked Example)

1. Review the acute myocardial infarction (AMI) assessment (Objective Structures Clinical Examinations [OSCE]).
   1.1. Recall learners you have taught to manage an AMI.
   1.2. Individually consider learners whose performance "bordered on mastery" (i.e., those who just passed the assessment or met the minimum safe level of competency).
   1.3. As a group discuss the characteristics of these learners and what they were and were not able to achieve. Develop "a common notion of a borderline learner"
2. Then as individuals identify the OSCE items indicative of borderline pass (e.g., in the AMI OSCE 27 nominal [yes/no] criteria). For example, was blood pressure recorded? Was a history taken? Was an ECG recorded? Which of these must (and are likely) to be achieved by a borderline candidate?
   2.1. Record and sum these individual scores and enter them in the table below.
   2.2. The sum score of the total possible is the designated pass-mark.

Expert Assessor	Characteristics	Score	Total
1.	Cardiac nurse 20 yr	17	27
2.	ER doctor 5 yr	14	27
3.	Unit manager 16 yr	15	27
4.	MET team leader 8 yr	22	27
5.	Cardiac nurse 15 yr	20	27
Total		88	135
Pass mark		Score/Total	65%

Source: Adapted from Ricker, K. (2006). Setting cut scores: A critical review of the Angoff and modified Angoff methods. *Alberta Journal of Educational Research, 52,* 53–63. Retrieved from http://hdl.handle.net/10515/sy54746z4

Feasibility can form part of the pilot testing procedures and, as described earlier, can incorporate technical, economic, operational, and schedule components. Feasibility studies should contain clearly articulated feasibility objectives that reflect the anticipated issues in the implementation stage. These may vary depending on the virtual simulation, the setting, and the audience. In the FIRST2ACTWeb program, for example, the following questions included: Did the program work well in some web browsers and less well in others? How well did the program run when internet connections were unstable or slow? Did users report that guidelines differed significantly in their home country? Was the program too practical to complete? Did the developed scales enable users to rate the design, completeness, and acceptability of the program? Feasibility studies typically focus on drug trials and are rarely published (Tickle-Degnan, 2013), with published trials of education interventions even more scarce (Bogossian, Broadribb et al., 2017). Given the resources involved in developing and implementing virtual simulation pedagogy, it is important that those involved contribute their experiences to the body of knowledge in the field by undertaking and publishing pilot and feasibility trials.

Following the trial phase, the implementation of a virtual simulation program requires a planned and supported approach. It is useful to roll out implementation in stages, during which sites and user groups are staggered. This approach not only means that site or user group issues can be quickly addressed, but also that specific issues do not become generalized in the wider context and user population, requiring the entire program to be shut down. Ideally, as part of the implementation plan, there should be at least one academic and one technical person able to support users or address technical glitches that may occur ad hoc or be identified through the evaluation processes.

Because virtual simulation is a relatively new learning modality and quality assessment and improvement are imperative, it is essential to include a formal evaluation. Evaluation provides data to make judgements about the value of the virtual simulation program. However, it is important to recognize that there may be different interests in an evaluation and that this may result in pluralist conceptions and multiple methods, measures, criteria, perspectives, and audiences (House, 1993, as cited in Mertens, 2010).

Mertens (2010) suggested that the steps in conducting evaluation parallel those of research projects but that in evaluation, steps vary based on the purpose of the evaluation, the status of the project, and the model of evaluation. Nonetheless, evaluation research methods need to be carefully considered and include cross-sectional (data from a specified point in time) or longitudinal (a sequence of exposures over time), cluster-randomized trials (group as opposed to individual randomization) or quasiexperimental (nonrandomized) approaches (i.e., preintervention and postintervention measurements; Cooper, 2016).

In education, randomized controlled trials (that are not clustered) are not necessarily the ideal approach; for example, there are limits to randomization—learners cannot be blinded, cross-contamination is possible, and the dynamics of a group change when it is split. Although a controlled trial improves **internal validity**, this approach reduces generalizability and **external validity** because the trial context does not mirror the real world (Cooper, 2016). Attempting to overcome these limitations in virtual simulation programs is likely to be impracticable, given the resource implications of establishing a control program.

What is important to virtual simulation evaluation is that there is a planned evaluation approach ideally drafted at the commencement of the project. This should include the focus of the evaluation (i.e., the items being evaluated, the purpose, stakeholders, constraints) and inform the development of evaluation strategies and selection of a model. The plan should be flexible but at minimum include details about data collection, analysis, interpretation, use, and management. Flexibility allows for the inclusion of additional unique evaluation elements that may emerge as the program is implemented and developed. For example, in the FIRST2ACTWeb program, as a result of being able to collect detailed "click data," we could evaluate the course of action of learners in the program (Cooper, Cant, Bogossian, Bucknall, & Hopmans, 2015), something we would not have clearly foreseen in the developmental phases.

Other evaluation considerations in virtual simulation programs include whether the evaluation should focus on broad, long-term intended effects (goals); the specific measurable effects of the program and its benefits to stakeholders (outcomes); and ways that the functions or procedures of the program (processes) contribute to the goals and outcomes (Suter, 2012). Evaluation is at risk of being the "Cinderella" of any education program development as a result of positioning at the end of the program cycle, when budgets are commonly depleted. However, in virtual simulation this risk is heightened by the rapid redundancy and replacement of technology.

Long-term effects and benefits to stakeholders are costlier to measure and require extended engagement. It is not surprising therefore that findings of a recent survey of simulation-based education (Bogossian, Broadribb et al., 2017), which were supported by a scoping literature review (Bogossian, Cooper et al., 2017), found outcome measures predominantly related to level 1, reaction (learner's degree of satisfaction) and level l2, Learning (changes in knowledge and skills) of Kirkpatrick's model of evaluation of educational outcome (Kirkpatrick Partners, 2017). Virtual simulation, because of its capacity to access users electronically, has the potential to extend evaluation to level 3, behavioral change (transfer of learning from the simulation to the clinical context/situation), and level 4, results (improvements in patient outcomes and/or organizational change; Kirkpatrick Partners, 2017). For example, in relation to eRAPIDS, level 2 and 3 impact was demonstrated (Liaw et al., 2015, 2016); for FIRST2ACTWeb, level 3 impact was demonstrated (Cooper et al., 2017).

Elements of rigor are equally important to guarantee the methodological quality of the evaluation and "avoid caveats such as contamination, high attrition rates and volunteer bias" (Al-Shorbaji et al., 2015, p. xvii). Therefore, it is important not only to conduct high-quality evaluation, but also to structure the evaluation to encourage learners to complete it. In the FIRST2ACTWeb program, users can access their course certificate only when the evaluation has been completed, resulting in high rates of completion of the evaluation. Over a four-year period, 15,952 users completed the last stage of the program, and 14,747 went on to complete the evaluation (92%). Conducting user evaluations online also has the benefit of rapid responsiveness so that critical issues, such as, password access faults, video accessibility, and software compatibility, can be addressed quickly.

Detailed in-depth quantitative evaluations also require high numbers of learners; for example, if you want to measure the **construct validity** of an assessment or rating tool, 100 or more learners are required for exploratory factor analyses. Detailed analyses of program outcomes also tend to require larger numbers; for example, we mapped the course-of-action of 367 FIRST2ACTWeb learners, identifying that only 18% took the "best course of action" (the right actions and timing), 70% took the right actions but in the wrong order, and 12% produced incomplete assessments/actions in the wrong order (Cooper et al., 2015)

FURTHER CONSIDERATIONS FOR VIRTUAL SIMULATION

Although it is possible to enhance validity and reliability in virtual simulation programs, there will always be limits. For international programs, matching all clinical guidelines is impossible, and international generic guidance is the accepted standard. Programming forms may also have limitations; for example, Flash cannot be used on all portable devices, and it works better on some web browsers than others.

It is also not possible to program a simulation to enable infinite variability, which will limit fidelity, and design and programming become increasingly complex with each new treatment outcome pathway that is added. For example, in earlier versions of FIRST2ACTWeb, users raised concerns that the patient did not "get better" even when treated correctly. In part, this was because the scenarios run for only eight minutes (not long enough to see the effects of most treatments), but this was also because multiple pathways would need filming and programming depending on treatment. In short, such programs are "screen based" and cannot completely mirror the real and complex world of clinical care.

There are, however, multiple benefits of virtual simulation, including ease of access to vast numbers of the population. Learners can repeat the program easily, and performance anxiety is also likely to be lower than in face-to-face settings, which may enhance learning (Ignacio et al., 2015; Leblanc, 2009). Fewer human resources are required, with significant reduction in costs over time compared with face-to-face instruction (Cooper et al., 2017), and when licensed and commercialized, programs may generate income to ensure their long-term sustainability.

KEY POINTS

- Rigor is key to designing and building a high-quality virtual simulation education program and assessment.
- Validity, reliability, and feasibility contribute to the rigor of virtual simulation education programs and assessment methods.
- Designing and developing virtual simulation requires a staged approach.
- Feedback and debriefing mechanisms are critical to any simulation program.
- What is important to virtual simulation evaluation is that there is a planned evaluation approach that is ideally drafted at the commencement of the project.
- There are multiple benefits of virtual simulation, including there is ease of access to vast numbers of the population, learners can repeat the program easily, performance anxiety is likely to be lower than in face-to-face settings, and fewer human resources are required, with significant reduction in costs over time compared with face-to-face instruction.

SUMMARY

Building a virtual simulation requires a five-stage approach. At each stage, there are opportunities to enhance the rigor of virtual simulation education programs and assessment methods. Application of elements of validity, reliability, and feasibility in determining aims and objectives, designing materials, performing real-life testing, and adapting materials to virtual simulation, followed by trialling, implementing, and evaluating, ensures the rigor of the program.

REFLECTIVE QUESTIONS

1. How is *reliability* defined in the context of an educational program? Can you also think of some examples of how it may be measured?
2. How is *validity* defined in the context of an educational program? Can you also think of some examples of how it may be measured?

REFERENCES

Al-Shorbaji, N., Atun, R., Car, J., Majeed, A., & Wheeler, E. (2015). *eLearning for undergraduate health professional education: A systematic review informing radical transformation of health workforce development.* Geneva, Switzerland: World Health Organization. Retrieved from http://whoeducationguidelines.org/sites/default/files/uploads/eLearning-healthprof-report.pdf

Bloxham, S. (2015). 4 November 2015: The multiple limitations of assessment criteria. Transforming Assessment Webinar Series. *Australasian Society for Computers in Learning in Tertiary Education.* http://transformingassessment.com/events_4_november_2015.php

Bogossian, F., Brodribb, W., Farley, R., Goodwin, H., Tin, A., & Young, J. (2017). A feasibility study to improve practice nurses' competence and confidence in providing care for mothers and infants. *Contemporary Nurse, 10*, 1–12. doi:10.1080/10376178.2017.1281087

Bogossian, F., Cooper, S., Kelly, M., Levett-Jones, T., McKenna, L., Slark, J., & Seaton, P. (2017). Best practice in clinical simulation education—Are we there yet? A cross sectional survey of simulation in Australian and New Zealand pre-registration nursing education. *Collegian.* doi:10.1016/j.colegn.2017.09.003

Cant, R., & Cooper, S. J. (2011). The benefits of debriefing as formative feedback in nurse education. *Australian Journal of Advanced Nursing, 29*(1), 37–47. Retrieved from http://www.ajan.com.au/Vol29/29-1_Cant.pdf

Cant, R., & Cooper, S. (2014). Measuring the non-technical skills of medical emergency teams: An update on validity and reliability of Team Emergency Assessment Measure (TEAM). *Resuscitation, 85*, 31–33. doi:10.1016/j.resuscitation.2013.08.276

Cooper, S. (2016). Simulation versus lecture? Measuring clinical impact: Considerations for best practice. *Evidence-Based Nursing, 19*(2), 55–55. doi:10.1136/eb-2015-102221

Cooper, S., Cant, R., Bogossian, F., Bucknall, T., & Hopmans, R. (2015). Doing the right thing at the right time: Assessing responses to patient deterioration in electronic simulation scenarios using course-of-action analysis. *Computers, Informatics, Nursing, 33*(5), 199–207. doi:10.1097/CIN.0000000000000141

Cooper, S., Cant, R., Sellick, K., Porter, J., Somers, G., Kinsman, L., & Nestel, D. (2010). Rating medical emergency teamwork performance: Development of the Team Emergency Assessment Measure (TEAM). *Resuscitation, 81*, 446–452. doi:10.1016/j.resuscitation.2009.11.027

Cooper, S., Kinsman, L., Chung, C., Cant, R., Boyle, J., Cameron, A., . . . Rotter, T. (2017). *The impact of face-to-face and web-based simulation on patient deterioration and patient safety.* ISBN 978-1-876851-972 (eBook). Retrieved from http://first2actweb.com/index.php/resources

Eldridge, S. M., Lancaster, G. A., Campbell, M. J., Thabane, L., Hopewell, S., Coleman, C. L., & Bond, C. M. (2016). Defining feasibility and pilot studies in preparation for randomised controlled trials: Development of a conceptual framework. *PLOS One, 11*(3), e0150205. doi:10.1371/journal.pone.0150205

Ignacio, J., Dolmans, D., Scherpbier, A., Rethans, J., Chan, S., & Liaw, S. (2015). Comparison of standardized patients with high-fidelity simulators for managing stress and improving performance in clinical deterioration: A mixed methods study. *Nurse Education Today, 35*(12), 1161–1168. doi:10.1016/j.nedt.2015.05.009

Kirkpatrick Partners. (2017). The Kirkpatrick model. Retrieved from http://www.kirkpatrickpartners.com/Our-Philosophy/The-Kirkpatrick-Model

Laerdal. (n.d.). The story of Resusci Anne and the beginnings of modern CPR. Retrieved from http://www.laerdal.com/gb/doc/2738/The-Story-of-Resusci-Anne-and-the-beginnings-of-Modern-CPR

Lancaster, G. (2015). Pilot and feasibility studies come of age! *Pilot and Feasibility Studies, 1*(1). doi:10.1186/2055-5784-1-1

Leblanc, V. (2009). The effect of acute stress on performance: Implications for health professional education. *Academic Medicine, 84*(10), s25–s234. doi:10.1097/ACM.0b013e3181b37b8f

Liaw, S. Y., Wong, L. F., Ang, S. B. L., Ho, J. T. Y., Siau, C., & Ang, E. N. K. (2015). Strengthening the afferent limb of rapid response systems: An educational intervention using web-based learning for early recognition and responding to deteriorating patients. *BMJ Quality & Safety, 25*, 1–9. doi:10.1136/bmjqs-2015-004073

Liaw, S. Y., Wong, L. F., Lim, E. Y. P., Ang, S. B. L., Mujumdar, S., Ho, J. T. Y., . . . Ang, E. N. (2016). Effectiveness of a web-based simulation in improving nurses' workplace practice with deteriorating ward patients: A pre- and post-intervention study. *Journal of Medical Internet Research, 18*(2), e37. doi:10.2196/jmir.5294

Mertens, D. M. (2010). *Research and evaluation in education and psychology: Integrating diversity with quantitative, qualitative and mixed methods* (3rd ed.). Los Angeles, CA: Sage.

Polit, D., & Beck, C. (2006). The content validity index: Are you sure you know what's being reported? Critique and recommendations. *Research in Nursing and Health, 29*, 489–497. doi:10.1002/nur.20147

Ricker, K. (2006). Setting cut scores: A critical review of the Angoff and modified Angoff methods. *Alberta Journal of Educational Research, 52*, 53–63. Retrieved from http://hdl.handle.net/10515/sy54746z4

Stone, C. (2016). Opportunity through online learning: Improving student access, participation and success in higher education. National Guidelines. National Centre for Student Equity in Higher Education and the University of Newcastle. Retrieved from https://www.ncsehe.edu.au/wp-content/uploads/2017/03/CathyStone_EQUITY-FELLOWSHIP-FINAL-REPORT-1.pdf

Strand, H., Fox-Young, S., Long, P., & Bogossian, F. (2013). A pilot project in distance education: Nurse practitioner students' experience of personal video capture technology as an assessment method of clinical skills. *Nurse Education Today, 33*, 253–257. doi:10.1016/j.nedt.2011.11.014

Suter, W. N. (2012). *Introduction to educational research: A critical thinking approach.* Los Angeles, CA: Sage.

Thabane, L., Ma, J., Chu, R., Cheng, J., Ismaila, A., Rios, L., . . . Goldsmith, C. (2010). A tutorial on pilot studies: The what, why and how. *Medical Research Methodology, 10*(1), 1–10. doi:10.1186/1471-2288-10-1

Tickle-Degnan, L. (2013). Nuts and bolts of conducting feasibility studies. *American Journal of Occupational Therapy, 67*(2), 171–176. doi:10.5014/ajot.2013.006270

Venkatesh, V., Morris, M., Davis, G., & Davis, F. (2003). User acceptance of information technology: Toward a unified view. *MIS Quarterly, 27*(3), 425–478. Retrieved from http://www.jstor.org/stable/30036540

SECTION III

STUDENT PERSPECTIVE—WORKING WITH STUDENTS TO IMPLEMENT VIRTUAL LEARNING STRATEGIES: MAXIMIZE LEARNING AND SUPPORT TRANSITION TO PRACTICE

The student influence portion of the model results from a diverse population of learners, some of whom are more mobile and technology savvy than previous generations and are not bound by time or place. From a student perspective, it is important to consider the transferable skills that can be gained by using a technology. Technologies must be intentionally selected to maximize learning and skills development. The new generations of students have different learning styles; therefore, integrating interactive technology helps meet the needs of students who are technology-savvy, team players gravitating toward group activities. Learning activities, including multiparticipant virtual learning environments, promote active engagement and offer preferred learning experiences to diverse learners. Students who are familiar with technology and thrive in a technology-rich culture are particularly equipped to be successful in simulation-based learning environments.

Four chapters in this section describe ways to improve communication between students and faculty, foster collaboration among students, and enhance social networking. It is important to maximize skills and support the transfer of knowledge to practice because the student perspective is an integral influence of the Faculty Administrators Students Technology Strategic Integration Model© (FAST SIM; Figure III.1) and may drive technology integration with curriculum, as well as its success or failure.

In Chapter 14, a student shares her personal experience, insights, and thoughts about beginning a virtual simulation. This author offers practical recommendations for other students and shares her journey from novice to comfortable user to expert.

Chapter 15 focuses on exploring the faculty role of mentor in virtual simulation–mediated learning. This author brings in her expertise as a mentor and discusses how she plans and evaluates her virtual environment activities. She provides mentoring goals in virtual simulation, provides tips and pearls for mentors working with students in virtual simulations, and presents two exemplars for guidance.

Chapter 16 describes nursing education and collaborative role playing with appropriate disciplinary professionals. Increasing realism is important for students, and it can be accomplished by enhancing experiential and immersive scenarios using interprofessional role players providing interdisciplinary elements. This authentic learning better prepares nurses for real-world practice. She includes two illustrative exemplars.

Chapter 17, stresses the need for nurse educators to prepare workforce-competent nurses for all settings but focuses on nursing informatics. The relationship between nursing and technology is integral to competent nursing practice; not cultivating this relationship leads to incomplete development of curricula. The author provides a description of an educational process used to develop and deploy a program of simulation to improve skills and knowledge for both students and faculty. Two exemplars are presented to meet faculty and student needs.

The student influence in the FAST SIM© is reflected in this section. Throughout these four chapters, the readers should reflect on how student influence in the model can be applied to the integration of technology in their specific teaching and learning context (Figure III.2).

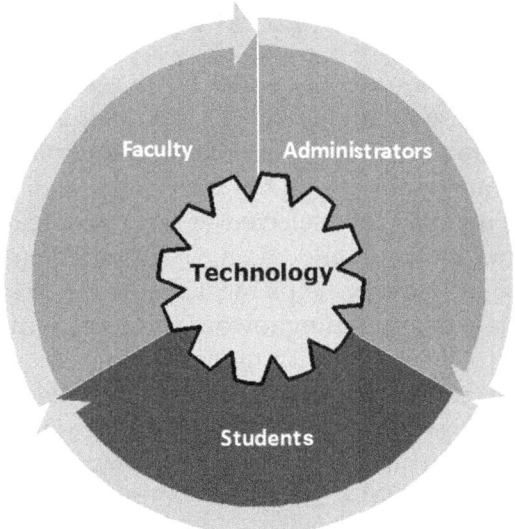

FIGURE III.1 Components of FAST SIM© (Faculty Administrators Students Technology Strategic Integration Model).

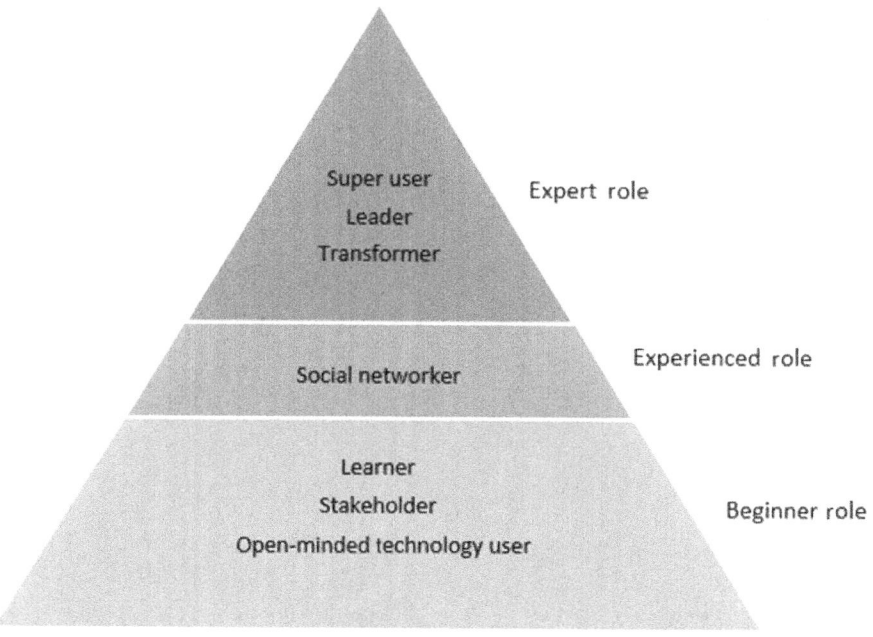

FIGURE III.2 Student roles.

CHAPTER 14

A Student's Journey Encountering a Virtual Learning Environment: A Pathway From Novice to Expert

KAREN WEST

LEARNING OBJECTIVES

Upon completion of this chapter, the reader will be able to:
- Assess different types of student interaction in virtual learning environments.
- Describe technology-supported educational opportunities.
- Explore the student role in the virtual learning environment.
- Appreciate technology as the central cog in the Faculty Administrators Students Technology Strategic Integration Model© (FAST SIM) conceptual model for students in education today.

KEY TERMS

Collaboration
Debrief
Network
Technology knowledge deficit
Three-dimensional (3D)
Virtual learning environment (VLE)

Every story has a beginning, and my story must begin with my decision to embrace the changes that technology brought to my practice as an RN. First, you must understand my lack of technology knowledge. I am a "baby boomer," the age group that did not grow up with technology as a part of childhood. I grudgingly learned what I needed to know about my computer system at work to be able to get my job done. I kept a basic cell phone for so long that it took my cell service provider to refuse to upgrade, because they had obsoleted my phone, to get me to change to a higher-functioning cell phone. My husband and I had a large base computer system (his, not mine), and I occasionally accessed the Internet to look around. I was technology shy through a self-imposed barrier of fear and very frustrated by my lack of knowledge. What I lacked was motivation, a stimulus to get out of my inertia and define my pathway to change. This was a strange place for me to be in because I was strongly involved in my nursing unit because I wanted change to happen there and I was willing to work to get it, but did that work involve me personally changing? Wow, I needed to go back to school. I always wanted to continue my education, so it was time for me to accept that challenge. I chose online learning instead of going back to my alma mater because I still had children at home and online learning was more flexible with my work–life schedule. I had to take on my **technology knowledge deficit** to become effective in that environment, and so my personal education challenge began. I struggled in the online environment, but failure wasn't an option, so I did whatever it took to succeed. I spent hours teaching myself the basics of technology through self-education with internet resources so that I could at least "dog paddle" in my learning environment. I reached out to IT support at the school and sent so many emails to my teachers that they probably groaned when they saw my name. I was a self-driven learner, and I did what it took not only to learn in this environment, but also to tap all the knowledge that I needed.

My encounter with the **virtual learning environment (VLE)** came in my next-to-last course as I worked on a Master of Science Nursing Degree in nursing Informatics (NI). I had accomplished my BSN, became enamored with the idea of NI, and had almost completed that degree. My option to come into the practicum component for NI in the VLE came as an offer to me after I had struggled for three months trying to find a mentor and work through the process of doing a practicum onsite at the facility where I work. Three weeks before the semester was scheduled to begin my mentor was not approved, and the paperwork process was delayed for more important issues at my facility. I was looking at a delay in my educational path and didn't know what to do. I called my practicum coordinator and explained my dilemma. After hearing the final update about my on-the-ground practicum, the coordinator talked to me about a voluntary option to do my NI practicum in the VLE. "Wow, great I would love to do that. Sign me up." I was relieved that there was an option so that I wouldn't have to delay my degree path. Little did I know that this encounter would be a pivotal moment in my career.

RELATION TO THE FAST SIM©

This chapter is related to the student influence. It demonstrates the journey from beginner role of learner and technology user through the ability to gain experience and social **network**, finally describing how learners reach the level of expert roles of transformer, leader, and super user. The student must be willing and motivated to consider the balance of educational opportunities and the transferable skills intended to be gained by using a technology. The student influence extends beyond their own situation and can impact the technologies specifically selected to maximize learning and skills development and may drive technology integration within the curriculum.

ENCOUNTER WITH THE UNKNOWN

Two weeks prior to the start of my practicum semester, my practicum coordinator sent me my learning contract for the VLE, which I signed and sent back to her. That was a little different, but it explained the "rules" of the environment and the fact that I would have a "mentor" in the VLE. Great, there is some help for me, yeah! I have already explained my path for my education, but I did not explain that tackling an unknown made me very anxious and nervous. I was afraid of failing in this environment I didn't know anything about. I believe that this is a leftover issue from the days of "pass or fail" in nursing. You realize, as old as I am, I feel like I could almost have been a classmate of Florence Nightingale. Have you ever heard of "fake it until you make it"? Well, this is how I felt about my knowledge in NI. I didn't want my professors to know that I still struggled with Microsoft Word, Excel, and PowerPoint. I had learned what I needed to know, but still, there was a fight between me and the technology (especially when new upgrades came out), and many times the technology won. This personal anxiety about my issues with technology colored my initial reactions and interactions in the VLE.

PREBRIEFING FOR MY VIRTUAL WORLD LEARNING EXPERIENCE

A week and a half before the beginning of this course I was sent a document that explained how to download Second Life® (SL), select a free avatar, and develop an appropriate name and password for my practicum. I read it through twice before I attempted. I was so nervous that after I selected my avatar I couldn't remember the naming process and was very unsure of how to get into my practicum class. I didn't think about windowing the SL screen and my Word document that explained how to do this, so I closed SL, found the document I needed, and printed it. Paper in hand is so much better for me. I opened SL again and found that I had to go through the initial process a second time. I spent some time looking at the avatars thinking, "Okay, who would I like to be today?" I chose an avatar that looked more conservative because I am more conservative, can be very quiet at times, and unsure of myself. Paper in hand this time I read the details about naming the avatar and finished the process and launched myself into SL. I landed at some place that looked like a beach and there were a lot of avatars there. Avatars kept coming and coming; some were talking to me but I didn't know how to make the avatar talks so I said, "I'm sorry," but they couldn't hear me. Whoops, I forgot to connect headphones to my computer. I logged off that day with a plan to get comfortable accessing SL and to buy some headphones. Before my orientation, I logged onto SL five or six times to get comfortable with the process, look at my avatar (if I could look like that in real life; oh well, I get to pretend for a while). I also have this problem with either being early or late. I could never seem to be somewhere exactly on time, so I developed the habit of being early. This logging-on process was my preparation work for my entry into the VLE for my practicum.

Week I

The first week in my practicum was very busy. On top of my regular class component, I had orientation parts one and two, a meeting with my faculty and SL mentor to discuss my project ideas, and a class meeting in the VLE at 5 p.m. Eastern time on Wednesday. I live in a state in Central time, so I had to figure out my meeting times in Eastern Standard Time and correlate them with my time zone. My first challenge: Internet, here I come. Finding a time zone converter is not difficult to do, so I mapped all those first appointment times in my Central time zone and put them on my cell phone calendar. (Yes, I even learned how to use a higher-level phone.) My VLE mentor was a professor that I had in a previous class (yea, someone I knew), but she might have looked at my name on the roster and thought, "oh no," because you remember that I sent a lot of emails to my professors.

Orientation Part One

Well, I had prepared for this right, so I was able to log in and get to "my beach," as I began to refer to it, and called the conference phone number that was supplied to me for orientation. I was a "little early" and was excited to hear a voice asking me, "Who is on?" I answered, telling her my name, and she asked me to give her my Avatar name. She sent me a floating sign that I saw, but then it disappeared. The woman said, "No problem." and sent it again. and I got it this time. I joined the group, and then another sign appeared, and she told me to click OK, I became a cloud and then appeared in this beautiful place. I was nervous but could concentrate enough to learn how to move my avatar somewhat and how to use voice to talk; with some effort, I got through the first two skill stations with the support specialist. Then I was on my own to finish the orientation trial. I did so with a lot of effort. I went back and forth, reread instructions to each skill station, and kept trying until I completed most of the skills (see Box 14.1). I finally achieved my orientation certificate! I did it, yeah!

BOX 14.1 Exemplar 1—Technology-Challenged Student in a Virtual Learning Environment

ABSTRACT

Virtual learning is a growing concept in education in general and healthcare education specifically. The nursing workforce has had many new challenges over the last 10 years as they watched their profession grow and change. Technology has had a role in evolving nursing practice. Nurses who are not ready to retire have to decide how to continue in their practice: continue with the status quo or identify their own personal knowledge deficits and make themselves functional in the new world of technology in healthcare. Answer the call of the American Nursing Association for higher education and become a member of progress in healthcare. This story is about one of those nurses who decided to answer the call and her personal challenges in acclimating herself into a virtual learning environment (VLE).

INTRODUCTION

The VLE is a new experience for many students. Along with traversing the unknown, anxiety, and the need to be punctual for meetings are driving forces for a new student. This seems like the "great divide" initially in this foreign environment. If the student has never played a game with an avatar, just being able to walk and talk are a challenge. Students' comfort zones and basic computer knowledge are a plus, but relating them to the software programming was an initial challenge, especially if they are afraid of breaking something. Moderate anxiety can be a stimulus to support learning, but high anxiety can interfere with understanding and learning.

(continued)

> **BOX 14.1 Exemplar 1—Technology-Challenged Student in a Virtual Learning Environment** (*continued*)
>
> Introduction into the VLE is done through an orientation process. I was one of three students being oriented on that day at that time. I had practiced entering Second Life 5 or 6 times, always worried that when my appointment time came, something would interfere with my getting in. I was the kind of person who was early or late, and couldn't seem to be somewhere exactly on time, so my habit was to be early. That left me, pacing, in front of my computer, phone in hand, in Second Life being run over by a lot of other avatars; some would speak to me, but I didn't know how to talk, so I would answer them to myself, "I'm sorry." The call to the support specialist I was meeting worked great, and she was so nice; she sent me some floating signs which I clicked on, and then I became a cloud and floated down in front of her. Wow," this place was so "cool! I was inside my Barbie's dollhouse that I had as a child. With practice, I got my avatar down to where the support specialist was, and we continued talking on the phone for a few minutes. When we all learned how to use our voice, we stopped the phone call. We reviewed walking again, and I figured out I was a "multiple clicker" when my avatar wanted to "run" away. The instructor was teaching me, but I was so nervous, I didn't remember most of what she said.
>
> "It is OK. I will come back and practice and figure out what I need to know," is what I told myself because I didn't want to look like an unexperienced person with this media even though I was. We went to the first orientation station. I clicked on the kiosk and accepted the sitting-in-a-chair tutorial. Of course, I didn't know where it went after I accepted it, it just disappeared. Well, I won't tell her that. With the support specialist's help and patience, I learned how to sit in a chair and get up. The next task was flying. I found out that I probably should have been born with wings if I was intended to fly. I kept on triple clicking and would wind up in the trees or high in the sky. After 5 tries, the support specialist walked me through this, making me do one click at a time, and I finally did it: no wings and I can fly at least once because after I get her on the ground, I probably won't do this again. What happens if I get too high? What if I can't get back down? Well, it is OK walking, so I will just have to fly when I learn how to do it well. It took me 5 hours to do the orientation trial, and the major hang-up point was that I was teleporting up to some place but couldn't figure out how to get down, so I exited Second Life and came back in at my home, which we had set at the beginning of my orientation. I bypassed the teleport station. I wasn't going to do that again. I finally finished my orientation, collected my certificate, and emailed it to the right person. Hoorah! I had done it, not well, but I had done it. Now for the second part of orientation.
>
> ## CHALLENGES
>
> 1. My lack of expertise in this environment made me very anxious.
>
> (*continued*)

BOX 14.1 Exemplar 1—Technology-Challenged Student in a Virtual Learning Environment (*continued*)

2. My self-esteem was shaky, and I was concerned about letting anyone know about my discomfort. What will they think of me as an online student who is having issues interacting in this environment?

STAKEHOLDER PERSPECTIVE

Student

1. As a student in this environment, it was important to learn what I needed to learn to effectively complete course outcomes.
2. Students need to be able to identify their technology knowledge deficit, learn about their resources, and effectively use them to correct their deficit.
3. Limiting myself to only what I needed to know decreased the full opportunity offered by this type of learning environment.

Resolutions

1. Satisfactions:
   a. Every new thing related to this technology that I learned increased my comfort and decreased my technology knowledge deficit.
   b. I felt that my role transition into a nurse informaticist could be a reality.
2. Frustrations:
   a. I had the wrong kind of headset, and it didn't always work "in world."
   b. During my first meeting with my mentor, I was given a teleporting address, and I had issues with doing this in orientation. My first class meeting, I was guided by my mentor using "in world" open chat and phone conference line. I had gotten lost and was late to my first class meeting.

SUMMARY

Many times, students limit their own knowledge by not reaching out for support or using their resources. These issues can lead to a less-than-optimal experience for the student and decrease actual learning knowledge in relation to the VLE. Hesitation by the student because of anxiety or "self-esteem" issues can be large stumbling blocks in this type of learning environment. "Having little experience in using the virtual classroom, students lacked knowledge to use it to its full potential" (Gedera, 2014, p. 100). Students must be able to identify their own technology knowledge deficit related to their learning environment and try to correct their deficit. Students must learn to ask questions, be able to say, "I don't know how to do this" or "I don't understand," identify their resources, and then use them.

(*continued*)

BOX 14.1 Exemplar 1—Technology-Challenged Student in a Virtual Learning Environment (*continued*)

LESSONS LEARNED

1. What worked?
   a. My computer and Internet access were up to date enough for me to access the VLE and interact effectively.
   b. I read my instructions for coming into the VLE more than once and was initially familiar with the process and my role.
   c. I could complete the initial orientation process even if I worked around teleporting.
   d. I read my class instructions for the VLE, called on the conference number, and had my mentor lead me to the meeting site when I couldn't find it.
   e. I remembered how to sit in a chair once I got to the auditorium and sat in the back row.
   f. I kept my sense of humor! I was able to laugh at myself even though I was stressed out.

2. What did not work?
   a. My cell phone had a quick time-out on my screen, and I had to try to dial the conference number several times before I could get through.
   b. My voice "in world" didn't work the third time in (I had my phone).
   c. I had problems with getting my avatar to walk the way I wanted her to because I kept triple clicking.

3. What would you do the same in the future?
   a. I would jump at the opportunity to come back into the VLE.
   b. I would continue my practice of reading all directions and associated information with my courses.
   c. I would have continued to use my mentor for support because she was an excellent resource.
   d. I practiced a lot with my avatar and interacted with things "in world." This was important for decreasing my knowledge deficit in this environment.

4. What would you do differently in the future?
   a. I would have researched VLE more.
   b. I would have asked more questions about my avatar and ways to use the programming for my course; I would have written down a way to interact with support specialists (e.g., email, phone).

(*continued*)

> **BOX 14.1 Exemplar 1—Technology-Challenged Student in a Virtual Learning Environment** (*continued*)
>
> 5. What will you take away from this experience?
>   a. Increase in my comfort zone in a VLE.
>   b. Knowledge of how some programs work with an avatar as a tool.
>   c. Increase in my self-esteem related to this type of technology (I can do this).
> 6. What advice would you offer to others in the same situation?
>   a. Read all information given to you about the VLE.
>   b. Write down your questions as you read this information and reach out to get your questions answered.
>   c. Research and read about VLEs.
>   d. Find out your personal resources (support specialist, orientation experts, and mentors) and use them.
>   e. Don't be afraid to look unknowledgeable or to ask questions (this is a learning environment).

First Meeting in the VLE With My Mentor and Other Virtual World Practicum Students

I arrived in my practicum world early this time and wandered around. Our meeting was in a specific place, so I was looking. I found the building but noticed it had several floors, so I was confused. I reached out to my mentor via email (hoping that would work) and told her I was in SL but lost and didn't know where to go. I got a quick response from her via email and she gave me a phone number. I connected to her via phone, and with some effort, she guided me to the meeting place. I was a little late, and a lot of other avatars were there already. I sat in the top row chairs excited to be able to sit my avatar down. I was so glad to be there! My voice was working, and I had made it to class.

Orientation Part 2

My second orientation required my avatar to ride a bicycle. Now that was interesting, and I fell off the bridge and landed in "no man's land." My orientation guide rescued me, and the bicycle and then put me back on it. This time I didn't get lost. This orientation was more comfortable for me, even with me getting lost again. I could focus because I had gotten through my first orientation and my anxiety was not as high. The "world" I was seeing was so cool that I had to keep refocusing on the guide. Believe it or not, I learned how to teleport and landmark areas in this world so that I could take my avatar back to them. I am a student in a VLE.

Challenge and Advantages of Using an Avatar

Manipulating an avatar initially was a challenge. Trying to get her to walk and talk. Working with the skills that I had been shown to develop some level of comfort and mastery. So, my plan of attack for this became spending a lot of time in the VLE.

- Practice, practice, practice!
- I came in that first weekend and spent hours walking around and trying to fly. After that weekend, I logged in every day. I learned how to change the avatar's clothes. I became braver and started looking at submenus and trying them out. I explored all four of the towns that I was told were a part of our practicum.
- I loved the beautiful avatar. She boosted my confidence because what people were seeing was her, not me. The uniqueness of this environment allows a person to change their avatar, but I found myself dressing my avatar as I would myself. So, if they saw my avatar, they still could see me in her. The avatar became my identity in the environment.
- I became comfortable with technology glitches. Technology can be impacted by many things: weather, Internet service providers, traveling, and programming issues. Several times I got logged off in SL, and I thought "uh oh, I did something wrong." My advice is, try and try again.

Find and Connect With Your Support

My support strength in this environment was my mentor. What I had neglected to do was to figure out how to contact support specialists who had oriented me because they would have been a great resource. I realized that I had access to my mentor and had multiple conversations about SL, as well as my practicum. I burned up her emails. She worked me through the first time I lost voice, recommended a better headset, explained technology glitches, log offs, losing voice, and so on. She gave me the knowledge I needed to build my comfort zone in this environment because I made a point to ask. I was here, I liked it, and I was determined to succeed.

Week 2

At the end of Week 2, I had learned a lot about my avatar skills and ways to maneuver. I still didn't understand the role that this "cool place" played in my practicum. Should I be doing something I wasn't doing? So, I had a repeat conversation with my mentor: What am I doing here? What should I be doing that I am not? I am spending time "in world" but surely walking around is not what I am supposed to be doing here. With great patience, my mentor explained the role of practicum experience here in this virtual world. I became aware that this wasn't the first time that I had heard this but I was so focused on my avatar and getting comfortable with the software that I did not understand my role here. This practicum had different specialty track educational offerings, the opportunity to collaborate with current peers in our track, and two other tracks, nurse executive and nurse educator. I could approach other mentors or students about my project and use them as a sounding board. I could become involved in another track's activities, which were developed for collaboration. Wow, the light went on! I found my comfort zone with my avatar and set about enhancing my learning experience.

Weeks 3, 4, 5, and 6

Week 3

I reached out to another NI student, and we met in the virtual world and discussed our projects. It was wonderful. Through verbalizing my project and showing her pictures, I realized I was bringing to life an idea of mine. The other student gave me positive support, and I did that for her as well. We both offered feedback on our respective projects.

After that, I made sure other NI students knew I was open if they wanted to meet.

Week 4

I went out and met some of the nurse educator students and the nurse executive track students. I just introduced myself and found out about them. I went and watched an educator track a scenario and was included by the mentor in the **debrief**.

Week 5

I became a volunteer for an executive nursing track scenario, developed a presentation for this, and gave it, pretending I was a CNIO. I met with an educator student about the education component that would accompany my project and got ideas.

Week 6

I took my project charter and scope to the executive track students as a group and presented it as I would in the "real world," answered their questions, and got approval with minimal proposed change.

Week 7

Now, I had to present my project to my group and participate in the debrief. During the debriefing for this first session of my practicum experience, I was asked for feedback on the experience, and they really wanted honest answers. It was during week 7 of my practicum experience that I was notified that my onsite practicum had finally been approved. I didn't want to go. I had learned how to effectively use this environment to meet my educational needs for my practicum, and I wanted to stay. I had gone from fear of the unknown to functional in this environment to being in love with this educational space and opportunity to learn among my peers.

This was an important decision that I needed to make about staying to complete my second practicum experience in the VLE or stepping out into the real world for practical experience as a nursing informaticist. I once again, my mentor and I had a conversation about what would be best for me. My mentor advocated for the onsite practicum because of the live experience of taking my project into the real world and being able to function in a NI working group—real world experience and what that would mean to me when I graduated. My mentor had been my lifeline initially in this environment and my rock until I learned how to walk. I saw the wisdom in her advice, but I was heartbroken about leaving the VLE.

BECOMING EFFECTIVE IN A VLE

Weaknesses

I let my anxiety and fear of this environment make it harder for me to be oriented.

1. I didn't show my lack of knowledge of my computer system and this software to the support specialist because I was afraid of looking inadequate as a student in the NI track.
2. I didn't ask the questions I needed to ask but struggled through on my own during orientation (missed some learning opportunities there).
3. I self-taught, as best I could, the submenu's in this software, and if I had reached out to a support specialist, I could have learned much more.

Strengths

1. I didn't give up. I was determined to succeed.
2. I did reach out to my mentor and used her as support for the VLE and my course.
3. I read all my material for the VLE (more than once) prior to coming in for orientation.
4. I researched virtual education and read some background prior to orientation.
5. I kept asking questions until I understood my role and the virtual education site component in my course.
6. I embraced the VLE, fully involving myself in the student role once I understood what that was.
7. I sought out learning opportunities and developed some to fit my practicum experience.

KEY POINTS

- Students need support when beginning a virtual simulation.
- Students should be provided with an alternate means to contact you outside of the virtual simulation.
- Students must know how to access support.
- Students should have plenty of time to practice and become comfortable in the virtual simulation environment.

SUMMARY

To document my path to learning in this VLE, I have chosen to share full insight to my thoughts, doubts, fears, and anxieties as a student in a new educational encounter. I have found that, personally, I can be my own worst enemy if strong fears are not addressed, and I have chosen to identify those fears and decrease them through a personal educational plan of action. Doing something, researching, reading, looking at different examples, and so on helped me focus on learning and decreased the strength of fear, self-doubt, and anxiety it causes as barriers to my learning (refer to Boxes 14.1 and 14.2). I hope my sharing has entertained you and helped

BOX 14.2 Exemplar 2—Tele-Sitter Project

ABSTRACT

In healthcare, there is a real issue of nursing shortage as baby boomers retire. This will impact healthcare not only by reducing the number of nurses, but also by creating a decreased level of expertise because new graduates need time to take learned skill and make it into working knowledge. This decrease in actual numbers is also accompanied by larger numbers of higher-acuity patients and increased safety issues as nurse-to-patient ratios increase (Lampert, 2016). Technology can assist on some levels with this significant safety issue.

INTRODUCTION

Tele-Sitter project is designed to increase safety for patients at risk because of decreased ability to communicate needs, confusion related to health processes or illness, unstable health status, or potential for self-harm. This project can offer an additional level of assessment (visual) to follow up on bed alarms and patient call lights and a brief assessment for a monitored change in vital signs. A call or page can be sent to relay information to the patient care nurse to go to the bedside with a request to check on the patient. (Tele-Sitter Project developed by Krystal Cunningham MSN RN student in a virtual world practicum, reproduced with permission of author.)

CHALLENGES

Developing a project idea can, at times, be very costly, and for a student, it can be prohibitive based on their project decision. As a result, in normal educational formats, the student is restricted to putting the idea on paper only.

STAKEHOLDER PERSPECTIVES

1. Administrative: Financial and other resources must be looked at from a full college perspective, and most institutions do not budget to help students develop graduate projects.
2. Faculty: Faculty want students to expand their thought processes and enhance their learning by thinking about and being able to bring multiple areas of expertise into their learning experience. Faculty directly impact student academic performance through their leadership and clear expectations (Tinto, 2012).
3. Students: At times, students have problems deciding on projects, depending on how restrictive their educational environment is. The financial impact of true project development can be prohibitive to students' ability to realize their full potential to bring innovative ideas

(continued)

> **BOX 14.2 Exemplar 2—Tele-Sitter Project (*continued*)**
>
> into the educational arena, which restricts progress in their field of study. A student's learning is greatly impacted by individual drive and educational goals (Tinto, 2012).
>
> ## RESOLUTIONS
>
> 1. This student worked with the virtual development specialist to script two different scenarios: (a) a patient getting out of bed and using the tele-sitter to talk with, and to visualize, the patient in his or her room while placing a call to the nurse or technician to respond to the patient room and (b) a patient's vital sign alarm and instant code white call for serious issue follow-up.
> 2. In a virtual environment, this could be set up in a three-dimensional (3D) format by placing an avatar in a hospital room environment to add authenticity, placing the program in an accessible location for students, and allowing other students to interact with the program and give feedback. This project was also role-played by students in the virtual learning environment (VLE) and debriefed for feedback. This student developed a survey on Survey Monkey to get feedback from multiple groups of students in the VLE.
>
> ## FRUSTRATIONS
>
> 1. This is a limited pilot because of the small number of students with access.
> 2. This pilot could not be done by students in real-life patient care situations.
>
> ## SUMMARY
>
> This student used all of her resources in a VLE, took her project idea, and developed it into a model for piloting in the VLE. Resources can be effective for learning impact only if they are used. This student's mentor in this environment helped connect her to the appropriate people to discuss her project and become working partners in its development. The VLE can become the doorway for student learning in strongly expanded ways but only if higher educational environments realize the potential. VLEs open access to these resources to students. Student learning can be impacted by bringing their imagination and applying themselves to their knowledge expansion. Therefore, learning can be limited only by the student's innovative imagination.
>
> ## LESSONS LEARNED
>
> 1. What worked? The pilot was successful from the perspective of the student being able to put her idea into a learning scenario. Students and mentors interacted with the program and gave the student feedback.

(continued)

> **BOX 14.2 Exemplar 2—Tele-Sitter Project (*continued*)**
>
> 2. What did not work? Some students did not click on the button to end the scenario, which created a situation in which other students had problems interacting. Also, it is a possibility that all the students to whom the pilot was open did not choose to try the program or give feedback through the survey.
> 3. What would you do the same in the future? Work with experts in this area to develop this type of pilot or another type. Visual stimuli plus active interaction promotes learning and understanding. Also, this process allows a more effective view of the project for evaluation.
> 4. What would you do differently in the future? Video development of the scenarios could be done so they could be used to present potential projects in the real world.
> 5. What advice would you offer others in the same situation? Find out what your resources are and how your project can be developed in a VLE.

you identify some of your own barriers to learning as you expand your knowledge through technology. If a "baby boomer" can do it, then you can do it. Take each encounter with technology, for education or otherwise, as a personal and professional challenge, knowing that you will succeed if you choose to do so.

Recommendations for Other Students

- Recognize and identify that you have a personal knowledge deficit related to this educational component.
- Write down what you do not know and work to eliminate that deficit (research, use the Internet, ask to speak with previous students who accomplished their course requirement, find out who your support specialists are and how to contact them with questions, and use your course mentor in this environment (their knowledge is large).
- Do not be afraid to ask for help. You are a student thus not expected to be a technology whiz.
- Do not wait until the last minute to prepare for your VLE course. Start early, plan, and read all the material given to you (more than once).
- Find out what technology you need to use for the course basics and plan to get those resources if you do not already have them. For example, if you need a higher-level laptop, find a center that can rent you one on a weekly basis.
- Learn software programs that you need to use to support your learning. Microsoft has education on all their products and YouTube has videos on many programs and other things that can support your learning; be your own best resource.

- Find out how you can do project development in your VLE and don't be afraid to think outside the box (pilot development, two-dimensional (2D) model, **three-dimensional (3D)** model, scenario, simulation, survey development). Give the project to your peers and the video development.
- Network and use your peer groups for collaboration. Seek out your peers for feedback and support; offer them the same.
- Do not be afraid to step or push yourself out of your comfort zone because if you are doing the pushing, you are ready to learn.

REFLECTIVE QUESTIONS

1. What is the computer technology required for your program of study or course? Do you feel these requirements are reasonable? Provide a detailed rationale for your answer. Discuss the ramifications for not meeting these technology requirements.
2. As you are introduced to the VLE, describe the course expectations and outcomes you feel could be met using this learning modality.
3. Assess what you can do as a student to maximize your learning opportunity in the VLE? Describe your role and that of your faculty member and/or mentor.
4. How can your project be made into a more visual or interactive project with the right resources? Elaborate on the resources necessary and describe how each one would be used.
5. Would being able to pilot and get feedback on your project help you decide to push your project into your work environment or craft it for publication? Describe in detail how you would begin the process of translating your project to your practice setting, as well as how you would craft it for publication.
6. As you consider your projects in higher education, describe in detail the resources that have been available to you. If you used a VLE, describe its impact on your learning; if not, describe the impact the VLE could have made.

REFERENCES

Gedera, D. (2014). Students' experiences of learning in a virtual classroom. *International Journal of Education and Development Using Information and Communication Technology, 10*(4), 93–100. Retrieved from https://files.eric.ed.gov/fulltext/EJ1059024.pdf

Lampert, L. (2016). Nurses storm the U.S. Capitol to demand safe staffing ratios. Retrieved from http://dailynurse.com/nurses-storm-u-s-capitol-demand-safe-staffing-ratios

Tinto, V. (2012). Enhancing student success: Taking the classroom success seriously. *International Journal of the First Year in Higher Education, 3*(1), 1–8. doi:10.5204/intjfyhe.v3i1.119

CHAPTER 15

Mentor Role in Virtual Simulation–Mediated Learning

REBECCA J. SISK

LEARNING OBJECTIVES

Upon completion of this chapter, the reader will be able to:
- Appreciate the role of the mentor in virtual learning.
- Apply the Faculty Administrators Students Technology Strategic Integration Model© (FAST SIM) to a three-dimensional (3D) virtual learning environment (VLE) practicum for graduate students in nursing education.
- Apply the NLN Jeffries Simulation Theory and a cultural diversity model to simulations in the 3D VLE.
- Analyze the role of authentic assignments in students' development of professional nursing roles and competencies.

KEY TERMS

Authentic	Plus-Delta debriefing
Authentic assignments	Presence
Cultural diversity	Scaffolding
Ecology of Culturally Competent Design model	Scripted simulation
	Second Life® Islands
Experiential learning	Simulation to Practice model
Fealty	Storyboard
Mentoring	Unscripted simulation
Mentees	Virtual simulation–mediated learning
NLN Jeffries Simulation Theory	Virtual world field trips (VWFTs)

NURSING EDUCATION PRACTICUM IN SECOND LIFE

Practicum experiences and capstone projects are commonly used at the end of graduate programs in nursing but could be applied in other professions. Students enrolled in online programs must sometimes find their own practicum sites and mentors where they reside. Sometimes this is a challenge because either the student lives in an area with few graduate nursing role models, or existing potential role models may be overburdened with other practicum students. Finding mentorships or preceptorships is likewise a challenge in teacher education and other fields (Hartley, Ludlow, & Duff, 2015).

The Faculty Administrators Students Technology Strategic Integration Model© (FAST SIM) provides an overall framework for faculty mentoring, administrative planning, and students' learning activities within a technology such as Second Life® (SL). The application of the FAST SIM© model to teaching and learning in a mentored virtual world practicum (VWP) is discussed in this chapter. The mentor's use of **authentic** assignments to help students meet professional role competencies and the application of social constructivist theory and other models related to simulation in three-dimensional (3D) virtual learning environment (VLEs) are covered. Two exemplars, "Peter the Service Dog" simulation and "Philippe the New Nurse" simulation, are described.

RELATION TO THE FAST SIM©

In the FAST SIM© model, faculty, administrators, and students together integrate technologies into the curriculum. Technologies are the tools faculty, administrators, and students use as designers and recipients of the curriculum. For example, in an SL graduate nursing practicum, faculty members can play the role of mentors, administrators typically provide the resources, and students participate and contribute to their own learning.

Technology

SL, a virtual world used by many educators, has been defined "as a computer-mediated, persistent and synchronous spatially based world that is inhabited by people represented through avatars and is highly interactive" (Fitzsimons & Farren, 2016, p. 11). 3D VLEs, such as SL, offer a platform for designing VWP for students. Faculty have used 3D VLEs for undergraduate nursing programs, but 3D VLEs can also be used for graduate nursing courses. For example, SL can be used for nurse executive, nurse educator, nursing informatics, nurse practitioner, and other MSN nursing programs with some planning. Conducting practicums in SL requires designers and programmers to develop SL parcels of land, also known as *Second Life® Islands*, designed with various purposes in mind and equipped with realistic buildings and furnishings. College buildings, hospitals, shopping centers, and clinics, as well as entire towns and various historical displays, can be built.

FACULTY AS MENTORS OF GRADUATE STUDENTS IN THE 3D VLE

Working in SL with nursing students involves developing mentoring skills. **Mentoring** can be described as "a broad caring role that encompasses formal or informal supporting, guiding, coaching, teaching, role modeling, counseling, advocating, networking, and sharing. Mentoring occurs within and/or outside the clinical setting and includes personal and career guidance" (American Nurses Association Massachusetts, n.d., para. 1). This definition implies that mentors in VWPs guide students in meeting their future nursing specialty competencies by (a) either constructing or working with designers to construct a virtual environment, (b) determining expected learning outcomes for students, (c) helping students select individual goals for their virtual experiences, (d) designing learning activities, (e) encouraging students to complete their goals, (f) role modeling professional practice, (g) providing feedback, and (h) collaborating with students.

Scarce information is available in the literature about mentoring students in SL. Gregg et al. (2016) studied mentoring for 188 disabled community college students over a five-year period and found that mentoring students in a virtual world motivated students to learn. Furthermore, Silva, Correia, and Pardo-Ballester (2010) described their mutual experiences as mentor–mentees, concluding that mentors helped **mentees** establish goals, taught them skills needed in SL, promoted a sense of community, designed activities, and collaborated with each other.

Mentors design opportunities for students to communicate and collaborate with one another and explore and interact within the virtual world. They teach how to build posters, models, and other artifacts, as well as participate in simulations. The faculty mentor uses **scaffolding** for the learning activities, guides students through these activities, and provides suggestions and feedback on student performance (Campbell & Cameron, 2016). In addition, mentoring facilitates the entry of graduates into a profession, socializes mentees to the values and beliefs of the profession, and teaches students collaboration and networking skills (Fountain & Newcomer, 2016). These mentoring goals are outlined in Table 15.1.

Role of Administrators and Staff

Administrators reflect the basic philosophy and goals of a college or university. An administration that supports the university's vision and mission by adopting instructional innovation facilitates the incorporation of technologies such as SL (Storey & Wolf, 2010). The decision to incorporate SL into the curriculum takes resources and careful planning (Box 15.1).

Although using open, public spaces in SL is possible, and perhaps necessary for an instructor who does not have funding, fee-based private islands are preferable for protecting students and faculty from avatar intruders. Where funding is available through the budget or through grants, administrators provide money to purchase parcels of virtual land, to purchase buildings and furnishings, and to hire staff. The staff either buys buildings and furnishings from various SL vendors or they design and build what is needed, according to their skill level.

In an early paper, Bhati, Mercer, Rankin, and Thomas (2009) described common administrative concerns when a university adopts teaching strategies in SL: The time required for training faculty, time taken out of course work to train students,

---

TABLE 15.1 Mentoring Goals in Virtual Simulation

- Develop learning objectives.
- Align activities with learning objectives and outcomes.
- Design opportunities for students to communicate and collaborate with one another.
- Encourage students to become fully immersed and engaged in the virtual environment.
- Guide and mentor students as they progress through learning activities.
- Provide feedback and evaluate performance.
- Socialize students to the values and beliefs of the profession.
- Teach students collaboration and networking skills.

the cost of using private islands in SL, and the cost of staff support for students and faculty—all must be considered. Multiple issues were described in a study by Coban, Karakus, Karaman, Gunay, and Goktas (2015), comparing challenges with using SL and OpenSim. These include technical issues related to computer equipment, the time required for developing the virtual world, inappropriately dressed and configured avatars, and the complexity required to design objects.

Roles of Students

Participants enter SL with avatars that they can select. The notion of operating in a body feels realistic, and learning and feeling are evoked by operating in virtual space (Fedeli, 2016). In fact, there is evidence that, while in a virtual world, students feel indistinguishable from their avatars (Pasfield-Neofitou, Huang, & Grant, 2015).

3D VLEs facilitate students' interaction within the virtual world to learn and create through communication and collaboration. Students are immersed in the virtual world as a community of scholars learning the roles and competencies of their chosen profession. 3D VLEs are thought to be more effective than traditional 2.0 web applications because participants are in a community with other participants in a virtual space and can use gestures and voice or chat to enhance communication (Minocha & Hardy, 2016). Pretending to be educators at a virtual college of nursing, we have assigned students to develop case studies, serve on a student affairs committee, complete item analyses, write **scripted simulations**, make presentations, evaluate their presentations, and network with colleagues. These are **authentic assignments**, designed to help students meet practicum course outcomes and competencies that lead to professional roles.

Led by mentors and building on prior knowledge, students experience the role of student, as well as the professional role they aspire to fulfill. Students learn as they are immersed in the virtual world and collaborate with one another, exemplifying the social constructivist theory (Storey & Wolf, 2010). In agreement with this learning theory, students work on individual and group projects in a virtual location, communicating and collaborating, exploring the environment, building posters and other learning objects/artifacts, and participating in simulations and role play. The sense of **presence** and the sense of being part of the virtual environment while learning contributes to students meeting learning outcomes (Fitzsimons & Farrin, 2016). Students are aware not only of the behavior and movement of their own avatars, but also of other avatars as they exist for the moment in a 3D VLE (Olasina, 2016).

Generally, students participate in four categories of mentor-led learning activities in SL, including communication and collaboration, building of objects, exploration, and simulation. *Communicating and collaborating* involves activities such as meetings, lectures, and mock interviews. Examples of *building* projects include structures, anatomical models, chemical equations, scientific displays, museum exhibits, and research posters. Once these projects are built, students can *explore* them, observe them, and write about them. For example, **virtual world field trips (VWFTs)** can take students to virtual displays of places they would never be able to go to in the real world (Fitzsimons & Farren, 2011). Finally, students can participate in virtual *role play and simulations*.

> **BOX 15.1 Tips and Pearls for Faculty as Mentors When Working in Second Life**
>
> - Exploring virtual houses, businesses, apartment buildings, clinics, universities, and hospitals can be fun, depending on the creativity of the designer. A tour of the environment can stimulate ideas on learning activities that relate to your students!
> - Some simulations are scripted; a situation or dilemma is dramatized through the use of a **storyboard**. Students act out the storyboard and then discuss the implications of the story and possible solutions to the problem while acknowledging how the story affected them emotionally and professionally.
> - Students must make a lot of decisions in an **unscripted simulation**. Similar to problem-based learning (PBL), they are given basic information about their task and need to figure out what they would do if they are the professionals solving the problem at hand. They clarify the issues, read about the topic, and derive solutions or products that meet the goals of the simulation.
> - Faculty mentors can provide VWP experiences without purchasing private islands and restricting access. However, finding public virtual environments that fit the experiences students need may be difficult, and the possibility of intruders makes private spaces more desirable.
> - An Internet search yields several opportunities to seek grant funding for VWPs.
> - SL offers mentors and students the opportunity to express attitudes and feelings using "gestures" and avatar behavior and conversation. Resulting simulations lead to lively debriefing sessions!
>
> Refer to Boxes 15.2 and 15.3.

KEY POINTS

- Mentoring can be formal or informal, occurring within and/or outside the clinical setting and includes personal and career guidance.
- Mentors design opportunities for students to communicate and collaborate with one another and explore and interact within the virtual world.
- Students should both develop and participate in VWP scenarios.

SUMMARY

This chapter focuses on exploring the faculty role of mentors in virtual simulation–mediated learning. Considering the importance of faculty, administrators, and students using a specific technology to enhance the curriculum, mentors working with students in a D VLE represent the faculty component of the FAST SIM$^{©}$.

> **BOX 15.2 Exemplar 1—*Peter and the Service Dog:* The Importance of Authentic Assignments**
>
> ### ABSTRACT
>
> *Peter and the Service Dog* is the title of a simulation produced by students in a graduate-level nursing education MSN course. The production of this simulation is an example of an unscripted simulation. Students were provided a goal, examples, and instructions on how they, as faculty members in a school of nursing or as nursing professional development specialists, would approach the problem of introducing service dogs to the healthcare system in a virtual world. However, the production simulation itself is an example of a scripted simulation because students use a storyboard consisting of the setting, the characters, the action, and the narrative, similar to, but simpler than, a script for a movie.
>
> ### INTRODUCTION
>
> Consistent with the Faculty Administrators Students Technology Strategic Integration Model© (FAST SIM), the graduate practicums in SL were developed for MSN students by the administration for students who, for a variety of reasons, cannot use a brick-and-mortar university or hospital for their practicum experience. Selected faculty members volunteered to serve as mentors. Thus, administration, students, and faculty collaborated for a successful experience in the SL platform.
>
> The nursing education graduate students go through an eight-week, 120-hour practicum focusing on their future faculty roles, including authentic assignments such as developing, delivering, and evaluating lectures; conducting and participating in small group discussions; conducting item analyses of an examination; making presentations; and designing simulations. Although students develop simulations in the practicum, the practicum itself is a simulation of what it is like to serve as a faculty member or nursing professional development specialist.
>
>> *[Tip/Pearl: The **NLN Jeffries Simulation Theory**, which provides a framework for designing simulation experiences that ensure that learning outcomes are met, is introduced to the student in the orientation and is followed in each practicum activity* (Jeffries, 2015). *An important concept in the NLN Jeffries Simulation Theory is "**fealty**," which represents the realism of the features of a simulation. In SL, the realism comes from being present and immersed in a community of scholars within a virtual world. Thus, using authentic assignments helps students successfully adopt the professional roles and competencies they hope to achieve.]*
>
> Virtual worlds are useful for authentic or **experiential learning** because students can develop the competencies they need as professionals (Farley, 2016; Fitzsimmons & Farren, 2016). Architecture students can build buildings,

(continued)

> **BOX 15.2 Exemplar 1—*Peter and the Service Dog*: The Importance of Authentic Assignments (*continued*)**
>
> art-appreciation students can view the classics, and law students can participate in a trial. Assessment using authentic assignments is a teaching method that "proposes providing real-world situations, using critical thinking to solve problems with multiple solutions, and transparency to learners about the competencies on which they are assessed" (Mattison, Schroeder, Sculthorp, & Zacharias, 2017, p. 189). Authentic assignments are thus designed to help students adopt the competencies and skills necessary in a profession.
>
> ## CHALLENGES AND RESOLUTIONS
>
> As an example of an authentic assignment, three nursing education students going through a practicum in SL were asked to design a scripted simulation related to a child entering the hospital as a patient with his service dog, Napa. The simulation they were developing is called "scripted" because the student wrote a brief story about what Peter, his mother, his dog, and the nursing staff experienced and wrote a story demonstrating the action with photographs taken within SL. They also wrote a script that provided the dialogue that they would incorporate into the simulation.
>
> We gave students instructions on scripted scenarios, as well as several examples. They were also instructed to apply the information provided in an article about service dogs by Krawczyk (2017). This article covers the definition of *service dog*, laws covering service dogs in the American Disabilities Act (ADA), access to healthcare for people with service dogs, and policies for caring for patients with service dogs. Students developed a story about what happened to Peter, his mother, and Napa during Peter's admission to the hospital, as well as what happened to the staff as they tried to implement care. Once students developed Peter's story, they were ready to make their storyboard.
>
> Storyboards consist of a series of images of the avatars in the 3D VLE hospital, showing where the action would take place, where character avatars should be placed in each scene, and what they should say. Learning how to take photographs in SL was part of the orientation to SL skills, but SL staff members helped with this and other technical tasks.
>
> Students, two in the Midwest and one on the East Coast, met one another periodically, either by phone or in SL. They also had access to WebEx for meetings. As they met, one assumed leadership. They completed their simulation and held a rehearsal that was videotaped by the VLE staff. Students rehearsed their simulation by playing out their story through their avatars, with the help of one faculty member and one staff member, and by following their storyboard. Subsequently, they tweaked their simulation based on feedback, and scheduled a final taping.

(continued)

> **BOX 15.2 Exemplar 1—*Peter and the Service Dog:* The Importance of Authentic Assignments (*continued*)**
>
> ### SUMMARY AND LESSONS LEARNED
>
> After the final taping, they debriefed, applying the **Plus-Delta debriefing** method. Using Plus-Delta, the facilitator/mentor asks just a few questions: "What went well?" and "What needs improvement" (Sawyer, Eppich, Brett-Fleegler, Grant, & Cheng, 2016, p. 214). The debriefing indicated a need for more specific simulation objectives, as well as some specific content. For example, one note was that the simulation did not point out that the family was responsible for meeting the service dog's needs. Faculty members and students in future practicums will further refine and test the *Peter and His Service Dog* simulation based on feedback.

> **BOX 15.3 Exemplar 2—Incorporating Cultural Diversity Issues in Virtual Simulations: *Philippe the New Nurse***
>
> ### INTRODUCTION
>
> In addition to *developing* simulations, students in the SL practicum also *participate* in scripted simulations related to nursing education practice, such as the cheating student, medication errors, or relationships with other professionals. In addition to writing simulations for future practicum groups, students play act and debrief simulations that have been developed by the students and mentor in the past.
>
> ### CHALLENGES AND RESOLUTIONS
>
> *Philippe the New Nurse* was developed in response to multiple issues in **cultural diversity** that students were encountering in practice and may encounter as educators. *Philippe the New Nurse* is an example of a scripted simulation. This simulation was originally designed by one of the graduate students in nursing education and was based on a real situation. In the original simulation, avatars were required to move from room to room frequently, which led to confusion and chaos at times. Through debriefing and improvement, the simulation was streamlined and otherwise updated. In addition, since the gender of SL avatars can be changed, we had gender flexibility: A female student or faculty mentor could become a male and play the role of Philippe if no male student was one of the mentees.
>
>   *Philippe the New Nurse* was designed to explore the effects of culturally diversity in hospital practice and to derive solutions to some of the dilemmas faced by people who are in the uncomfortable position of being different from a

(continued)

BOX 15.3 Exemplar 2—Incorporating Cultural Diversity Issues in Virtual Simulations: *Philippe the New Nurse* (continued)

homogeneous group in some way. Philippe is a new BSN graduate from Puerto Rico who arrives in a small rural hospital in Louisiana to begin his first job as a registered nurse. However, he is nervous: How will the staff treat him? Does he have enough skills under his belt? What if no one talks to him? What if he makes a mistake? He enters the nursing station and encounters sexism, ridicule for his accent, and bullying. He is assigned a patient load that is too heavy for a new graduate nurse and receives little help from his preceptor.

Philippe the New Nurse was developed based on the Games and Bauman (2011) **Ecology of Culturally Competent Design model**, which offers a framework for incorporating cultural diversity into a simulation, adding depth and breadth to the story it tells. The Ecology of Culturally Competent Design model can be applied to any type of diversity because "culture" does not apply to race alone; simulations related to characteristics such as gender, gender identity, or disability can be depicted.

When designing Philippe, the four factors in the Ecology of Culturally Competent Design model were applied.

- *Activities*—Phillippe reports for duty timidly and acts frustrated when he cannot get help. The nurses with whom he will be working whisper as he goes by and ridicule his accent.
- *Context*—The context of the simulation is important. This is demonstrated in *Philippe the New Nurse* by a racially homogenous staff; few people who are not part of the culture work in the medical center where Philippe works. For examples, pictures hanging on the wall depict only Caucasian nurses. This is an advantage of using SL: The environment can be designed to be as diverse or not diverse as preferred. In addition, it appears that Philippe's preceptor is not eager to help him. Is it possible that she was assigned rather than volunteered to be a preceptor?
- *Characters*—Cultural issues can be displayed with the attitudes of the characters. Philippe is fearful, but staff nurses are sarcastic about his new BSN. His mentor lets him "sink or swim," and the staff talk behind his back.
- *Narrative*—Cultural issues can be incorporated into a virtual simulation through narratives or conversations. Philippe plaintively asks for help from his preceptor while the staff says mean and prejudicial things to him, such as "Didn't they teach you anything in the barrio?"

We also follow the **Simulation to Practice model** by Bauman (2013) when playing out simulations. In this model, students are assigned study material for preparation prior to the simulation. As students work through the story, they begin to reflect on what is going on (reflection-in-action); they sometimes go off script as they react to the action. When the story ends, they begin debriefing;

(continued)

> **BOX 15.3 Exemplar 2—Incorporating Cultural Diversity Issues in Virtual Simulations:** *Philippe the New Nurse* (*continued*)
>
> this phase is called *reflection-on-action*. We use the Plus-Delta debriefing questions and discuss participants' reactions to what went well and how the simulation and their interactions could be improved. While debriefing, students display the desired learning outcomes by exploring their feelings and discussing administrative and educational interventions to support Philippe. Often, an English as second language (ESL) student provides vivid descriptions of what they have experienced because of their accents. In the future, we plan to work more on taping simulations and practicing and critiquing various debriefing techniques to further develop the simulation.
>
> ## SUMMARY
>
> The *Philippe the New Nurse* simulation has been an excellent tool for practicum students to address cultural issues in hospitals and universities. The discussion is lively, but just as important, students gain an understanding of how to develop scripted simulations and apply educational models to their teaching.

Using the resources provided through administrative support, faculty mentors plan and evaluate student learning activities appropriate for 3D VLEs such as SL. The application of the FAST SIM© in the virtual environment for graduate nursing students in nursing education was described in this chapter.

REFLECTIVE QUESTIONS

1. Reflect on a learning experience that could be developed into a scripted scenario for a virtual simulation. What are the first three steps you would complete to begin to develop this virtual simulation?
2. Consider a learning experience that you would not want to script. Why would you choose to not script this virtual simulation? What is the main outcome that would be achieved by this learning experience because it is unscripted?
3. Critically think about the role of mentor in a virtual world. Describe all of the ways that it is similar to and different from the mentor role in the real world.
4. Thinking about a topic you typically teach, what kind of authentic assignment would be appropriate? How could students use SL to complete that assignment collaboratively?
5. What experiential learning could you assign for your students in SL?
6. What are the advantages of using SL instead of in-person settings for authentic learning?
7. Thinking about cultural diversity, what stories have you experienced that could be turned into a simulation for your organization? For your students?
8. What debriefing questions would you suggest when discussing cultural issues in your organization?

REFERENCES

American Nurses Association Massachusetts. (n.d.). Mentoring definitions. Retrieved from http://www.anamass.org/?61

Bauman, E. B. (2013). *Games-based teaching and simulation in nursing and health care.* New York, NY: Springer Publishing.

Bhati, N., Mercer, S., Rankin, K., & Thomas, V. B. (2009). Barriers and facilitators to the adoption of tools for online pedagogy. *International Journal of Pedagogies and Learning, 5*(3), 5–19. doi:10.5172/ijpl.5.3.5

Campbell, C., & Cameron, L. (2016). Scaffolding learning through the use of virtual worlds. In S. Gregory, M. J. W. Lee, B. Dalgarno, & B. Tynan (Eds.), *Learning in virtual worlds: Research and applications* (pp. 242–259). Edmonton, Canada: AU Press, Athabasca University.

Coban, M., Karakus, T., Karaman, A., Gunay, F., & Goktas, Y. (2015). Technical problems experienced in the transformation of virtual worlds into an education environment and coping strategies. *Educational Technology & Society, 18*(1), 37–49. Retrieved from http://www.jstor.org/stable/jeductechsoci.18.1.37

Farley, H. S. (2016). The reality of authentic learning in virtual worlds. In S. Gregory, M. J. W. Lee, B. Dalgarno, & B. Tynan (Eds.), *Learning in virtual worlds: Research and applications* (pp. 129–149). Edmonton, Canada: AU Press, Athabasca University.

Fedeli, L. (2016). Virtual body: Implications for identity, interaction, and didactics. In S. Gregory, M. J. W. Lee, B. Dalgarno, & B. Tynan (Eds.). *Learning in virtual worlds: Research and applications* (pp. 67–85). Edmonton, Canada: AU Press, Athabasca University.

Fitzsimons, S., & Farren, M. (2016). A brave new world: Considering the pedagogical potential of virtual world field trips (VWFTs) in initial teacher education. *International Journal for Transformative Research, 3*(1), 9–15. doi:10.1515/ijtr-2016-0002

Fountain, J., & Newcomer, K. E. (2016). Developing ad sustaining effective faculty mentoring programs. *Journal of Public Affairs Education, 22*, 483–506. Retrieved from http://www.jstor.org/stable/44113751

Games, A. I., & Bauman, E. B. (2011). Virtual worlds: An environment for cultural sensitivity education in the health sciences. *International Journal of Web-Based Communities, 7*(2), 189–205. doi:10.1504/IJWBC.2011.03951

Gregg, N., Wolfe, G., Jones, S., Todd, R., Moon, N., & Langston, C. (2016). STEM e-mentoring and community college students with disabilities. *Journal of Postsecondary Education and Disability, 29*(1), 47–63. Retrieved from https://files.eric.ed.gov/fulltext/EJ1107474.pdf

Hartley, M. D., Ludlow, B. L., & Duff, M. C. (2015). Second Life®: A 3D virtual immersive environment for teacher preparation courses in a distance education program. *Rural Special Education Quarterly, 34*(3), 21–25. doi:10.1177/875687051503400305

Jeffries, P. (Ed.). (2015). *The NLN Jeffries simulation theory.* New York, NY: Wolters Kluwer.

Krawczyk, M. (2017). Caring for patients with service dogs: Information for healthcare providers. *Online Journal of Issues in Nursing, 22*(1). doi:10.3912/OJIN.Vol22No01PPT45

Mattison, K. M., Schroeder, H., Sculthorp, S. L., & Zacharias, J. (2017). A return to doing: How authentic assessment changes higher education. In K. Rasmuusen, P. Northrup, & R. Colson (Eds.), *Handbook of research on competency-based education in university settings* (pp. 186–209). Hershey, PA: IGI Global.

Minocha, S., & Hardy, C. (2016). Navigation and wayfinding in learning spaces in 3D virtual worlds. In S. Gregory, M. J. W. Lee, B. Dalgarno, & B. Tynan (Eds.), *Learning in virtual worlds: Research and applications* (pp. 3–42). Edmonton, Canada: AU Press, Athabasca University.

Olasina, G. (2016). Exploratory study of collaborative behavior in Second Life®. *British Journal of Educational Technology, 47*(3), 520–527. doi:10.1111/bjet.12447

Pasfield-Neofitou, S., Huang, H., & Grant, S. (2015). Lost in Second Life®: Virtual embodiment and language learning via multimodal communication. *Education Technology Research and Development, 63*, 709–726. doi:10.1007/s11423-015-9384-7

Sawyer, T., Eppich, W., Brett-Fleegler, M., Grant, V., & Cheng, A. (2016). More than one way to debrief: A critical review of healthcare simulation debriefing methods. *Simulation in Healthcare, 11*(3), 209–217. doi:10.1097/SIH.0000000000000148

Silva, K., Correia, A. P., & Pardo-Ballester, C. (2010). A faculty mentoring experience: Learning together in Second Life. *Journal of Computing in Teacher Education, 26*(4), 149–159. Retrieved from https://files.eric.ed.gov/fulltext/EJ893873.pdf

Storey, V. A., & Wolf, A. A. (2010). Utilizing the platform of Second Life® to teach future educators. *International Journal of Technology in Teaching and Learning, 6*(1), 58–70. Retrieved from https://www.researchgate.net/profile/Valerie_Storey/publication/228795748_Utilizing_the_Platform_of_Second_Life_to_Teach_Future_Educators/links/0deec518e49f0ee515000000.pdf

Creating Interprofessional Simulation Scenarios in Virtual Learning Environments

ELLEN JAKOVICH

LEARNING OBJECTIVES

Upon completion of this chapter, the reader will be able to:
- Assess the difference between skill-based and collaboration-based interdisciplinary assignments.
- Explore the two types of interprofessional involvement in simulation development.
- Describe ways to encourage interdisciplinary professionals to volunteer in simulation development.

KEY TERMS

Collaboration
Collaboration-based
External involvement
Interdisciplinary
Internal involvement
Interprofessional
Skill-based

Today's healthcare services are provided within the construct of a business, so that nurses can expect to be called on to collaborate with business and information technology (IT) professionals. Nurses may find themselves working with accountants, finance officers, lawyers, marketing professionals, IT specialists, and others. At a minimum, nurses should understand enough about these professions for collaboration to be effective. Even more likely is that nurses may require basic skills in business or IT as part of their job descriptions (Jain, 2015; McGonigle, Hunter, Sipes, & Hebda, 2014). As we strive to develop a more experiential and immersive nursing curriculum through virtual simulations, an opportunity arises. We can increase the realism and effectiveness of these simulations by including interprofessional skills and collaborations that nurses can expect to encounter in actual practice.

RELATION TO THE FAST SIM©

If the Faculty Administrators Students Technology Strategic Integration Model© (FAST SIM) is viewed as a revolving gear with administrators, faculty, and students each representing one third of the gear, any of these three can bring the mechanism to a standstill simply by refusing to budge. In that respect, the model requires each of the three to advance in the same direction, at the same time, and at the same speed. If they cooperate, the gear will turn. Working together, they drive the speed and direction of the technology rather than being pushed along by force or not moving at all.

Where is the development of **interprofessional** virtual simulations reflected in the model? Today's nurses collaborate with professionals in accounting, finance, law, insurance, project management, and other fields. Developing a realistic simulation depends on input from professionals who are experts in their fields. This interprofessional **collaboration** functions as the "grease" in the technology wheel. It improves the operation and functionality of the entire gear by making it move more smoothly. The gear would still revolve without it, but it would require more effort to make it turn. A simulation involving interprofessional skills but lacking interprofessional input could certainly work, but its implementation and operation is bound to encounter sticky spots that could have been avoided.

IDENTIFYING INTERPROFESSIONAL VIRTUAL SIMULATIONS

It is not a question of whether incorporating interprofessional skills and collaborations into immersive virtual simulations enhances the effectiveness and depth of student learning (Caylor, Aebersold, Lapham, & Carlson, 2015; Nicely & Farra, 2015; Owen, Shaw, & Mitchell, 2015). It is more a question of how to identify viable proposals for interprofessional virtual simulations. Should we start by brainstorming ideas for simulations? We could quickly be overwhelmed with great ideas only vaguely associated with curriculum goals. Perhaps the best approach is not to start from scratch. Nursing courses are replete with fully developed assignments already based on course learning objectives. These are the perfect place to start. Not every assignment lends itself to immersion, and in some cases, the addition of technology can distract students from learning. Each existing assignment and activity should be reviewed with an eye toward answering the question: "Would this assignment's learning objective(s) be understood and/or retained better if conducted in an immersive environment?" This review will likely lead to only a handful of assignments suitable for development as virtual simulations. This pared-down list of assignments serves as the starting point for a second review. The purpose of a second review is to identify assignments that contain—or we would like to contain—interdisciplinary elements. These **interdisciplinary elements** can be present in two ways, skill based and collaboration based.

Skill Based

A **skill-based** interprofessional element is present if an assignment requires students to perform tasks typically associated with another profession. Skill-based interprofessional elements are generally measurable and, as a result, are easier to quantify and code into a simulation than collaboration-based interprofessional elements. The virtual skill-based interprofessional simulation can place the learners in roles of practicing, interacting, performing, and/or behaving based on another profession while they are gaining knowledge or learning about this profession.

An initial, cursory search is likely to result in a negative finding simply because nursing assignments are generally designed by, conducted by, and evaluated by nurses. Even if interdisciplinary skills are present in an assignment, they are not likely to be identified as such. It takes an open mind and a fresh perspective to see the "hidden" interdisciplinary elements contained within an assignment and then track them to the related profession. Does the assignment involve forecasting project costs? Perhaps a financing officer or project manager could assist. If an assignment involves ratio analysis or past revenues and costs, an accountant could help. Does the assignment require developing ways to increase sales? Ask a marketing professional to weigh in. Does the assignment require protecting confidential patient data? Perhaps it is time to call either a lawyer or an IT specialist.

Collaboration Based

If interprofessional collaboration is already part of an assignment, it is easily identified because the assignment specifically mentions nurses working with an accountant or another professional. However, most nursing assignments are designed to teach a specific nursing skill apart from the interprofessional collaborative environment in which the skill will be performed. As a result, it may become necessary to add some aspect of interprofessional collaboration to an existing assignment. Expanding an assignment in this way requires imagining the environment in which the tasks would be carried out in practice and then modifying the scenario to include interactions with other professionals. It can work to recall actual events in which interprofessional collaboration took place and then develop an assignment around that situation. However, because collaboration by its very nature is person-to-person and nonquantifiable, coding a **collaboration-based** simulation presents a real challenge. Furthermore, collaboration-based simulations require the real-time participation of a professional from another field to interact with students, and this poses other challenges. Unless the professional works for the university, availability and accountability may be an issue.

LEVELS OF INTERPROFESSIONAL INVOLVEMENT

Whether developing a skills-based or a collaboration-based virtual simulation, it is necessary to involve a professional from an appropriate field from the very beginning. Once simulation development is underway, making a change becomes increasingly expensive due to rework and delays. However, if the professional can weigh-in on the simulation's initial design, expensive redevelopment costs and delays can be avoided. Interprofessional involvement can be internal or external to the simulation.

Internal Involvement

Internal involvement is when the professional works from within the simulation and is an integral part of the activity. It occurs after the simulation is live and students are actively participating. The interdisciplinary professional works with students within the immersive environment to simulate interdisciplinary collaboration in the real world. Internal interprofessional involvement more often relates to collaboration-based simulations.

External Involvement

External involvement occurs before and during simulation development. The professional assists in the development of the simulation to create realistic scenarios but plays no role inside of the simulation. External involvement by the interdisciplinary professional is helpful to both skills-based and collaboration-based simulations; however, it is critical to avoid costly errors in simulation development in skill-based simulations.

FINDING AN INTERPROFESSIONAL VOLUNTEER

Identifying assignments to turn into interprofessional virtual simulations is only half the battle. Finding a professional in a discipline outside of healthcare willing to dedicate time and effort on a nursing simulation is the other half. The obvious place to start searching for volunteers is at the university. Universities employ professionals from many disciplines. Because these professionals are already involved in education to some extent, they may be more open to assisting. If this search is unsuccessful, extend the search to personal contacts from former jobs, conferences, and committees. What if no one wants to play?

Sometimes just asking is not enough. It may become necessary to sell the idea. In a time when most professionals are already overextended, offering something of value in exchange for their time may pique interest. Several nonmonetary incentives can be suggested. Does the professional want to be published or speak at conferences? This effort is a unique collaborative effort that lends itself to publication and presentations. Need recognition? Agree to send a letters of appreciation to the person's direct supervisor on each milestone reached. Looking for a resume boost? Quantify the achievements in which the professional would participate. Sell the invitation to participate as a rare chance to be part of something futuristic that will set the persons apart from peers.

KEY POINTS

- Nurses are required to work with professionals from fields outside of healthcare, so nursing education should incorporate activities with an interdisciplinary component.
- Virtual simulations with interprofessional involvement create a more realistic immersive environment that better prepares nursing students for practice.
- Appropriate interdisciplinary volunteers are scarce, so simulation designers/developers should be prepared to offer nonmonetary incentives for involvement.

SUMMARY

Today's healthcare environment increasingly requires nursing practitioners to collaborate with professionals from other disciplines. One way to prepare nursing students for this eventuality is to incorporate immersive virtual simulations containing skill-based or collaborative-based interdisciplinary elements (refer to Boxes 16.1 and 16.2). Development of such simulations requires identifying potential assignments for the simulation, determining whether interprofessional involvement should be internal or external to the simulation, and finding an interdisciplinary professional with the appropriate background willing to volunteer for the effort.

REFLECTIVE QUESTIONS

1. Consider the interprofessional collaborations that can be made at the student level. What are the collaborations made at the professor's level?

2. What arguments could be made that would successfully defend the professor's inclusion of virtual worlds in a course?

3. When beginning to explore using virtual worlds in education, what preparations should the professor do in advance? How far in advance must the professor prepare? How could the professor obtain buy-in?

4. Critically think about implementing an interprofessional simulation. What obstacles might be encountered? How would you handle each one?

5. Should a committee approve the development of virtual simulations, knowing that resources are limited? Why or why not?

BOX 16.1 Exemplar 1—The Students Succeeded; the Professor Failed

After discovering an innovative and technological solution, a professor allows excitement and expediency to bypass collaboration, learning a professionally embarrassing lesson in the process.

I remember the exact day I was introduced to virtual worlds. It was December 21, 2006, and I was on my winter break from teaching. My husband surfed the headlines, while I mentally debated which would be less painful: teaching my upcoming senior project course in an undergraduate college of business program or sawing off my toe with a butter knife. Then my husband piped up "Have you ever heard of Second Life®?" The online article he ad found kicked off my exploration of virtual worlds, along with a frenzied rework of my entire course from scratch.

The overarching goal was to merge the lessons from each stove-piped course in accounting, finance, marketing, operations, writing, speaking, and so on, into a cohesive, interdisciplinary practical application of skills in a realistic business situation. My colleagues had mentioned how past efforts to involve students with actual businesses and real-life challenges had generally resulted in students being assigned to meaningless issues or even secretarial work. As a result, the assignment in the senior project course had devolved into a dull and ineffective case study. Despite practically turning cartwheels in class to generate enthusiasm, my students were not invested, did the minimum, and just wanted to be done and graduate. After teaching the course twice, I was desperate to try a different approach, and the virtual world of Second Life (SL) seemed like a heaven-sent solution. It was not only home to numerous progressive companies, it was also fun! I doggedly powered through SL's steep learning curve, inspired by visions of virtual worlds as the future of business collaboration.

Two weeks later:

"Hello everyone! You have made it to your senior project course! This course is unlike any course taken so far. There is no textbook, homework, examinations, or lectures. However, you WILL have deliverables, deadlines, and responsibility

(continued)

> **BOX 16.1 Exemplar 1—The Students Succeeded; the Professor Failed** (*continued*)
>
> for your team's performance. It is time to apply what you have learned in your degree to a real business problem . . . in a virtual world."
>
> I paused for effect and smiled while the students exchanged questioning glances with each other. I went on to explain that in teams, they would form service-based businesses of their choice: website development, marketing, whatever. Then, each student business-team would develop an unsolicited proposal detailing improvements to the virtual operations of a real-life company in SL.
>
> The proposals were to involve collaboration with the target company when possible, and would describe the proposed operation as if it already existed. Each team would produce a portfolio containing several detailed business analyses such as cost-benefit, staffing, and required infrastructure, as well as a final presentation inside of the virtual world. Several students looked at me as if I had spoken in some alien language, so I simplified it: "Find a challenge to some business in SL, research what it would take to fix it, write up your solution, and present it."
>
> As the students learned to log in and create and personalize their avatars, their enthusiasm grew. To be part of something futuristic was exciting! Within days, they were holding virtual meetings under water, in space, or while sipping virtual martinis and dancing on the deck of the Titanic. It took about a week before problems started to surface. The learning curve was steep, and our limited class time was not enough to address all the hurdles they ran into. Several did not have home computers able to handle the advanced graphics of SL. A few students started to grumble about the project—it was not realistic; it was too hard; it was childish. I ignored this, because in every class some students complain, and I was certain they would come around as they became more familiar with the platform. Although this outlook eventually came back to bite me, most of the students remained enthusiastic, and from these sprouted dozens of innovative business proposals, including:
>
> - A student Television Script Writing/Filmmaking Company collaborated with the Food Channel to develop and market an upcoming TV cooking show with an 8-week pilot of the show in SL using a fully animated avatar of the chef.
> - A student company doing custom website development collaborated with "The Knot," a wedding-planning company, to link SL to their existing website for click-to-order custom cakes, napkins, and other items for a wedding in the real world. (This ability has since been developed.)
> - A student travel agency worked with small local museums to create historically accurate back-in-time tours and immersive experiences based on lesser-known historical figures and towns.
>
> Perhaps the most successful collaboration was between a student marketing company and the Centers for Disease Control and Prevention (CDC). The

(*continued*)

> **BOX 16.1 Exemplar 1—The Students Succeeded; the Professor Failed** (*continued*)
>
> students' proposed idea was simple enough to be achievable and innovative enough to be effective. More than that, the CDC participated in the effort, making the team's learning experience much more robust.
>
> The CDC's sim was a standard layout of plain buildings and informative posters that drew little to no traffic. Occasionally, the site was used for meetings, which saved on their travel budget, but most of the time, it sat empty (A. Casanova, personal communication, March 3, 2017). The students' proposal was to inform and better promote the CDC's mission and services to the global public by making their site more interesting, interactive, and educational for visitors. The premise was if the site was fun to visit, more avatars would stop by and learn about diseases and health-related issues. Visiting avatars could click on "disease poseballs" and watch their avatars progress, cartoon-style, through the various symptoms and stages of an illness, with dropdowns explaining each stage. The proposal was met with genuine interest and led to direct collaboration between the students and the Senior Technology Associate at the CDC. He helped refine the proposal and attended the students' senior project presentation in SL (A. Casanova, personal communication, March 3, 2017).
>
> All in all, the revised course was a success. It did not seem to matter whether a student team's proposal was accepted, rejected, or ignored by the target company. The students became more comfortable reaching out to business personnel both in the virtual and real worlds to request and conduct meetings, ask questions, offer solutions, and obtain feedback. The students learned to create project timelines with deliverables, testing schedules, and detailed budgets for a real opportunity for a real client. Even when the actual clients would not participate, the projects were still realistic because unsolicited proposals are generally developed without participation from the target company anyway. In addition, students discovered how even a great idea will not sell unless it is pitched professionally, with confidence, enthusiasm, and an in-depth understanding of all aspects of the project.
>
> In hindsight, I should not have overlooked the complaints of those few unhappy students. It took just one student complaining directly to the campus president before I found myself in the unenviable position of trying to explain the virtues of SL to someone convinced it was no more than a game. My experience had been that administration was interested in what topics were taught, not in how they were taught. Yet standing there, it was apparent I had overstepped a boundary. Earlier, I had informed my program administrator of the course revision as a courtesy, but the information had not made its way to the campus president. Furthermore, because I had developed the revised course so quickly, it never occurred to me I might have to defend the educational value of virtual worlds to anyone. Accordingly, my response was more a surprised splutter than a convincing defense. I realized that although my students were deeply involved with cross-collaboration between their student businesses and the real businesses, I had failed to collaborate with my own university administration. I felt my face get hot as I realized I would have flunked my own course.

> **BOX 16.2 Exemplar 2—No Money, No Time, No Questions, No Simulation**
>
> An accounting and finance professor with experience in Second Life collaborates with the nursing college to add realism to a nursing simulation, yet higher priorities and a hesitation to ask questions put the project on a permanent back-burner.
>
> I do not recall who contacted whom first, but I found myself volunteering to work with a committee of technologically open-minded nurses who taught for an online college of nursing program. One of the many initiatives the committee was involved in was the creation of immersive nursing experiences and education via the virtual world of SL. I am not a nurse though. I am a business professor teaching accounting and finance. However, I do bring several years of experience working with virtual worlds to the table.
>
> It had been a few years since I had worked with virtual worlds, so it was nice to be surrounded by like-minded professionals who saw the possibilities inherent in the technology. I realized I had little to offer the committee beyond generic suggestions that centered around SL itself. Since I do not teach nursing courses, I had no knowledge of each course's objectives. Even if I had been granted full access to the nursing curriculum, most of it would be pure mishmash to me. Brainstorming ideas for nursing simulations was out of my league.
>
> It did not take me long to bring it up to the committee leader:
>
> Me: I am quite good at holding this chair down, but I am not sure I add much else of value to these committee meetings. Do you perhaps have any courses that require nurses to manage money?
>
> Committee Leader: Actually, we do—our Advanced Nursing Practicum course! The course centers on developing a plan for a postcardiac wellness clinic. The nurses come up with a plan, forecast expected revenues and costs, and see if they can make it break even. I would love to turn that into a simulation!
>
> Me: Email me the project and some sample student work. I will get back to you on what I find!
>
> The project write-up was detailed, and the concepts were well developed. It required a team of nursing students to develop a plan for a postcardiac wellness clinic. The computations the nurses were required to do did not easily lend themselves to a virtual simulation because most were analytical rather than visual. And then I saw it—two key areas had been left open-ended. Although the project identified an existing trailer on the hospital grounds for the clinic, the size and configuration of the trailer were not specified, nor was there a realistic limitation on the budget. Students could assume the trailer was the size of a football stadium if they desired, and they were granted practically all the money they might need. I smiled to myself. THIS is the simulation!
>
> I could hardly wait to hear what the committee would say! At the next meeting, I explained the discovery and proposed a simulation in which student teams were given a set budget and a fixed-size trailer in SL. These limitations

(continued)

BOX 16.2 Exemplar 2—No Money, No Time, No Questions, No Simulation (*continued*)

would add realism to the project, pushing the students to make critical trade-offs between services provided, space available, and cost. The simulation would allow students to change the trailer's configuration to meet their needs, but each change would have an associated cost. An automated budget display would keep a running balance. Once students determine what services to provide based on available space and cost, the virtual simulation part of their project would be complete. The information from the simulation would be the basis for their projected revenues and costs, as well as the foundation for their overall plan.

The idea went over well, so I started working with the SL programmer on the committee to get the simulation out of my head, onto paper, and into virtual reality. Over the next few months, we identified and refined the requirements, and then our programmer attempted to hire an amateur programmer to take on the project under his guidance. This was when the project began to fizzle. For the miniscule amount the committee could pay, no one was interested. Our programmer, extremely busy with other tasks levied on him by the committee, did not have the time to work this project himself (P. Woodcock, personal communication, February 23, 2017). At the same time, I was traveling and teaching overseas. When I returned months later and attended another committee meeting, no one mentioned the project, and I was not certain I should either. The committee was obviously working on several other high-priority efforts, and I was worried that by bringing it up, I might inadvertently put our hard-working programmer on the spot. It took a few more meetings, but eventually I simply had to know. Trying my best to sound nonchalant, I asked "So, whatever happened to the nursing practicum project?" Awkward silence. Then the programmer shrugged, grinned, and explained how the project simply died a low-priority death (P. Woodcock, personal communication, February 23, 2017).

I should have been disappointed, but all I felt was relief! Like our programmer, I was very busy, and this was one project officially off my plate. My involvement had introduced a different perspective to the committee, so overall, my purpose for participating had been achieved.

I realize now that as a volunteer, I was hesitant to ask pointed questions. It felt presumptuous and downright rude to ask, "Who will work on this project? How much time will be dedicated to this project each week? How much funding is available? Is there a deadline? Do we have the support of management?" Because these questions were not addressed, we wasted valuable time and effort. However, just as I was hesitant to ask questions, the committee was hesitant to tell their enthusiastic volunteer that the idea was not a priority! Sometimes, politeness is the enemy of efficiency.

REFERENCES

Caylor, S., Aebersold, M., Lapham, J., & Carlson, E. (2015). The use of virtual simulation and a modified TeamSTEPPs™ training for multiprofessional education. *Clinical Simulation in Nursing, 11*(3), 163–171. doi:10.1016/j.ecns.2014.12.003

Jain, S. (2015). *Harvard Business Review* leadership development: The skills doctors and nurses need to be effective executives. Retrieved from https://hbr.org/2015/04/the-skills-doctors-need-to-be-effective-executives

McGonigle, D., Hunter, K., Sipes, C., & Hebda, T. (2014). Why nurses need to understand nursing informatics. *Association of Operating Room Nurses Journal, 100*(Special Focus Issue), 324–327. doi:10.1016/j.aorn.2014.06.012

Nicely, S., & Farra, S. (2015). Fostering learning through inter-professional virtual reality simulation development. *Nursing Education Perspectives, 36*(5), 335–336. doi:10.5480/13-1240

Owen, S., Shaw, J., & Mitchell, C. (2015). What's going on? The effectiveness of communication in undergraduate inter-professional education: The student experience. *Australian Nurse Teacher's Society e-Bulletin, Peer Review Section, 7*(3), 5–15. Retrieved from http://www.ants.org.au/ants/pluginfile.php/36/mod_page/content/80/ANTS_ebulletin_October2015c.pdf

CHAPTER 17

Advancing Nursing Informatics Knowledge and Skills Using a Virtual Learning Environment

CAROLYN SIPES

LEARNING OBJECTIVES

Upon completion of this chapter, the reader will be able to:
- Discuss correlation of nursing informatics (NI) and applications in simulation.
- Assess how NI skills are used in virtual learning environments (VLEs) to increase knowlege and advance competencies.
- Describe four skills needed to "work and practice" in the VLE/simulation environments.
- Evaluate barriers to learning NI skills using VLE/simulation.
- Appreciate how the Faculty Administrators Students Technology Strategic Integration Model© (FAST SIM) can inform curriculum development in nursing informatics.

KEY TERMS

American Nurses Association (ANA)
American Association of Colleges of Nursing (AACN)
American Medical Informatics Association (AMIA)
Immersion
Institute of Medicine (IOM)
Informatics nurse specialist (INS)
Nursing Informatics (NI)
Quality and Safety Education for Nurses Initiative (QSEN)
Virtual learning environments (VLEs)
Simulation
Second Life® (SL)
TIGER-based Assessment of Nursing Informatics Competencies (TANIC)
Technology Informatics Guiding Education Reform (TIGER)

Today, faculty's goal should be to create a workforce competent in applying technology in practice in all settings and areas of nursing. The **Technology Informatics Guiding Education Reform (TIGER)** (2009) initiative was one of the first organizations to recognize the need for nurses to become more competent using technology such as electronic information tools and devises. The **American Nurses Association (ANA), American Association of Colleges of Nursing (AACN), American Medical Informatics Association (AMIA),** and **Institute of Medicine (IOM)** are the major driving forces for mandating the advancement of competencies in the use of technology in the healthcare industry.

These professional organizations and accrediting bodies such as the **Quality and Safety Education for Nurses Initiative (QSEN)** (2014) require informatics skills as part of today's workforce preparation. Findings in the literature indicate and define expectations that all nursing faculty must possess **nursing informatics (NI)** competencies to support graduates in developing skills demanded in today's workforce (Darvish, Bahramnezhad, Keyhanian, & Navidhamidi, 2014; IOM, 2010). Yet, according to Hunter, McGonigle, and Hebda (2013), gaps remain in nursing curricula not only in the preparation of nursing graduates (Farokhzadian, Khajouei, & Ahmadian, 2015), but also in the knowledge and skill sets of the graduate faculty. To further appreciate these gaps in context, it is imperative to first understand what NI is, as defined by the ANA's *Nursing Informatics: Scope and Standards of Practice* (2015). According to the ANA:

> Nursing informatics (NI) is the specialty that integrates nursing science with multiple information management and analytical sciences to identify, define, manage, and communicate data, information, knowledge, and wisdom in nursing practice. NI supports nurses, consumers, patients, the interprofessional healthcare team, and other stakeholders in their decision-making in all roles and settings to achieve desired outcomes. This support is accomplished through the use of information structures, information processes, and information technology (pp. 1–2).

These national organizations identified certain skills and knowledge as inadequate or missing for both students and faculty. When faculty do not have the skills or knowledge, it leads to unsatisfactory and ineffective development of curricula. Early on, national organizations, such as QSEN, the National League for Nursing (NLN), ANA, and AACN, mandated that students need to have informatics competencies and now require that educators have competencies as well (Lilly, Fitzpatrick, & Madigan, 2015; McGonigle, Hunter, Sipes, & Hebda, 2014; Rajalahti, Heinonen, & Saranto, 2014; Sipes et al., 2015). With the advent of **virtual learning environments (VLEs)** and virtual simulation, there is a greater need for faculty to develop informatics skills and competencies. In addition, academia has a responsibility to support faculty attainment of the skills needed to teach and assess NI competencies in their faculty to meet the requirements of the technology-driven healthcare industry today.

RELATION TO THE FAST SIM©

This chapter addresses the influence of the student role, especially in relation to students studying NI. The NI student's influence moves beyond the beginner roles and should be in the expert role. As students learn about NI, they also explore emerging technologies that provide opportunities for student-to-student collaboration. To construct knowledge, educators acknowledge the need to foster social interaction through collaboration. Students' influence is evident in their desire for more control of the learning experience, as well as when and how they use it, which influences their educators to change outdated practices that no longer serve the needs of highly mobile, technology-savvy students.

MEETING NEEDS THROUGH VLE AND VIRTUAL SIMULATION

These days, the integration and deployment of technology using VLE and **Second Life® (SL)** concepts are now considered the norm for all nursing curricula regardless of practice area. Simulation can be enormously beneficial and transformative when used to develop basic knowledge and skills and used in specific specialty areas such as NI, where there may be no opportunities to advance competencies in an area. Whereas the Faculty Administrators Students Technology Strategic Integration Model© (FAST SIM) is used as a framework to explain *how* important simulation is in education today, Exemplars 1 and 2 (Boxes 17.1 and 17.2) explain *why* using the functionality of NI also applies to the overall concept informing nursing curriculum development.

BOX 17.1 Exemplar 1—MSN Graduate Core: Fundamentals of Nursing Informatics Skill Development for Students Using Simulation

Exemplar 1: Process to Meet Needs and Requirements for Students
The simulation model used to develop or advance current NI skills for students in the first graduate core course was Second Life.

- During the initial assessment week, take the pre–**TIGER-based Assessment of Nursing Informatics Competency (TANIC)** skills to identify gaps in competencies.

- During week 2, start orientation to a virtual learning environment (VLE) of an activity to begin to explore the simulation environment; create an avatar, and begin to complete basic activities in the VLE (i.e., log in, walk in a specific environment, find a building where additional activities need to be completed).

- Move to more complex activities that include completing a number of physical activities such as walking, finding the College of Nursing and the lecture hall, then completing course assignments and posting them in the correct area for grading.

- As activities become more complex, find community and government leadership areas required in the course assignments; complete a health policy activity (e.g., defining what is needed to address an infectious disease issue, such as the Zika virus).

- Move to the next level of complexity starting website exploration to find a relevant topic for research, developing a paper to support the research, and justifying the potential impact on practice or a perspective on practice in the future.

- Complete an additional skill-development requirement by creating a PowerPoint presentation with narration of the concept; share it, and publish the presentation in a threaded discussion section to share with peers.

(continued)

> **BOX 17.1 Exemplar 1—MSN Graduate Core: Fundamentals of Nursing Informatics Skill Development for Students Using Simulation (*continued*)**
>
> - After completing these activities, during Week 7, complete another self-assessment of competencies by using the TANIC.
> - The final reflection is on the VLE/simulation experience; students need to justify how each activity they completed met course and program outcomes and aided new knowledge discovery.

> **BOX 17.2 Exemplar 2—MSN Graduate Faculty: Fundamentals of Nursing Informatics Skill Development for Faculty with Planned Immersion Using Simulation**
>
> **Exemplar 2: Process to Meet Needs and Requirements for Faculty**
> The simulation model to advance current nursing informatics (NI) skills for faculty through immersion in the Fundamentals of Nursing Informatics graduate core course was Second Life.
>
> - Similar to the development plan for students, faculty's initial assessment began by taking the pre–TIGER-based Assessment of Nursing Informatics Competency (TANIC) skills to identify gaps in competencies needed to support students.
> - During step two, faculty start an orientation to NI by participating in two American Association of Colleges of Nursing (ANCC) webinars entitled, "*Informatics in Academia: Incorporating an Emerging Specialty into the Curriculum*," and "*Maximizing Nursing Informatics Competencies in the Curricula*," which also provides continuing education units. These courses/webinars were developed by informatics nurse specialist (INS) specialty faculty at the college who oversee the development of NI curricula based on American Nurses Association (ANA, 2015) *Nursing Informatics: Scope and Standards of Practice*.
> - After the initial webinars are completed, faculty participate in an immersion process in a virtual learning environment (VLE)/simulation with activities in which they begin to explore a simulation environment just as the students did; they develop an avatar and begin to complete basic activities in the VLE such as:
>   - Logging in
>   - Walking in a specific environment
>   - Finding a building where they need to complete additional activities
>   - Moving to more complex activities that include completing a number of physical activities such as walking, finding the College of Nursing

(continued)

> **BOX 17.2 Exemplar 2—MSN Graduate Faculty: Fundamentals of Nursing Informatics Skill Development for Faculty with Planned Immersion Using Simulation (*continued*)**
>
> and lecture hall, and completing the assignments for the course, posting them and worksheets in the correct area for grading.
>
> - Increasing the level of complexity, they have to find community and government leadership areas required in the course assignments and complete a health policy activity such as defining what is needed to address an infectious disease issue such as the Zika virus.
> - Moving through various activities with increased complexity, faculty then have to demonstrate skills in navigation, which is tracked on a spreadsheet by the VLE staff, automatically updating as activities are completed. A note also appears above the avatar's head when activities are completed.
> - After completing all activities, with successful debrief by VLE staff, faculty reassess competency and skill levels using the TANIC tool.
> - After successful sign-off by VLE staff, faculty are assigned to teach an NI course, which includes many VLE/simulation activities.

EDUCATION OF FACULTY AND STUDENTS

There are many advantages of using VLE/SL to develop overall curricula to improve basic skills through active learning for both faculty and students. One frequent use is to develop specific programs such as NI, including more advanced skills in which there may be a lack of skilled and knowledgeable faculty in the specialty area. Faculty can take advantage of the same VLE/SL activities as the students to become competent in teaching these courses.

Advantages for students include VLE/SL simulation of a laboratory or clinical setting, such as an urgent care center, to use when no clinical site is available. Additional examples of VLE education strategies include ability to develop essential skills needed to perform as an **informatics nurse specialist (INS)**. An innovative VLE can provide simulated experiences as a solution to address gaps where there is a lack of availability of venues for skill development.

EXEMPLARS AND STUDENT FEEDBACK

Table 17.1 includes a discussion of where skill development is needed, and Tables 17.2 through 17.5 include students' comments regarding the value of using a VLE/SL.

Although the FAST SIM© is used as a framework for explaining *how* important simulation is in education today, Exemplars 1 and 2 (Box 17.1 and 17.2) tie in the relevance of *why* using the functionality of nursing informatics applies to the overall concept informing nursing curriculum development. Comments from students before and after completing the core Fundamentals of Nursing Informatics course,

TABLE 17.1 Using Simulation to Meet the Needs for Skill and Knowledge Development

Venues Where Skill Development Is Needed: Simulation Is the Method Used to Develop NI and Technology Skills

- Faculty need to develop skills in education facilities, colleges, and universities.
- Students need to develop skills in the workforce through education facilities, colleges, and universities.
- Administrators, managers, and directors need to develop skills in healthcare organizations and the industry to meet current technology demands.
- The use of simulation can provide alternative clinical sites and experiences for students and faculty in education, colleges, and universities; for administrators, managers, and directors for staff in healthcare organizations and the industry.

including the pre– and post–self-assessment of skills/competencies using the TANIC and four weeks of VLE/SL activities are included in Tables 17.2 through 17.5.

Exemplar 1 (Box 17.1) emphasizes how the FAST SIM© can be used as a framework for explaining how to integrate technology into curricula. Using the FAST SIM©, the course design took into consideration faculty, administrators, and students using technology of simulation as the core (refer to Box 17.1). VLE/SL provides an environment for students to explore and develop necessary skills. For example, they move through and perform certain activities designed to bring them from initial and simple activities, such as logging into an island after they create their avatar then learning to "walk" with gradually more complex activities such as taking a "selfie" with the mayor in the city administration building. This is all completed in the safe simulation environment with opportunities to

TABLE 17.2 Student Self-Assessment Prior to Taking a Basic Nursing Informatics Course Using Simulation

Graduate Students' Knowledge of Nursing Informatics and Simulation Prefundamentals of Nursing Informatics Core Course

Before this class, I did not know about informatics or Second Life (SL).

. . . the assignment was unrelated to anything I had previously done in a master's level course, but when I reflect on how the virtual environment can be tailored to what is being taught at the moment, it is very exciting to see and use.

. . . was not thrilled at the idea of SL being set-up like a game as I do not play video games, but now appreciate the concept more—it was fun to explore while learning. Nursing informatics (NI) plays a major role in healthcare with technology, which is constantly evolving; it is relevant and necessary for the INS to collaborate now, as it can be used to educate nurses.

Before taking this class, I had no knowledge of what informatics roles in nursing consisted of. . . .

Completing the TIGER-based Assessment of Nursing Informatics Competencies (TANIC) self-assessment on the first assignment, I now realize that there are more informatics skills required of the professional nurse than I had thought. . . .

17: ADVANCING NURSING INFORMATICS KNOWLEDGE AND SKILLS

TABLE 17.3 TIGER-based Self-Assessment of Nursing Informatics Competencies (TANIC) Used in Course Week 1

Competency Self-Assessment using TANIC: *Pre-TANIC* **Self-Assessment Knowledge of Skills**

Using the TANIC self-assessment assignment, I realized how many areas and skills I am missing, mainly basic computer competencies. This class is challenging with new skill opportunities I previously had not known—had no idea.

The TANIC self-assessment helped to clarify those areas that need improvement and now realize there are few more areas for improvement that I did not know about.

After completing the pre-TANIC self-assessment and participating in the various discussion posts in SL, my current skill level has improved—now that I am more aware of what I do and what is required.

TABLE 17.4 Student Self-Assessment After Taking a Basic Nursing Informatics Course Using Simulation

Graduate Students Knowledge of Nursing Informatics and Simulation *Post-*Fundamentals of Nursing Informatics Core Course

Nursing informatics (NI) is so much more than I ever expected . . . did not realize until this course how much informatics is used in everyday nursing . . . first impressions of Second Life (SL) reminded me of the computer games kids play, and was skeptical about the advantages in a graduate program but after learning to navigate my avatar during orientation it was a fun way to learn.

I was surprised to learn at how significant informatics is to everyday nursing practice. Now, it is hard to imagine not having it available in practice; it has changed communication and managing the care of patients. . . .

Many of us did not understand the significance of how NI plays a significant role in nursing practice until taking this course

Today, informatics is helping nurses—especially with the electronic medical records documentation—but originally thought it was so silly because I did not understand what it was but now understand the benefits of using it in many areas of our practice.

I was surprised to learn about informatics and how important it is in advancing the nursing discipline—the more I learn about it the more I appreciate it.

I am surprised at all that informatics affords us in our healthcare practices—I never thought about this before this class. I now have a better appreciation of all that informatics can assist us with clinical documentation, including such tasks as creating care plans to tracking medication administration.

SL immersion into a VLE helps students increase and develop the use of technology skills. Students' interactions through the use of the activities and tasks in this course led to the need to find specific information that encouraged the need for further research.

SL was an enjoyable experience, with the ability to improve clinical experiences, critical thinking, and collaboration using simulation. With the incredible amount of information and knowledge in this class, can now see how NI and information technology tie together; It is obvious now that nurses must be well prepared in information technology and NI to have a successful practice.

The activities completed in SL helped improve my computer skills at work—I am constantly looking for more ways to use my new skills at work and also to see how it will be used in my next courses.

TABLE 17.5 TIGER-based Self-Assessment of Nursing Informatics Competencies (TANIC) Used in Course Week 7

Competency Self-Assessment Using TANIC: *Post-TANIC* Self-Assessment and Knowledge
Initially wondering what this course was about and what we had to do, then eventually realized how nursing informatics is used in almost everything nurses do, now understand the need for NI better. It is the common communication and tool used in everyday documentation when patients first come through the ER, and if admitted throughout the entire stay—even on follow-up in the OP clinics. In Second Life (SL)/virtual learning environment (VLE), having to use the keyboard more in all of our activities, as well as having fun, was able to see and apply to real life situations which made it more enjoyable.
The Nursing Informatics class was inspiring and motivating and fun. The weekly threaded discussions reinforced and met my expectations of the course requirements, as well as SL, TANIC self-assessment, scavenger hunt activities. Other course requirements included a PPT and health IT paper we had to develop.

make and correct mistakes. The environment is also supported by VLE staff who encourage students as they move through the different activities.

Exemplar 1 (Box 17.1) defines steps used, including an initial assessment of competencies, then describes activities and education used to develop skills through the core course, Foundations of Nursing Informatics. The TIGER-based Assessment of Nursing Informatics Competencies (TANIC) tool was used to evaluate both the student and faculty skills.

Exemplar 2 (Box 17.2) defines steps used, including an initial assessment of competencies using the TANIC consistent with what students experienced, then describes activities and education used to develop skills through the core course immersion, Foundations of Nursing Informatics (refer to Box 17.2). The TANIC tool was used to evaluate both prefaculty and postfaculty skills.

EVALUATION PROCESS

The VLE/SL simulation process is evaluated through student feedback in a variety of ways. In Week 8 of the course, each student is asked to reflect on how they personally met and applied each one of the course outcomes in the threaded discussion area for that week. They are also graded using the structured process of a grading rubric each week; they complete formal written assignments as they progress through the different stations in SL. The VLE/SL process is evaluated informally by the course instructors because they are the frontline responders to students' complaints. This information is sent to the course leader (designer of the course) for resolution.

Both the instructors and students are supported by the VLE/SL staff who have helpline phone numbers and office hours posted for issues such navigating through the SL Islands and completing the assignments if they get "stuck." The VLE/SL staff created a complete orientation program with directions posted in Week 1 of the course so that students and interested faculty can develop avatars and then practice logging in and navigating through the islands as they complete simple tasks such as walking, sitting, and flying. Other issues such as content, grading issues and questions from instructors are addressed by the course leader/designer of the course. The course leader also serves as the mentor for faculty to help them understand the different processes and rationale for specific activities and the way that these apply to and meet program outcomes. Overall, the role of course leader/designer/mentor is enhanced by functioning in the instructor role, working closely with both students and faculty to ensure that they have a great experience.

CHALLENGES OF THE PROGRAM

There were obstacles to the full implementation of the program for faculty but not students. Some of the challenges include the following:

- After an initial **immersion** with the ANCC webinars on the basics of NI, developed by NI expert faculty, participants indicated "lack of time to take on additional tasks."
- There was a lack of interest in and understanding of NI and simulation.
- The perceived view was that NI is "difficult/too hard" based on anecdotal feedback and analysis after TANIC-based self-assessments.
- There was a lack of understanding of *where and how* simulation, but more so for NI, can be used in all nursing practice, in part due to lack of engagement in the orientation process.
- The perceptions were that NI is only about "data collection and analysis," is based on original and early literature, and "does not apply" to education programs.
- Insufficient stakeholder/leadership support was provided.
- Not all faculty are comfortable or "have time" to go through the VLE/SL orientation or learn the "new methodology."

Overall, the process of developing an innovative educational program with the integration of simulation, NI, and technology had few early adopters but more information and a greater understating of future needs provided many opportunities for additional education programs. Faculty understand better what is needed to be an effective teacher; students have an improved understanding of the value of simulation and the way that nursing informatics and technology are used in everyday practice.

KEY POINTS

- There are misconceptions of what and how a simulation environment can improve skills and knowledge when other opportunities are not available.
- After initial lack of understanding by students, NI core courses are a success, are well received, and are models for using simulation and technology as educational tools.

- Comments from students now expect it in "upcoming courses" and "excited to see how SL will be used in the future."
- The course example described here is an impressive example of the integration of simulation, NI, and technology as educational tools.
- As nurses in all healthcare settings become more familiar with technology, NI, and simulation being integrated in their practices, it will lead to a better understanding by faculty as they understand the skills needed to teach effectively.

SUMMARY

This chapter provides a description of an educational process used to develop and deploy a program of simulation previously lacking in the graduate program and now used to improve NI skills and knowledge for both student and faculty. The foundations and framework for this project are based on needs and mandates identified by industry, healthcare, and professional organizations such as the ANA, QSEN, and NLN.

REFLECTIVE QUESTIONS

1. How does NI impact simulation or simulation impact NI?
2. How is the FAST SIM© model used to integrate simulation, NI, and technology?
3. How do each—faculty, administrators, and students—impact the use of simulation, NI, and technology?
4. What are barriers or challenges to implementation of an education program that integrates simulation, NI, and technology?

REFERENCES

American Nurses Association. (2015). *Nursing informatics: Scope and standards of practice* (2nd ed.). Silver Spring, MD: Author.

Darvish, A., Bahramnezhad, F., Keyhanian, S., & Navidhamidi, M. (2014). The role of nursing informatics on promoting quality of health care and the need for appropriate education. *Global Journal of Health Science, 6*(6), 11–18. doi:10.5539/gjhs.v6n6p11

Farokhzadian, J., Khajouei, R., & Ahmadian, L. (2015). Information seeking and retrieval skills of nurses: Nurses' readiness for evidence based practice in hospitals of a medical university in Iran. *International Journal of Medical Informatics, 84*(8), 570–577. doi:10.1016/j.ijmedinf.2015.03.008

Hunter, K., McGonigle, D., & Hebda, T. (2013). The integration of informatics content in baccalaureate and graduate nursing education: A status report. *Nurse Educator, 38*(3), 110–113. doi:10.1097/NNE.0b013e31828dc292

Institute of Medicine. (2010). The future of nursing: Leading change, advancing health. Retrieved from http://iom.nationalacademies.org

Lilly, K., Fitzpatrick, J., & Madigan, E. (2015). Barriers to integrating information technology content in doctor of nursing practice curricula. *Journal of Professional Nursing, 31*(3), 187–199. doi:10.1016/j.profnurs.2014.10.005

McGonigle, D., Hunter, K., Sipes, C., & Hebda, T. (2014). Why nurses need to understand nursing informatics. *Association of Operating Room Nurses Journal, 100*(3), 324–327.

Quality and Safety Education for Nurses Initiative. (2014). Graduate KSAs. Retrieved from http://qsen.org/competencies/graduate-ksas

Rajalahti, E., Heinonen, J., & Saranto, K. (2014). Developing nurse educators' computer skills towards proficiency in nursing informatics. *Informatics for Health & Social Care, 39*(1), 47–66. doi:10.3109/17538157.2013.834344

Sipes, C., McGonigle, D., Hunter, K., Hebda, T., Hill, T., & Lamblin, J. (2015). Operationalizing the TANIC and NICA-L3/L4 tools to improve informatics competencies. Full paper presented at 13th International Congress in Nursing Informatics, Geneva, Switzerland.

Technology Informatics Guiding Education Reform. (2009). TIGER Informatics Competencies Collaborative (TICC) Final Report. Retrieved from http://tigercompetencies.pbworks.com/f/TICC_Final.pdf

SECTION IV

ADMINISTRATIVE PERSPECTIVE—NAVIGATING THE CHASM WHEN A PROFOUND DIFFERENCE EXISTS AMONG STAKEHOLDERS, VIEWPOINTS, AND FEELINGS REGARDING VIRTUAL SIMULATION

The administrator influence in the Faculty Administrators Students Technology Strategic Integration Model© (FAST SIM; Figure IV.1) is reflected in this section. While viewing this section, readers should reflect on how the administrator's influence in the model can be applied to the integration of technology in their specific teaching and learning context (Figure IV.2). Technologies, including virtual simulation, should reduce the administrative burden on faculty, thus allowing teachers to manage their workload more efficiently and give more time to individual student's educational needs.

Chapter 18 outlines the use of virtual simulation from an administrative perspective of the FAST SIM©. Administrators, such as deans, directors, and chairs of nursing schools, advocate to provosts and presidents for access to innovative teaching modalities. This chapter discusses the advantages and disadvantages of simulation integration, strategic planning, support and barriers to integration, and faculty requirements associated with technology integration and maintenance, and it offers ideas for developing and leveraging partnerships. Identifying the impact of incorporating virtual simulations to the nursing program and curriculum to the overall organization is critically important. Recognizing the fit with the faculty and students' vision, mission, and values depends on leadership to allow for time to reflect and integrate new methods.

Chapter 19 explores the financial, ethical, and legal implications that impact technological systems and curriculum. Administrators should be adaptable and innovative because their role is influenced by the educational environment. The administrator's role in technology integration includes being the strategic partnership organizer and industry champion, advocator, collaborator, team developer, budgeter, director, stakeholder, and technology user. Administrators can foster technology integration by providing faculty with support and training that are necessary to adopt new teaching modalities. The authors of this chapter illustrate the administrator's role with an insightful and relatable vignette.

IV: ADMINISTRATIVE PERSPECTIVE

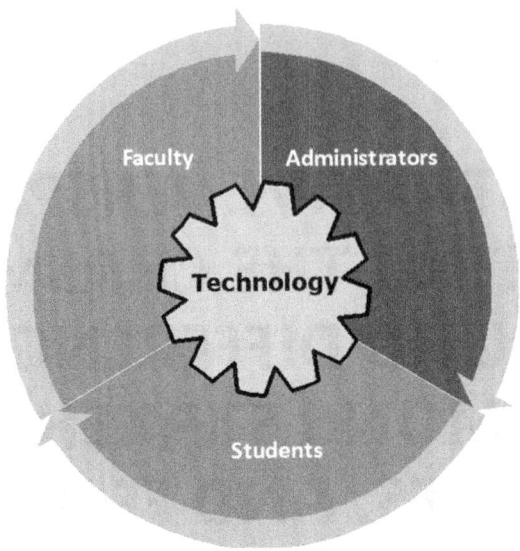

FIGURE IV.1 Components of FAST SIM© (Faculty Administrators Students Technology Strategic Integration Model).

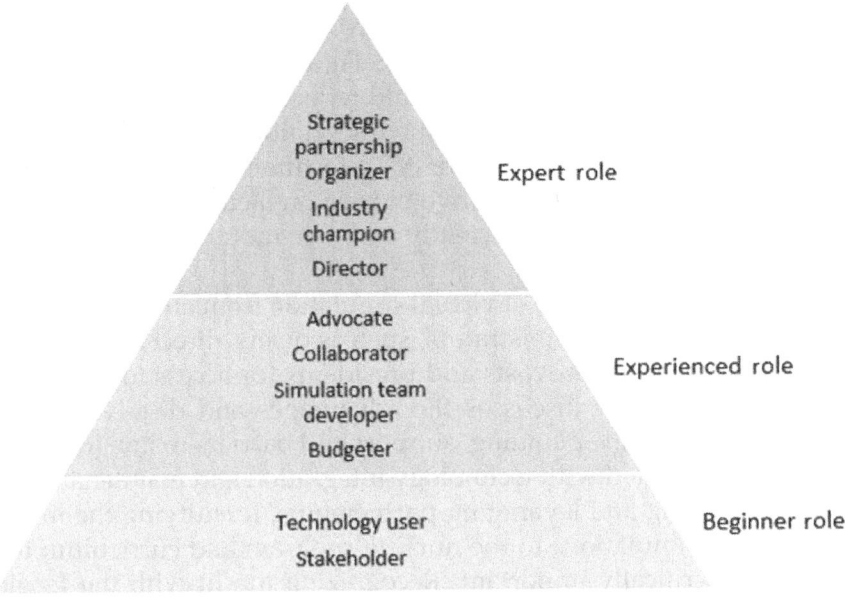

FIGURE IV.2 Administrator roles.

CHAPTER 18

Administrative Perspective

SUZANNE HETZEL CAMPBELL

LEARNING OBJECTIVES

Upon completion of this chapter, the reader will be able to:

- Recognize and outline increased pressures on higher education for the incorporation of innovative teaching methodologies.
- Assess the costs associated with integration of new technologies in both physical and human resources.
- Explore the challenges to incorporation of virtual simulation and similar technologies.
- Analyze options for faculty development and capacity building.
- Appreciate the hidden costs in time, expertise, and human resources.
- Formulate possible methods for adequate program planning and budget setting given this new and innovative way of teaching.

KEY TERMS

Faculty Learning Communities
Faculty professional development
Flexible Learning
Human patient simulators (HPS)
Innovative learning methodologies
Simulation-based-education
Virtual education
Virtual patient nursing activity model (vpNAM)
Virtual patients (VPs)
Virtual simulation

Higher education is transforming every single day, and the leaps and bounds we have experienced in nursing and health professional education in the past 10 to 15 years have been extensive. We have gone from classroom PowerPoint lectures and technical skills laboratories on static body parts to engaged education with high-fidelity simulation, learner-centered experiential teaching, and simulated and standardized patients, helping students learn to think, act, and reflect like nurses (Campbell, 2012; Campbell & Daley, 2017). Amid these changes in teaching methods and innovation has been a technological explosion that many nursing faculty struggle to keep up with and seek to incorporate and understand because their students demand a different way of teaching and learning. This has placed increasing demands on the expenses of providing higher education.

RELATION TO THE FACULTY ADMINISTRATORS STUDENTS TECHNOLOGY STRATEGIC INTEGRATION MODEL© (FAST SIM)

According to the model, the administrator at the beginner role should be able to assume the role of technology user and stakeholder. As administrators become more experienced in their role and with technology, they can assume the roles of simulation team developer, budgeter, and advocate. At the expert level, the administrator can act as a champion and strategic partnership organizer. Nurse administrator should ensure that the financial, ethical, and legal implications are considered while they reduce the administrative burden on educators so that educators can give more time to individual student's educational needs. Once a technology such as virtual simulation is adopted, the administrator must inform student services, advisers, marketing, faculty, and students so they are aware of the simulation goals and rationales for integration strategies.

SIMULATION-BASED EDUCATION

There is no argument that simulation-based education has a favorable effect on skill acquisition of health care professionals, confirmed initially in 1997 to have a large effect and larger metasyntheses of over 418 studies demonstrating a statistically significant ($p < .05$) stabilized small effect size (Cook, 2014). The evolution of the use of simulation in nursing has led to best practice standards (International Nursing Association for Clinical Simulation and Learning [INACSL], 2016), simulation standard guidelines for integration into nursing pedagogy and curriculum (Alexander et al., 2015), and a repository for instruments to use in research on simulation (INACSL, 2015). One area that is often not acknowledged is the cost in maintaining these programs and the cost of developing faculty with new skills for experiential learning, perhaps best served by developing consortiums (Jeffries et al., 2013) and memos of understanding between academic and practice institutions (BC Provincial Simulation Coordination Committee [BCPSCC], 2013; McDougall, 2015). We see a wide gap between the resources provided to various schools for clinical learning areas, even within our own states and provinces—and yet because of the dwindling clinical placement opportunities, acuity levels of patients, and high expectations of our new graduates, these clinical learning and simulation centers have become necessary. It is apparent that practicing clinical scenarios in high-fidelity situations, where vital signs, bodily functions, and voice responses assist students to critically think through situations and provide simulated care with physiological and "human" responses, leads to improved learning that is sustainable over time (Hayden, Smiley, Alexander, Kardong-Edgren, & Jeffries, 2014).

Virtual reality simulation has gained popularity (Foronda, Godsall, & Trybulski, 2012) and has been used for medication administration (Vottero, 2014), decontamination (Ulrich, Farra, Smith, & Hodgson, 2014), diagnostic reasoning (Duff, Miller, & Bruce, 2016), disaster triage (Foronda et al., 2016; Olson, Scheller, Larson, Lindeke, & Edwardson, 2010), and nontechnical skills such as empathy (Bearman, Palermo, Allen, & Williams, 2015).

Similarly, virtual education is occurring with the use of Second Life® (SL); care of virtual communities (Aebersold, Fenske, & Gonzalez, 2012) and multiple examples of the use of avatars for nursing education, including mental health, inclusivity, and team training (Aebersold, Tschannen, Stephens, Anderson, & Lei, 2011; Caylor, Aebersold, Lapham, & Carlson, 2014; Hermanns & Kilmon, 2011; Honey, Connor, Veltman, Bodily, & Diener, 2011; Irwin & Coutts, 2015; Kidd, Knisley, & Morgan, 2012; Sweigart, Burden, Carlton, & Fillwalk, 2013; Sweigart & Carlton, 2009; Tiffany, 2011; Tiffany & Hoglund, 2013; Tiffany & Hoglund, 2016; Tschannen, Aebersold, McLaughlin, Bowen, & Fairchild, 2012). A systematic review of the use of SL in undergraduate nursing programs concluded that although evaluation research is at an early stage, initial studies demonstrate a positive learning outcome with the use of Second Life (Irwin & Coutts, 2015).

Finally, our knowledge of the neuroscience behind learning continues to grow; interconnections between the body's biological, chemical, and physiological dynamics increase our awareness of interconnections between circuits in the brain and biochemical reactions that can affect cognition and learning. Early work by Seigel (2007) proposes a neurobiological theory based on the integration of right and left brain function, values combining memorization with learning to create new neural pathways and increase significant learning. Other authors purport how the brain learns (Sousa, 2011) by considering mindful learning and an examination of neuroscience and simulation (Cardoza, 2011). Simulation, virtual or real, has the ability to promote cognitive (i.e., critical thinking) and metacognitive (i.e., reflective thinking) skills, thereby integrating right and left brain functioning and leading to learning experiences that shape the growth of the nursing student from novice to expert (Benner, 1982).

The complexity of the clinical environment, barriers in place for clinical education, and silos between academic and practice continues—might online education and virtual simulation be part of the answer?

ADMINISTRATIVE SUPPORT ROLE

The most important roles of academic administrators are managing the expectations and fears of faculty, staff, and students and creating a safe environment for teaching and learning. When it comes to virtual simulation and technology-enhanced teaching and learning, the fears can be many and vary, given the age and background of both faculty and students. In the framework for simulation learning in nursing education (Daley & Campbell, 2009, 2017a), the "digital culture" and individual experiences that students bring to the learning situation are important considerations. This goes for faculty as well. In managing faculty fears, it is important to look at some key areas that faculty express fears about, including the following:

- Issues surrounding their continued employment, own professional development, and informatics literacy:
  - I'll be replaced.
  - I'll never get the hang of it.
  - I don't have the time to change the way I teach.
  - What about all the "content" I have to cover (content focus vs. concept focus)?

- Issues related to the development of innovative learning experiences:
  - What if the technology doesn't work?
  - What if students do something unanticipated?
  - How do I react, debrief, and guide the discussion/interaction back on track?
  - How do I assess/evaluate learning (formative vs. summative, tasks vs. skills, and clinical decision making)?
  - How will I balance the extra work (development, assessment, on-line presence)?
- Issues related to career trajectory:
  - Who owns the intellectual property of created scenarios and learning experiences?
  - Author credit and recognition—how do they count?
  - What is the impact on tenure and the promotion process?
  - What about student evaluations?

An integrative review of barriers and enablers to using high-fidelity human patient simulators (HPS) in nurse education found that "lack of time, fear of technology, and workload issues were among the top-10 barriers (Al-Ghareeb & Cooper, 2016). In contrast, educators in this integrative review, and those this author has worked closely with in the past 10 years on three editions of *Simulation Scenarios for Nursing Educators: Making it Real* (3rd ed.) (Campbell & Daley, 2017), found themselves enabled to use this new technology when they were provided professional development, felt supported by administration, and had a dedicated simulation coordinator (Al-Ghareeb & Cooper, 2016).

- Faculty hopes for the use of simulation include the following:
  - Student outcomes will improve.
  - Students will enjoy the experience and realize how much they know.
  - Students will become curious, find it fun, and be satisfied with their learning while increasing their confidence in their emerging role as a professional nurse.
  - I will be able to work *smarter* and not *harder* and accomplish my goal of educating the next generation of nurses.

In a provincial report on the use of simulation in British Columbia, Canada, responders were asked the level of importance of human resources and support. Findings identified that "leadership support for simulation events and/or centre was recorded as the highest priority after funding. Technician support and train-the-educator sessions were ranked in the top 5 out of 14 in terms of priority" (BCPSCC, 2013, p. 17).

Faculty and staff professional development, especially for those who may be uncomfortable with new technology and new ways of teaching, is of the utmost importance and requires involving such faculty in the process, providing support for changes (e.g., funding, professional development opportunities), and helping them marshal forward with recognition of champions and successes.

Similarly, students share misconceptions and fears that need to be managed. These include the following:
- Misconceptions—informatics literacy and course requirements:
  - I'm a computer whiz. (Just because they can play video games and post on Facebook and Instagram does not mean they have the informatics literacy necessary for course management systems or professional use of informatics for education and health care practice.)
  - Faculty will be available 24/7; therefore, I deserve an immediate response.
  - Why am I paying for a course if I have to do all the work myself?
  - Online courses are less work, and I don't need to do any prep.
- Fears related to actual simulated learning experiences follow:
  - What if I don't know the answer?
  - Will this be graded?
  - What happens if I submit my answers and they disappear, the computer crashes, or my Wi-Fi cannot handle the bandwidth for the lesson?
  - Will it be videotaped/audio-recorded and end up on YouTube?
  - What if others laugh at my responses?
  - What if I fail?

Orientation to the platform for virtual simulation education, similar to the pre-briefing and preparation for in-person simulations, is necessary. Incorporating a short quiz to help students identify areas where they need assistance or increased skills, creating a list of frequently asked questions, walking students through a virtual simulation in the classroom [and allowing them to follow along on their own devices if feasible] are just a few options for increasing student comfort. Clear guidelines should be provided in the course syllabus regarding the role of virtual simulations: where they fit in the grading scheme, how the assignment will be graded (i.e., a rubric with clearly identified learning outcomes and expectations); what the faculty role is; and what the student role is. This will allay some of the faculty's and students' angst and lead to increased comfort with the new technology.

TECHNOLOGY EXPLORATION: VIRTUAL TECHNOLOGY MEDIATED LEARNING

Virtual technology and mediated learning is not new. In 2001, authors were describing the use of the software SimCity® for examining community health priorities by exploring environmental issues in the real world (Bareford, 2001). Gaming research has demonstrated the present generation's fascination with video games and ways that the critical thinking/problem solving of this methodology can make a difference in student learning. Serious games are on the horizon, as described in Chapter 11, and provide a version of virtual simulation that teaches both health care practitioners and students, as well as parents, about care for premature infants (Fonseca et al., 2014, 2015). Some of the other components of flexible learning include creating online modules for preparatory learning (reading, videos, instructor delivered lectures), so that when students are present in the classroom, the teaching involves more case-based learning, small group discussions, and/or demonstration of what is learned (Campbell, MacPhee, & Ryan, 2017). All of these opportunities address the different ways that students are socialized into a profession, learn the foundational skills so that they can incorporate them in real-life situations, and combine knowledge gained from a variety of sources: reading, practicing, and vicarious observation. Virtual simulation allows for a similar format of learning and, depending on how it is presented, provides opportunities for innovation, growth, and transfer of knowledge into the behaviors and attitudes expected of professional nurses.

TECHNOLOGY INTEGRATION ACROSS THE CURRICULUM (CREATING TECHSAVVY PRACTITIONERS PREPARED TO HANDLE THE CURRENT AND FUTURE TECHNOLOGY CHALLENGES AND INITIATIVES)

Integrating simulation across nursing curriculums is not a new concept (Daley & Campbell, 2017b), yet the research on "simulation education" has leaned towards high-fidelity simulators and laboratory-controlled scenarios. Simulation also includes virtual simulation and virtual patients (VPs), used to develop clinical reasoning skills within the nursing paradigm. Some of the advantages and challenges of virtual simulation follow.

Advantages
- Student outcomes and confidence are improved.
- Students/faculty are engaged in the learning process; It's made fun.
- Student curiosity is renewed.
- The classroom is connected to clinical experience.

Challenges
- Technology fails.
- Students behave in unexpected ways.
- Content is missing.
- Time and location scheduling are needed for running the virtual simulation.
- Administrative support is required.

Historically, nursing education programs have used simulation in a variety of ways to teach both technical and nontechnical skills (i.e., assessment and communication); clinical reasoning, prioritization, and delegation; and development of critical thinking for problem solving and teamwork. Simulation has been integrated pedagogically in a variety of ways, including integration throughout the curriculum, in preclass preparation, at the start of class observation and debriefing, or for specific scenarios for courses with leveled objectives. Simulation has been used for competency-based testing at various stages to assess student mastery of competencies individually or in teams. The evaluation can be formative, giving feedback for enhanced mastery, or summative, such as an Objective Clinical Structured Evaluations (OSCE) for end-of-program competency testing. This second form is also referred to as *high stakes testing*. Another way simulations have been used is by developing scenarios by concept so that they fit a variety of specialties and can be leveled by student capabilities.

Virtual simulation is one way of teaching and learning professional skills, without waiving patient safety, to supply knowledgeable, up-to-date, and skilled professionals without overwhelming educators or learners (Georg & Zary, 2014). The development of a virtual patient Nursing Activity Model (vpNAM) allowed adapting VPs to the nursing paradigm for the development of clinical reasoning skills in students and provided a basic template for systematically developing different types of VPs from a common model, allowing for shared pedagogical designs across technical solutions (Georg & Zary, 2014). This computer-based simulation referred to as *virtual patients* has been proposed to assist with the integration of acquired scientific knowledge, theory, and practice to promote clinical reasoning and critical thinking (Georg & Zary, 2014). Areas where the use of virtual simulation has been especially useful include those dedicated to psychiatric and mental health nursing. Low-cost, narrative-based VP simulation techniques for this population have been reportedly used as a web-based pilot course (Guise, Chambers, & Välimäki, 2012). Promotion of essential skills, including critical thinking, communication, delegation, and decision making, were amenable to e-learning environments, and the authors suggested that they may be advantageous when multilingual simulations are necessary (Guise et al., 2012).

As a starting point, it is suggested that virtual simulation can "enhance lecture or web-based courses, replicate high-risk clinical experiences, act as clinical makeup, foster intra-disciplinary and interdisciplinary education, and address practical challenges and barriers to contemporary nursing education" (Foronda & Bauman, 2014, p. 412). High-fidelity simulation is also pointed to as the answer for skill and behavior mastery for competent health care practitioners, deliberate practice, and integrated teaching methods such as simulation to bridge theory to actual patient care in clinical environments. Practice of critical skills, including communication, conflict management, and priority setting, are feasible via virtual simulation, and knowledge transfer from classroom to clinical setting is possible. Benefits include lower costs for virtual simulation compared with high-fidelity simulation; practice of nontechnical skills, including communication, teamwork, clinical judgment, and leadership skills; and overall improved student performance (Tschannen et al., 2012).

STRATEGIC PLANNING

Identify: Support and Barriers for Integration

Supporting faculty and staff for innovative teaching requires that identification of supports and barriers and a strategic plan for success be paramount. Cost-effectiveness of simulation programs has been hard to prove, and a systematic review demonstrates infrequent and incomplete reporting of costs when instructional approaches are compared (Adamson & Prion, 2016; Zendejas, Wang, Brydges, Hamstra, & Cook, 2013).

- Create a budget plan and university support for a variety of options:
  - Development of virtual simulations in house
  - Development of videos, learning modules, and foundational provisions

- Unknowns: number of students/class and actual faculty time in marking, emailing, providing insight, and guiding students
- Changing costs of technology: As universities change platforms, will the new platform allow the flexibility and needs of the virtual simulation environment?
- Identify a faculty professional development strategy.
    - Create in-house faculty learning communities (Cox, 2004).
    - Collaborate with regional schools of nursing and share resources for workshop development.
    - Locate endowment funds for sending faculty to conferences.
    - Purchase online learning resource licenses for use by all faculty.
- Identify the challenges:
    - Refer to the hidden costs in time, expertise, and human resources.
    - Identify methods for adequate program planning and budget setting, given this new and innovative way of teaching.
- Identify the opportunities:
    - Analyze options for faculty development and capacity building.
    - Create in-house resources.
    - Build capacity—create administrative foundation for success.
    - Identify a budget that considers all of the costs for implementing a high-quality program.
    - Develop collaborative partnerships.
        - Consortiums (Jeffries et al., 2013)
            - Venues for health care and educational institutions with shared goals to pool knowledge, monies, and labor covering a geographic area
            - Individual organizations that collaborate and develop strategic planning goals to transform clinical education and improve patient care
            - Collaborate and network with others to overcome common barriers
        - Memorandum of understanding (MOU or MoU; BCPSCC, 2013; McDougall, 2015)
            - Sharing of space and resources
            - Team planning—crisis resource management for trauma or emergency care (i.e., disaster preparedness)
            - Performance of in situ or planned interprofessional simulations virtually (i.e., medication reconciliation)

Buy-In

The beginning step is to identify champions. Champion educators tend to demonstrate an innovative teaching style, they recognize the use of a variety of methods to meet the various learning styles of the students, and they often are early adopters of new technology and methods. For champions in the area of simulation, it helps if they recognize how case studies can be used to incorporate themes such as communication, end-of-life care, and social justice. Helping faculty share even simple, first steps toward innovation encourages others to join, and getting students involved (i.e., writing cases, evaluating their peers, exploring new technologies) is a good way to expand the enthusiasm and joy of learning. For example, students' assistance in developing cases from learned experiences in clinical environments and incorporating the necessary technology leads to excellent learning opportunities.

In developing a strategic plan for the incorporation of innovative teaching methods, it is important to remember that faculty cannot do it all. Specialized support for information technology (IT), laboratory assistants, and a director of the simulation/clinical learning center is important. One example can be hiring "tech-rovers," work/learn students who work with faculty on developing their virtual simulations tied to their course objectives and outcomes.

Another important component of the strategic plan needs to include a way of measuring outcomes and evaluation, especially return on investment. It may be necessary to configure laboratory fees that include some of these expenses, and this can be difficult in systems where there are freezes on tuition costs or student fees. There is no doubt that it is more expensive to educate health professional students than other students. For nursing, this is related to the clinical-faculty ratios required for clinical supervision and is increasingly related to the costs of simulated and clinical learning environments.

Ongoing Faculty Professional Development

Professional development for faculty and staff have been identified as top priorities for most simulation programs. This can include conference attendance, workshop days, curricular planning and integration as new curriculums are rolling out, even webinars and online learning. Locally, finding a way to have champions' showcase what they are doing in a nonthreatening way helps to encourage others to try something new. Providing peer-mentoring and evaluation can also assist. Having prepared simulation scenarios that can provide templates and guidelines for scenario development can also help (Campbell & Daley, 2017; vSim, 2015). Having students help in the creation of simulations or forming consortiums to bring together academic and practice partners to work together to prepare shared, clinically relevant simulations are strategies for building capacity.

Providing regional conferences and Simulation User Networks (SUNs) is another way for professional development and building capacity. Finally, the centers for teaching and learning, educational excellence, and education department colleagues within your institution should be used to determine out what services are offered and if there is any funding for course development and transition will also help. Recognizing that initial development of a course incorporating simulation takes more time and energy, especially if the faculty and staff are new to it, means calculating carefully the workload and creating a realistic estimate of input/output. Creative ideas, such as using teaching assistants (TAs), can help with the development of new simulations for a course; other approaches are assigning co-teaching, two faculty working together, and pairing of faculty with skill sets in different areas that will complement each other and provide the least amount of burden for all.

Student Orientation and Socialization Into the Profession of Nursing and the Role of Technology

Nursing education is about orienting and socializing students into the profession of nursing. Through the use of simulation, opportunities for the use of electronic health records, policy and protocol search technology, and credible resources are available to students so that they can learn to search for what they need. Virtual simulation provides an opportunity for many creative methods to be incorporated for student learning. Creating methods for assessment and evaluation that provides students with timely feedback and support is of utmost importance.

Organizational Impact

It is important to identify the impact of incorporating virtual simulations into the nursing program and curriculum and to the overall organization. Recognizing the fit with the faculty and students' vision, mission, and values depends on leadership that allows for time to reflect and integrate new methods. Taking small steps and celebrating victories is important. Creating opportunities for fun—video competitions, community or patient-naming options, team competition for most efficient and patient-centered resolutions for virtual simulations/VPs and communities—is also important. A few highlights to map the organizational impact include the following:

1. Strategies for success: viability, scalability, and sustainability
2. Incorporation of innovative teaching including virtual simulation (Foronda & Bauman, 2014) into the strategic plan, with identified resources, budgets, staff, and support
3. Incorporation of research, including return on investment (ROI), transfer of knowledge, and reality of worthiness of method (i.e., how much is enough, how much can be substituted, is mastery of competencies still being demonstrated?)
4. Funding, including maintenance, updates, research, and professional development

The success of integration of new technology into teaching the next generation of nurse leaders relies in part on administrators who can support faculty's innate curiosity and sense of fun in creating opportunities for playful, educational, and knowledge-translating learning. The benefits are real for faculty, students, and most importantly, patients.

KEY POINTS

- Higher education is transforming every day, and there is no argument against simulation-based education having a favorable effect on skill acquisition of healthcare professionals.
- Virtual simulation could provide a solution for, while addressing the complexity of, the clinical environment, barriers in place for clinical education, and silos between academic and practice.
- The most important roles of academic administrators are managing the expectations and fears of faculty and providing professional development for faculty and staff, especially those who may be uncomfortable with new technology and new ways of teaching.

- Virtual simulation is one way of teaching and learning professional skills without waiving patient safety to supply knowledgeable, up-to-date, and skilled professionals
- Beginning steps are to identify champions and plan for the incorporation of innovative teaching methods.
- It is important to remember that faculty cannot do it all, and professional development should be identified as top priority for most simulation programs.
- The success of integration of new technology into teaching the next generation of nurse leaders relies in part on administrators who can support faculty's innate curiosity and sense of fun in creating opportunities for playful, educational, and knowledge translating learning.

SUMMARY

This chapter explored the use of virtual simulation from an administrative perspective. Nursing education is moving from PowerPoint lectures and technical skills laboratories on static body parts to engaged learning with high-fidelity simulation, learner-centered experiential teaching, and simulated and standardized patients, all of which help students learn to think, act, and reflect like nurses. Virtual simulation is one way of teaching and learning professional skills, assisting with the integration of acquired scientific knowledge, theory, and practice to promote clinical reasoning and critical thinking.

As administrators, we can either participate and lead or observe and follow the transformative changes occurring in higher education today. It is imperative that we take an active part in this transformative process. Administrators, deans, directors, and chairs of nursing schools must consider how they can advocate to their provosts and presidents for access to innovative ways of learning such as virtual simulation. Administrators must also keep faculty and students in mind. Amid these changes in teaching methods and innovation, there has been a technological explosion that many nursing faculty are struggling to keep up with, and faculty are seeking to incorporate and understand because their students mandate a different way of teaching and learning. This has placed increasing demands on the costs of providing higher education. This chapter explored ways in which administrators can support faculty and students while enhancing the educational experience at their institutions. It is important that administrators manage faculty and student expectations and needs while assessing university support for a variety of options; they must address the challenges and opportunities, including consideration of all the costs for implementing a high-quality program, and explore ideas for leveraging support by developing partnerships. Administrators must assume responsibility for their roles because they are in a position to influence the success or failure of innovative virtual simulation learning experiences.

REFLECTIVE QUESTIONS

1. When you are looking at the big picture, how do you conceptualize and plan for the integration of technology, especially virtual worlds? What are the top-2 priorities you must keep in mind?
2. How do you explain virtual simulations to your administrators, staff, faculty, and students? Is it one message, or should you create targeted messages addressing each group's needs, concerns, and benefits?

3. As the administrator of 50 full-time faculty members who do not like technology and state it openly, how would you plan to incorporate virtual simulation into your curriculum? Provide a rationale for each plan of action you would take.
4. Describe in detail how virtual simulation can address the complexity of the clinical environment. With whom would you share this information at your institution? Explain why you would choose this person.

REFERENCES

Adamson, K. A., & Prion, S. (2016). Making sense of methods and measurement: Cost-effectiveness research. *Clinical Simulation in Nursing, 12*(2), 49–50. doi:10.1016/j.ecns.2015.10.009

Aebersold, M., Fenske, C., & Gonzalez, L. (2012). Using virtual communities as context for education. *Clinical Simulation in Nursing, 8*(8), e386–e387. doi:10.1016/j.ecns.2012.07.005

Aebersold, M., Tschannen, D., Stephens, M., Anderson, P., & Lei, X. (2011). Second Life: A new strategy in educating nursing students. *Clinical Simulation in Nursing, 8*(9), e469–e475. doi:10.1016/j.ecns.2011.05.002

Al-Ghareeb, A. Z., & Cooper, S. J. (2016). Barriers and enablers to the use of high-fidelity patient simulation manikins in nurse education: an integrative review. *Nurse Education Today, 36*, 281–286. doi:10.1016/j.nedt.2015.08.005

Alexander, M., Durham, C. F., Hooper, J. I., Jeffries, P. R., Goldman, N., Kardong-Edgren, S. S., . . . Tillman, C. (2015). NCSBN simulation guidelines for prelicensure nursing programs. *Journal of Nursing Regulation, 6*(3), 39–42. doi:10.1016/S2155-8256(15)30783-3

Bareford, C. G. (2001). Community as client: Environmental issues in the real world: A SimCity computer simulation. *Computers in Nursing, 19*(1), 11–16.

BC Provincial Simulation Coordination Committee. (2013). *BC simulation current state report.* Retrieved from http://med.ubc.ca/files/2014/01/PSCC-Current-State-Report-2013-12-04.pdf

Bearman, M., Palermo, C., Allen, L. M., & Williams, B. (2015). Learning empathy through simulation: A systematic literature review. *Simulation in Healthcare, 10*(5), 308–319. doi:10.1097/sih.0000000000000113

Benner, P. (1982). From novice to expert. *American Journal of Nursing, 82*(3), 402–407.

Campbell, S. H. (2012). Role-playing: An underutilized tool for teaching students to think, act, and reflect like a nurse. *Clinical Simulation in Nursing, 8*(7), e261–e262. doi:10.1016/j.ecns.2011.05.001

Campbell, S. H., & Daley, K. (Eds.). (2017). *Simulation scenarios for nursing educators: Making it real* (3rd ed.). New York, NY: Springer Publishing.

Campbell, S. H., MacPhee, M., & Ryan, M. (2017). Innovative approaches to simulation-based faculty development. In S. H. Campbell & K. Daley (Eds.), *Simulation scenarios for nursing educators: Making it real* (3rd ed., pp. 37–46). New York, NY: Springer Publishing.

Cardoza, M. P. (2011). Neuroscience and simulation: An evolving theory of brain-based education. *Clinical Simulation in Nursing, 7*(6), e205–e208. doi:10.1016/j.ecns.2011.08.004

Caylor, S., Aebersold, M., Lapham, J., & Carlson, E. (2014). The use of virtual simulation and a modified TeamSTEPPS™ training for multiprofessional education. *Clinical Simulation in Nursing, 11*(3), 163–171. doi:10.1016/j.ecns.2014.12.003

Cook, D. A. (2014). How much evidence does it take? A cumulative meta-analysis of outcomes of simulation-based education. *Medical Education, 48*(8), 750–760. doi:10.1111/medu.12473

Cox, M. D. (2004). Introduction to faculty learning communities. *New Directions for Teaching and Learning, 97*, 5–23. doi:10.1002/tl.129

Daley, K., & Campbell, S. H. (2009). Framework for simulation learning in nursing education. In S. H. Campbell & K. Daley (Eds.), *Simulation scenarios for nurse educators: Making it real.* (2nd ed., pp. 287–290). New York, NY: Springer Publishing.

Daley, K., & Campbell, S. H. (2017a). Framework for simulation learning in nursing education. In S. H. Campbell & K. Daley (Eds.), *Simulation scenarios for nursing educators: Making it real* (3rd ed., pp. 13–18). New York, NY: Springer Publishing.

Daley, K., & Campbell, S. H. (2017b). Integrating simulation-focused pedagogy into curriculum. In S. H. Campbell & K. Daley (Eds.), *Simulation scenarios for nursing educators: Making it real* (3rd ed., pp. 19–26). New York, NY: Springer Publishing.

Duff, E., Miller, L., & Bruce, J. (2016). Online virtual simulation and diagnostic reasoning: A scoping review. *Clinical Simulation in Nursing, 12*(9), 377–384. doi:10.1016/j.ecns.2016.04.001

Fonseca, L. M. M., Aredes, N. D. A., Dias, D. M. V., Scochi, C. G. S., Martins, J. C. A., & Rodrigues, M. A. (2015). Serious game e-Baby: nursing students' perception on learning about preterm newborn clinical assessment. *Revista Brasileira de Enfermagen, 68*(1), 9–14. doi:10.1590/0034-7167.2015680102i

Fonseca, L. M. M., Dias, D. M. V., Góes, F. D. S. N., Seixas, C. A., Scochi, C. G. S., Martins, J. C. A., & Rodrigues, M. A. (2014). Development of the e-Baby serious game with regard to the evaluation of oxygenation in preterm babies: contributions of the emotional design. *Computers, Informatics, Nursing, 32*(9), 428–436. doi:10.1097/CIN.0000000000000078

Foronda, C., & Bauman, E. B. (2014). Strategies to incorporate virtual simulation in nurse education. *Clinical Simulation in Nursing, 10*(8), 412–418. doi:10.1016/j.ecns.2014.03.005

Foronda, C., Godsall, L., & Trybulski, J. (2012). Virtual clinical simulation: The state of the science. *Clinical Simulation in Nursing, 9*(8), e279–e286. doi:10.1016/j.ecns.2012.05.005

Foronda, C. L., Shubeck, K., Swoboda, S. M., Hudson, K. W., Budhathoki, C., Sullivan, N., & Hu, X. (2016). Impact of virtual simulation to teach concepts of disaster triage. *Clinical Simulation in Nursing, 12*(4), 137–144. doi:10.1016/j.ecns.2016.02.004

Georg, C., & Zary, N. (2014). Web-based virtual patients in nursing education: Development and validation of theory-anchored design and activity models. *Journal of Medical Internet Research, 16*(4), e105. doi:10.2196/jmir.2556

Guise, V., Chambers, M., & Välimäki, M. (2012). What can virtual patient simulation offer mental health nursing education? *Journal of Psychiatric and Mental Health Nursing, 19*(5), 410–418. doi:10.1111/j.1365-2850.2011.01797.x

Hayden, J. K., Smiley, R. A., Alexander, M., Kardong-Edgren, S., & Jeffries, P. R. (2014). The NCSBN National simulation study: A longitudinal, randomized, controlled study replacing clinical hours with simulation in prelicensure nursing education. *Journal of Nursing Regulation, 5*(2), C1–S64. Retrieved from http://mtcahn.org/wp-content/uploads/2015/12/JNR_Simulation_Supplement-2015.pdf

Hermanns, M., & Kilmon, C. (2011). Second Life® as a clinical conference environment: Experience of students and faculty. *Clinical Simulation in Nursing, 8*(7), e297–e300. doi:10.1016/j.ecns.2011.04.002

Honey, M., Connor, K., Veltman, M., Bodily, D., & Diener, S. (2011). Teaching with Second Life: Hemorrhage management as an example of a process for developing simulations for multiuser virtual environments. *Clinical Simulation in Nursing, 8*(3), e79–e85. doi:10.1016/j.ecns.2010.07.003

International Nursing Association for Clinical Simulation and Learning. (2015). Repository of instruments used in simulation research. Retrieved from http://www.inacsl.org/i4a/pages/index.cfm?pageID=3496

International Nursing Association for Clinical Simulation and Learning. (2016). Standards of best practice: Simulation. *Clinical Simulation in Nursing, 12*, S48–S50. doi:10.1016/j.ecns.2016.10.001

Irwin, P., & Coutts, R. (2015). A systematic review of the experience of using Second Life in the education of undergraduate nurses. *Journal of Nursing Education, 54*(10), 572–577. doi:10.3928/01484834-20150916-05

Jeffries, P. R., Battin, J., Franklin, M., Savage, R., Yowler, H., Sims, C., . . . Dorsey, L. (2013). Creating a professional development plan for a simulation consortium. *Clinical Simulation in Nursing, 9*(6), e183–e189. doi:10.1016/j.ecns.2012.02.003

Kidd, L., Knisley, S., & Morgan, K. (2012). Effectiveness of a Second Life: Simulation for undergraduate mental health nursing students. *Clinical Simulation in Nursing, 8*(8), e408. doi:10.1016/j.ecns.2012.07.072

McDougall, E., M. (2015). Simulation in education for health care professionals. *BCMJ, 57*(10), 444–448.

Olson, D. K., Scheller, A., Larson, S., Lindeke, L., & Edwardson, S. (2010). Using gaming simulation to evaluate bioterrorism and emergency readiness education. *Public Health Reports, 125*(3), 468–477. doi:10.1177/003335491012500316

Seigel, D. (2007). *The mindful brain: Reflection and attunement in the cultivation of well-being*. New York, NY: W. W. Norton.

Sousa, D. A. (2011). *How the brain learns*. London, UK: Corwin, Sage Co.

Sweigart, L., Burden, M., Carlton, K. H., & Fillwalk, J. (2013). Virtual simulations across curriculum prepare nursing students for patient interviews. *Clinical Simulation in Nursing, 10*(3), e139–e145. doi:10.1016/j.ecns.2013.10.003

Sweigart, L., & Carlton, K. H. (2009). Volunteer clients and Second Life virtual experiences change the landscape of health appraisal across the lifespan. *Clinical Simulation in Nursing, 5*(3), e152. doi:10.1016/j.ecns.2009.04.079

Tiffany, J. M. (2011). Second Life®: An innovative strategy for teaching inclusivity to nursing students. *Clinical Simulation in Nursing, 7*(6), e265–e266. doi:10.1016/j.ecns.2011.09.075

Tiffany, J. M., & Hoglund, B. A. (2013). Teaching/learning in Second Life: Perspectives of future nurse-educators. *Clinical Simulation in Nursing, 10*(1), e19–e24. doi:10.1016/j.ecns.2013.06.006

Tiffany, J. M., & Hoglund, B. A. (2016). Using virtual simulation to teach inclusivity: A case study. *Clinical Simulation in Nursing, 12*(4), 115–122. doi:10.1016/j.ecns.2015.11.003

Tschannen, D., Aebersold, M. L., McLaughlin, E., Bowen, J., & Fairchild, J. (2012). Use of virtual simulations for improving knowledge transfer among baccalaureate nursing students. *Journal of Nursing Education and Practice, 2*(3), 15–24. doi:10.5430/jnep.v2n3p15

Ulrich, D., Farra, S., Smith, S., & Hodgson, E. (2014). The student experience using virtual reality simulation to teach decontamination. *Clinical Simulation in Nursing, 10*(11), 546–553. doi:10.1016/j.ecns.2014.08.003

Vottero, B. A. (2014). Proof of concept: Virtual reality simulation of a pyxis machine for medication administration. *Clinical Simulation in Nursing, 10*(6), e325–e331. doi:10.1016/j.ecns.2014.03.001

vSim. (2015). *vSim for nursing: Medical-surgical*. Wolter Kluwer Health/NLN/Laerdal. Retrieved from https://thepoint.lww.com/book/show/446600#/CoursePointContent/Show/c7c81e79-b0cd-4128-865b-375a0103c8c4?forceView=False&viewMode=Student&productAssetId=c7c81e79-b0cd-4128-865b-375a0103c8c4&behavior=Display&groupby=learningactivity&ts=1481871147507

Zendejas, B., Wang, A. T., Brydges, R., Hamstra, S. J., & Cook, D. A. (2013). Cost: The missing outcome in simulation-based medical education research: A systematic review. *Surgery, 153*(2), 160–176. doi:10.1016/j.surg.2012.06.025

CHAPTER 19

Administrator Role

DEE McGONIGLE AND RANDY M. GORDON

LEARNING OBJECTIVES

Upon completion of this chapter, the reader will be able to:
- Assess the role of the administrator in relation to the success or failure of technology integration strategies.
- Explore ways in which the administrator can facilitate technology integration.
- Investigate and garner support for opportunities to integrate simulation within the nursing curriculum.

KEY TERMS

Advocates
Budget
Collaborative
Direct costs
Elevator pitch
Indirect costs
Pitch
Stakeholders
Strategic partnership
Technology
Virtual simulation

Administrators must be adaptable and creative because their role is rapidly changing in the international educational ecosystem. Higher education is experiencing dwindling funding, and the need to maintain competitive tuition further limits the amount of money available. As administrators struggle to prioritize needs in relation to financial constraints, they must be able to acquire the resources necessary to maintain the continuous advances, innovation, and change essential for their institution to remain viable and even flourish in this highly competitive educational marketplace. In the midst of this environment, the successful administrator must be able to encourage faculty to actively participate in the efforts to integrate **technology** across the curriculum to transform courses to meet learning outcomes and enhance the program. According to the Office of Educational Technology (2017),

> Institutions and faculty should continue to explore engaging learning experiences that leverage technology to reduce instructional costs for the institution and cost of tuition and fees for students. Institutions and researchers should work together to provide technology-enabled interventions that lower costs for students and apply evidence-based strategies to improve learning outcomes (p. 70).

Administrators must make a decisive, purposeful, realistic, and practical allocation of resources to lead and support the effort to adopt new, cost-effective, and learning enhancing instructional technologies (see Box 19.1). To set the stage for the integration of technology, especially virtual technology solutions, the organizational culture must change, and the necessary investments must be made for acquiring the resources to support the effort. According to Li, Lin, and Lai (2016), administrators can generate an innovative teaching and learning milieu that expects competence in instructional technology. Administrators must model, support and encourage

> **BOX 19.1 Creative Resource Acquisition and Allocation**
>
> In our financially constrained times, we must be creative in identifying, acquiring, and using resources other than money. Even though it is terrific if we have money available, allocating other resources can be just as or more important than locating the money necessary to fund a request. We typically talk about personnel, in-kind, time, money, and setting resources when we are trying to launch technology integration such as virtual simulation. The administrator must leverage personnel, other resources (in-kind), time, money, and settings to integrate technology to improve learning.
>
> **Personnel** are designated to technology integration project; the amount of time being purchased, donated, or exchanged per day, week, month, or year should be stipulated. Of course, we all would like to be able to receive donations. The astute administrator would develop and deploy the human resources available in a pragmatic, prescriptive way.
>
> **In-kind** means services, expertise, or products that would be provided to the project in lieu of money. This is a creative challenge since in-kind could refer to software or other resources that can be used to springboard your effort. Typically, a monetary value is placed on the services or products. You can barter for programming time by offering access to other services or products. You could exchange or trade talent or personnel skills for other talents/skills needed for this project. Some external grants allow you to provide in-kind resources and indicate the amount of money those services would be worth. Internal funding areas might also ask for in-kind, including infrastructure and expertise. You could list a new faculty's expertise in virtual simulation as in-kind and place a monetary value on this resource based on the number of hours allotted to the proposed project.
>
> **Time** is the amount of time that will be allocated to the project. The administrator must designate and accurately account for everyone's time in relation to the project, as well as make sure that the milestones or deadlines are met, with any associated deliverables being completed as promised. This is when the administrator must make sure that the project not only comes in on **budget** but also on time.
>
> **Money** refers to the direct allocation of money. The amount of money allocated must be sufficient to properly fund the project through its completion.

(continued)

> **BOX 19.1 Creative Resource Acquisition and Allocation (*continued*)**
>
> **Setting** refers to the location where the project will be completed. The administrator must be able to secure the location; they might need to dedicate a computer laboratory or room or another brick-and-mortar space. The setting might be virtual and include supporting or extending infrastructure access to remote personnel. One of the challenges with any team-related project is maintaining communication, sharing deliverables, and sustaining project momentum; these challenges are intensified when working with or remotely or with virtual teams.
>
> Administrators must also identify and appropriately allocate direct and indirect costs associated with the integration of technologies such as virtual simulation. **Direct costs** relate to a particular cost event or object; cost events or objects might be specific projects, products, or academic units. The materials used to develop the project and the labor costs are considered direct costs.
>
> **Indirect costs** are not associated with a specific product or project but reflect the day-to-day operational costs that reflect the company's cost of doing business or providing services—in the case of an academic institution, providing educational episodes. These are the costs incurred after the direct costs are calculated and are sometimes called the *real costs* of doing business or providing a service. As costs are assessed, everything that is a cost item must be calculated. Think of things that keep the doors open, such as utilities, rent, or mortgage payment, office equipment (including phones and computers, office supplies, even cleaning supplies). Indirect costs reflect anything and everything that has a cost associated with conducting the company's business. The administrator must be able to clearly show how direct and indirect costs relate to specific projects such as developing virtual simulation.

a cultural change that enhances the prescriptive integration of technology. The administrator must therefore strategically interface the financial resources, faculty, infrastructure support, staff members, other administrators, and stakeholders, and of course, students, to facilitate the successful transformation of the educational setting with technology.

RELATION TO THE FACULTY ADMINISTRATORS STUDENTS TECHNOLOGY STRAGIC INTEGRATION MODEL© (FAST SIM)

Nursing education administrators facilitate faculty development and active engagement in the area of **virtual simulation** and the use of technology in the teaching–learning process. The nurse administrator's role is to ensure that technological systems are transformed effectively and that financial, ethical, and legal implications are considered (Lucas, 2016). As technologies are explored, their advantages and disadvantages must be assessed. Technology tools should reduce the administrative burden on teachers and allow teachers to manage their workload more efficiently, and then be able to give more time to individual student's learning needs. Administrators must form **strategic partnerships** with student services, advisers, marketing, financial services, faculty, and students to develop rationales for the appropriate integration strategies to successfully meet the simulation goals.

ADMINISTRATOR'S ROLE IN TECHNOLOGY INTEGRATION

Strategic Partnership Organizer and Industry Champion

The administrator must enact organizational culture change by partnering and working with all internal and external **stakeholders** to develop a shared vision in relation to expectations for technology use that is aligned with the institution's mission, vision, and strategic plan. Based on this shared vision, a cooperative, collective, technology-enhanced plan is developed that is evidence-based and promotes institution-wide effective technology integration practices for other administrators, faculty, and students. This shared vision is critical to garner support for a sustained effort related to technology use.

The recognition and reward system within the institution must acknowledge the innovative and cost-savings efforts resulting from technology integration. Learning new technologies can require steep learning curves that can be time intensive. Typically, faculty are rewarded for publishing, presenting, and receiving funding, and they focus their efforts on these pursuits to attain tenure. As they prioritize their time, they cannot risk diluting their efforts by exploring and implementing innovative technologies that will not help them achieve their goal of tenure. Once tenured, these faculty have an established program of research and service that they must attend, and many do not deviate from their routine. The faculty who are hired without the possibility of tenure, designated as nontenure track faculty, are not motivated to adopt technologies for fear of poor student evaluations that could result in their termination. Without changing this rigid, restrictive reward system, innovative technology applications will not be explored willingly by the faculty.

Advocate and Collaborator

Administrators must lead the entire process of technology integration because they are responsible and accountable for developing and upholding a policy that is inclusive and supportive. Lucas (2016) believed that administrators are key to the adoption of instructional technology. "They have to encourage adoption and organizational change in as many ways as possible: appointing associate deans for classroom innovation, investments in technology and instructional designers, and by rewarding those who step forward to participate" (Lucas, para. 14). Innovative administrators establish a process to cultivate, develop, execute, monitor, maintain, evaluate, and replace or upgrade a systemic, total integrative technology plan to realize the shared vision; **advocates** for internal and external funding; makes informed decisions about the technology plan based on data and information; facilitates learner-centered technology integration in a **collaborative** culture of sharing, teaming, and supported educational opportunities for the stakeholders, faculty, and students; showcases technology integration successes and failures, instilling the project management process to capture these processes and lessons learned; and establishes and supports collaborative teaching and learning communities that empower faculty and students to transform learning.

Simulation Team Developer

Administrators must judiciously allocate the resources (e.g., financial, equipment, personnel, space or remote access, infrastructure) to ensure complete and sustained implementation of the shared vision's technology plan and innovative initiatives; foster continuous quality improvements to existing technologies while exploring new technologies and preparing for future technology integration based on the technology and implementation plan; and facilitate integrating and framing technology in the learning processes to prepare nursing students who are ready to work in technology-laden healthcare environments.

Director, Stakeholder, and Technology User

Administrators must ensure that the technology plan has robust assessment and evaluative components that are managed appropriately; make sure that the technologies are assessed and evaluated based on financial ramifications, access issues, privacy, security, learning, social, ethical, legal, communication, and applicable stakeholder productivity impact using multiple modalities; and role model the integration of technology when gathering data and information, analyzing and synthesizing the faculty and student comments, interpreting the results, and disseminating the findings to enhance teaching practice and student learning opportunities that are realized, as well as missed.

KEY POINTS

- Administrators play a critical role in how thoroughly, effectively, and comfortably technology is integrated and used in their institutions.
- The administrator must strategically and creatively interface with financial resources, faculty, infrastructure support, staff members, student services, other administrators, stakeholders, and, of course, students to develop rationales for the appropriate integration strategies to successfully meet the virtual simulation goals and facilitate the technological transformation of the educational setting.
- The recognition and reward system within the institution must acknowledge the innovative and cost-savings efforts resulting from technology integration.
- Administrators must lead the entire process of technology integration because they are responsible and accountable for developing and upholding a policy that is inclusive and supportive.
- The innovative administrator establishes a process to cultivate, develop, execute, monitor, maintain, evaluate, and replace or upgrade a systemic, totally integrative technology plan to realize the shared technology integrated vision.

SUMMARY

Technology is everywhere in our society, including in the educational arena. The administrator enacts diverse roles that can either facilitate or hinder the adoption of virtual simulation. In this chapter, we focused on the positive aspects of the administrator's roles as they relate to the integration of virtual simulation. The roles described provide a brief overview of the influence administrators can have on their institution's technology plan, faculty's willingness to engage in technology integration, and student learning. Visionary administrators are able to inspire, motivate, and support their faculty and students while paving the path to a smooth transition into virtual simulation integration. At times, the logistically and operationally minded constraints of their role might inhibit their role as visionaries and create an ambivalent environment (see Box 19.2).

> **BOX 19.2 A Snapshot in the Life of an Administrator**
>
> **8:00 a.m.**   You just get into the office and sit behind your desk.
>
> Your secretary tells you that a student is waiting to see you.
>
> You are ready to say "send him in" when the phone rings.
>
> The campus president is asking to meet with you at your earliest convenience. You explain that you have a student to see and you will be right over after that meeting.
>
> The student enters your office. Her complaints center around the technology she is asked to use in one of her courses, and the other three courses do not require additional technologies. She wants to know if she could have an alternate assignment and not comply with the faculty request to enter a virtual world and complete orientation.
>
> **WHAT WOULD YOU DO?**
>
> **What would your response be to this student?**
>
> **Would you notify the faculty member?**
>
> **8:30 a.m.**   You walk into the president's office, and he looks upset. He wants to know why there is a line item in the budget for ZZY Technology. Who approved this $5,000.00 disbursement? You explain that it was an internally funded request that was approved by the technology **integration team**. The president asks you to explain what this technology is all about.
>
> **WHAT WOULD YOU DO?**
>
> **What information should you be able to quickly impart?**
>
> **Would you contact the lead faculty for the technology integration team for assistance?**
>
> **9:00 a.m.**   Your president wants more information to share with the board of directors this evening. He wants to know what the return on investment will be and the number of students who will be exposed to this innovation, as well as other financial milestones. He wants to examine how these monies will be translated into actions that meet the articulated educational goals and objectives. You leave his office and go to the faculty member's office who is leading the technology integration team.

(continued)

BOX 19.2 A Snapshot in the Life of an Administrator (*continued*)	
	This lead faculty member has office hours at 10 a.m. and you plan to return then.
9:30 a.m.	After entering your office, you try to gather the necessary information from the reports that you were given. However, you notice that the financial statements are not robust enough to address all of the president's information needs.
10:00 a.m.	You arrive at the lead faculty's office.
	WHAT WOULD YOU DO?
	How would you approach this faculty member to gain the necessary information for your president?
	Would you suggest that the lead faculty schedule an immediate meeting with the team?
	Would you suggest that the lead faculty schedule an immediate meeting with the president?

TIPS/PEARLS

- Administrators must construct a vision where technologies play a critical part or function in the enhancement of teaching and learning. One of the best ways to get stakeholders on board is by attaching the financial considerations and the tipping point where they would realize a return on investment.
- As the technology plan is developed to integrate technologies, it is paramount to incorporate the assessment and evaluative schema, along with a solid research methodology to validate their use.
- Administrators must update and maintain their knowledge and skills related to instructional technologies. Visionary administrators are the ones who realize their deficits in relation to the technology and seek to understand the placement and use of these tools in their curricula.
- If you choose to approach your administrator outside of a scheduled meeting time, remember the idea of an **elevator pitch**. You want to make your key points in under a minute. You will most likely need to follow any **pitch** with a written proposal (refer to Appendix B).

REFLECTIVE QUESTIONS

1. You are an administrator of a medium school of nursing. You have five faculty interested in incorporating technology A and five other faculty interested in integrating technology B. You have only enough funding to grant one of the requests. How would you decide which one to fund?
2. A faculty member approaches you in the hall and asks if he could pilot a technology tool for a specific course. What should your initial response to this faculty member be and why would you choose this response?

3. A student enters your office, exasperated. He states that he really likes the virtual simulation in the virtual world but feels that his faculty member does not fully understand the tool and is not leveraging its potential. How do you respond to this student? What do you do next after the student leaves your office?

REFERENCES

Long, L., Canchu, L., & Guolin, L. (2016). Technology sensemaking by university administrators, faculty and staff: Unity and divergence. *International Journal of Technology in Teaching & Learning*, 12(1), 1–16.

Lucas, H. (2016). The higher education technology paradox. Retrieved from https://edtechmagazine.com/higher/article/2016/05/higher-education-technology-paradox

Office of Educational Technology. (2017). Reimagining the role of technology in higher education. Retrieved from https://tech.ed.gov/files/2017/01/Higher-Ed-NETP.pdf

EPILOGUE: FACULTY ADMINISTRATORS STUDENTS TECHNOLOGY STRATEGIC INTEGRATION MODEL©: ANALYSIS, SYNTHESIS, AND APPLICATION

As technologies emerge and administration and faculty pioneer, the learning landscape will continue to change dynamically. We have a collective responsibility to ensure that educational activities we associate ourselves with are conducted to the highest ethical standards. The convenience, the potential for innovation, and the opportunities to expand education in new and exciting ways are all temptations to fall into the trap of justifying the means with the ends. Throughout this text, you were challenged to reflect on your current learning setting and learning tools. It is important that we continually assess how we approach teaching and learning so that we can explore and integrate new instructional technologies.

The process of technology integration is continually shifting. Successful integration of technology with nursing curriculum is contingent on a myriad of contributing factors, not the least of which is that technology and curriculum continue to develop. A growing trend in nurse educator literature is the need to transform nursing education to include technology as a fundamental educational tool. The Faculty Administrators Students Technology Strategic Integration Model© (FAST SIM) provides a framework for the development of effective communication, as well as guidance, for the technology integration process. To achieve successful integration of technology with the nursing curriculum, the FAST SIM© posits that equal appreciation and recognition must be given to faculty, administrators, and students as significant contributors to the technology integration process. As stakeholders, all contributors find relevance in applying the model from their individual perspective and particular needs. Preparing the instructional environment for simulation requires attention to the key components of the FAST SIM©.

Opportunities for the use of virtual simulation in nursing education are vast, and the advantages for this teaching pedagogy are clear. The use of virtual simulation for clinical practicum hours, clinical experience consistency, standardized feedback, virtual patient assessment, deliberate practice of clinical skills, remote collaboration, and interprofessional education has been explored and is supported. Virtual simulation is a creative approach that provides interactive, engaging instruction. Whereas practice environments have become more complex, educational delivery methods have remained stagnant. Innovative technologies provide opportunities to enhance nursing student learning and help nursing programs become more responsive to changes in the practice environment; however, obstacles may hinder successful implementation. Concerns about cost, staffing, or the fit of the technology with the program's current culture may inhibit administrative support. Students may lack the interest or resources necessary to engage with nontraditional teaching strategies. The rapid pace of technological change, as well as the absence of research support for some educational technologies, may lead to hesitation about the adoption of technological tools, particularly virtual simulation.

All the stakeholders need sufficient knowledge and understanding of simulation appropriate to their role to successfully learn with this educational approach. Legal and financial issues can shape the way in which the simulations are designed and delivered. The faculty time involved to prepare simulations is an often overlooked but important factor. Access issues to the Internet may impact faculty and students who participate in simulation from remote locations. Despite the challenges, the rewards that come from learning through virtual simulation make it well worth the resources devoted to preparing this instructional environment. Concepts of fit, just-in-time, and anytime–anywhere learning were discussed within the context of the educational digital paradigm.

Virtual gaming simulation (VGS) is a novel pedagogical tool and a type of virtual simulation that combines gaming features in a simulated learning experience. These types of virtual gaming pedagogies provide deep-rooted learning in which the primary goal is education. In the past, games were used for education to create a climate of fun and excitement, encouraging students' sense of competitiveness and curiosity. Today, with advanced technology and various devices becoming popular even in developing countries, serious games (SGs) are an upcoming trend. Researchers using virtual games recognize that player characteristics, game features, and the context of play variables all have an influence on game outcomes and require further study.

The use of simulation in nursing is one of many methods used for teaching students. Teaching and learning in a virtual learning environment has many advantages for administrators, faculty, and students. Some of the advantages include the use of other disciplines to help create or participate in a virtual world learning experience. Virtual worlds provide faculty with a way of presenting possible real-life scenarios without risk of injury to participants. Flexibility in creating learning experiences in a virtual world has the advantage of providing variation for students as well.

Building a virtual simulation requires a five-stage approach. At each stage there are opportunities to enhance the rigor of virtual simulation education programs, and assessment methods. Application of elements of validity, reliability, and feasibility in determining aims and objectives, designing materials, performing real-life testing, and adapting materials to virtual simulation, followed by trialing, implementing, and evaluating, ensures the rigor of the program.

Working in Second Life® (SL) with nursing students involves developing mentoring skills. Mentoring can be described as a broad caring role that encompasses formal or informal supporting, guiding, coaching, teaching, role modeling, counseling, advocating, networking, and sharing. Mentoring occurs within and/or outside the clinical setting and includes personal and career guidance.

Virtual simulations that touch on interdisciplinary areas are effective training tools and benefit from having a professional in an appropriate discipline actively participate in the simulation and/or weigh in on the simulation's design. Difficulty in finding an interdisciplinary professional to volunteer may need to be addressed, but the increased realism stemming from inter-professional involvement in simulation design, development, and operation makes it worth the effort. Today, faculty's goal should be to create a workforce competent in applying technology in practice for all settings and areas of nursing.

Higher education is transforming every day, and the leaps and bounds we have experienced in nursing and health professional education in the past 10 to 15 years have been extensive. We have gone from classroom PowerPoint lectures and technical skills laboratories on static body parts to engaged education with high-fidelity simulation, learner-centered experiential teaching, and simulated and standardized patients helping students learn to think, act, and reflect like nurses. Amid these changes in teaching methods and innovation, there has been a technological explosion that many nursing faculty struggle to keep up with and seek to incorporate and understand as their students demand a different way of teaching and learning.

Technology is everywhere in our society including in the educational arena. The administrator enacts roles that can either facilitate or hinder the adoption of virtual simulation. Visionary administrators are able to inspire, motivate, and support their faculty and students while they pave the path to smooth transitioning into virtual simulation integration. At times, the logistically and operationally minded constraints of their role might inhibit their role as visionaries and create an ambivalent environment.

Virtual simulation provides solutions to many issues in nursing education, yet it also leaves us with questions. Because of the constant changes in the learning landscape, the need to evolve and innovate is ever present. Faculty, administrators, students, and the technology all need careful consideration, or the cog will not turn to create the momentum needed to carry out simulation-based learning experiences.

APPENDIX A: SIMULATION INTEGRATION STRATEGIES

DATA, INFORMATION, KNOWLEDGE, WISDOM (DIKW) PATHWAY IN EDUCATION USING THE PREBRIEF, ENACTMENT, DEBRIEF, ASSESSMENT (PEDA) APPROACH

Prebrief

What data and information will be provided?

Enactment

What activities are necessary for the learner to complete to acquire the necessary data and process it into meaningful information?

What activities are necessary for the students to demonstrate knowledge?

What activities are necessary for the students to demonstrate wisdom?

Debrief

How will you help the learners:

    Reflect on their learning?

    Assess the knowledge they gained?

    Reflect on their wisdom?

Assessment

How will the learners be assessed?

How will you know what information or knowledge they gained through this activity?

How will you assess their wisdom?

TIPS AND STRATEGIES TO IMPROVE TECHNOLOGY INTEGRATION FROM AN INSTRUCTIONAL DESIGN PERSPECTIVE

- Dream big! An instructional designer can quickly conjure up simulation scenarios that outstrip the organization's technical capabilities. However, some seemingly ambitious approaches are more achievable than one might think. Start with designing a simulation that would be ideal. Next, consult with technical experts to determine how the dream could become a reality, and adjust the design accordingly.

- Start small. The instructional designer may have a brilliant idea for simulation but may be unsure how it will impact the organization. Undergoing a pilot test can produce evidence needed to convince decision makers to make a larger commitment to technology integration.
- Learn the lingo. Communication is improved if the instructional designer and the technologist are speaking the same language. Ascertaining basic technology-related terms and their meaning helps both sides gain a deeper understanding of what the instructional designer has requested and what the technologist determines should be expected. Also, teaching the technologist a few terms may help them better comprehend what is desired, especially when working with graphic designers and software engineers.
- Anticipate technology change. Technology innovation is moving at a rapid pace. When designing simulation, plan for what technology will be in place when the simulation is launched, and do not limit the design to what is present today.
- Study economics. The instructional designer who has a grasp of the economics at work in an organization can optimize and prioritize the use of resources devoted to simulation. Knowing, for example, who makes the budget, when requests need to be submitted, and how to fill in applications enables the instructional designer to seek funds for the technology necessary to conduct the types of simulations that are planned.

APPENDIX B: PROPOSAL STRATEGIES

ELEVATOR PITCH EXAMPLE

Elevator pitch is one way to conceptualize the *pitch*; you should be able to completely summarize the virtual simulation concept, educational outcomes, and return on investment in less than a minute, about the time you might spend in an elevator during a chance encounter with a stakeholder or decision maker, hence the term *elevator pitch*.

Guide to Writing an Elevator Pitch

Define the problem	"Fragmented technology systems are not being used consistently across programs and colleges."
Describe your solution	"We can centralize and integrate technology tools and support and barter expertise for equipment."
Know the stakeholders	"Students, faculty, and administrators all have a part in this solution."
Use evidence-based validation	"The technology vendor has validated research to support the inclusion of this educational technology based on research and publications."
List who is on your team	"I have support from my Dean, but I am seeking additional support from academic leadership."
Provide a financial summary	"The initial investment would $10,000 for the start-up, with a break-even in 12-months and a 5% return on investment in 18-months."
Show traction with milestones	"We will integrate the technology with core nursing classes, then coordinate between departments in 6 months and move towards college-wide adoption in a year."

WRITTEN PROPOSAL OUTLINE EXAMPLE

Creating a budget plan and university support for a variety of options:

- Development of virtual simulations in house
- Development of videos, learning modules, and foundational provisions
- Unknowns: number of students/class and actual faculty time in marking, emailing, providing insight, and guiding students
- Changing costs of technology: As universities change platforms, will the new platform allow the flexibility and needs of the virtual simulation environment?

Identify a faculty professional development strategy to:

- Create in-house faculty learning communities.
- Collaborate with regional schools of nursing and share resources for workshop development.
- Locate endowment funds for sending faculty to conferences.
- Purchase online learning resource licenses for use by all faculty.

Identify the challenges:

- Refer to the hidden costs in time, expertise, and human resources.
- Identify methods for adequate program planning and budget setting, given this new and innovative way of teaching.

Identify the opportunities:

- Analyze options for faculty development and capacity building.
- Create in-house resources.
- Build capacity and create an administrative foundation for success.
  - Identify a budget that considers all of the costs for implementing a high-quality program.

Develop collaborative partnerships.

- Consortiums
  - Venue for health care and educational institutions with shared goals to pool knowledge, monies, and labor covering a geographical area
  - Individual organizations to collaborate and develop strategic planning goals to transform clinical education and improve patient care
  - Collaboration and networking with others to overcome common barriers
- Memorandum of understanding (MOU or MoU)
  - Sharing space and resources
  - Team-planning: crisis resource management for trauma or emergency care (i.e., disaster preparedness)
  - Performing in situ or planned interprofessional simulations virtually (i.e., medication reconciliation)

VIRTUAL LEARNING LABORATORY PROPOSAL EXAMPLE

Overview

Over the past year, several barriers that have precluded the integration of new technologies with family nurse practitioner (FNP) courses have been identified. Perhaps the greatest challenge has been trying to incorporate technologies and virtual learning tools into courses that are already written, courses not currently undergoing revision, or courses that are being taught successfully without the technologies. Mandatory training to learn to use the technology, coupled with the burden of a technology that is not intuitive for novice users, have left many full-time FNP faculty resistant to new technologies. Although the FNP program is taught exclusively online with the use of internet-based teaching platforms and virtual classrooms, the faculty members of the FNP program have agreed to be against the forceful inclusion of new virtual learning modalities without thoughtful consideration and evidence to support their benefit. The lack of available clinical sites and preceptors is a growing concern. Hundreds of FNP students are without an approved clinical site, which means they are unable to progress in their clinical courses.

Proposal

For any student without an approved clinical site or preceptor, the Virtual Learning Laboratory (VLL) will serve as an optional clinical site for one clinical course during concurrent enrollment in the clinical courses.

Competency-Based Education

The scope of a competency-based curriculum focuses on knowledge, attitudes, and skills that encompass professional nursing practice. The VLL will use competency-based assessment tools to evaluate student performance and outcomes. Learning activities completed in Shadow Health provide progressive clinical competency development and data analytics. Shadow Health incorporates metrics to assess competency. It uses a validated framework to measure six discrete components of clinical reasoning: therapeutic communication, subjective data collection, objective data collection, information processing, documentation, and self-reflection. These components of clinical reasoning are assessed as students interact with virtual patients and are used to provide automatic scores using standardized grading rubrics. Students must also complete a reflection following the activity to facilitate critical thinking and promote comprehension.

Self-Directed Learning

Shadow Health learning activities provide individualized feedback, showing students how their questions, interpretations, and decisions compare to those of an expert. These activities can be completed asynchronously and do not require separate faculty feedback. This instructional method has been shown to promote clinical reasoning and decision making and encourage learning.

Practicum Clinical Hours

Students will be offered virtual clinical hours for their participation in problem-based learning activities conducted in the virtual environment. The number of clinical hours is contingent on the amount of time spent in meaningful interaction completing activities with simulated patients. The twelve (12) case study simulations and four (4) concept laboratories in Shadow Heath allow students to practice interview and assessment skills without the need for a synchronous faculty or preceptor. Shadow Health offers the following conversion formula to compare time spent completing virtual patient care activities in Shadow Health to actual on-site clinical hours:

1 hour of virtual patient experience = 3 hours of actual patient experience

This calculation is based on the richness and quality of the virtual patient experiences with respect to the "downtime" that occurs in a traditional clinical setting (e.g., waiting for patients to be brought to rooms, breaks, low patient census). The activities in Shadow Health comprise **18.25** hours of virtual patient experience, which is equivalent to **54.75** hours of actual patient experience according to the conversion formula. The four concept laboratories require approximately 2 hours to complete (in total). This assumes that a student attempts each learning activity only once and achieves a satisfactory student performance score. However, most students will need to repeat learning activities to be successful, which requires additional time. Students will be given a total of three attempts to achieve satisfactory performance scores. Not including the concept laboratories that are not graded, if a student requires three attempts for each graded assignment to achieve a satisfactory performance score, the student will have completed **146.25 hours.**

Student Performance Evaluation

Student performance will be provided to the course instructor using the current evaluation method in eLogs. The VLL faculty will complete the midterm and final evaluation forms.

TALKING POINTS EXAMPLE A

Advantage of Simulation Compared With Actual Clinical Experience

- Reduces training variability and increases standardization
- Guarantees experience for every student
- Can be customized for individualized learning
- Allows reflective learning
- Is student-centered learning
- Allows independent critical thinking, decision making, and delegation
- Allows Immediate feedback
- Offers opportunity to practice rare and critical events
- Can be designed and manipulated
- Allows calibration and update
- Can be reproduced
- Occurs on schedule
- Offers opportunities to make and learn from mistakes

- Is safe and respectful for patients
- Allows deliberative practice
- Also uses the concept of experiential learning

Limitations of Simulation Compared to Actual Clinical Experience
- Not real
- Limited realistic human interaction
- Students may not take it seriously
- No/incomplete physiological symptoms

TALKING POINTS EXAMPLE B

Pros
- The case study simulations and concept laboratories in Shadow Health (SH) are **interactive, realistic,** and **asynchronous,** allowing students to practice interview and assessment skills without the need for a synchronous faculty member.
- Shadow Health that allows students to use their **own words to ask questions and organize their interview** with virtual patients, which **promotes critical thinking and decision making.**
- **Automatic scoring and feedback is preformatted and standardized,** is immediate, and will save time for faculty if used for a graded assignment (e.g., documentation shows a "Model Note"). This will assist with consistency among multiple faculty who are teaching the course. Also, **feedback can be modified** to suit the expectations and needs of the course faculty.
- Students must **provide their rationale for clinical decisions** throughout the simulation, specifically in the Clinical Decision Making assignment (i.e., why do you need xyz lab?).
- Shadow Health incorporates **postsimulation questions** and **self-reflective journaling**.
- The various layers of feedback will allow faculty to see the **growth of individual students** throughout the program, as well as to compare the performance of sections/cohorts on a larger scale (Shadow Health provides feedback on the individual student and the sections).
- SH allows students to **self-populate** into their **course sections**. This means that faculty **do not** need to manually enroll students into the digital clinical experience, which will save a lot of time and confusion.
- Faculty are provided **instructor accounts, training, and instructional design support free of charge.**

Cons
- We **cannot create additional case studies** or **build cases to match the current case studies** in clinical courses, as compared to Second Life (SL).

- Shadow Health **does not** offer a forum for **group discussion and/or interaction with faculty** within the virtual learning environment platform (only SL offers this feature to students).
- Depending on state regulations, the time spent with Shadow Health may or may not be applied toward clinical practicum hours.
- **Results** from practice activities are **not** generated into a **downloadable report**. Therefore, students cannot upload their activity results as a document in the learning management system. It is possible to use a screenshot of their notes.
- **Faculty** must be **trained** to use Shadow Health. Training is handled by Shadow Health in both live and asynchronous online formats and takes **45 minutes**.

ABBREVIATIONS

2D	two dimensional
3D	three dimensional
AACN	American Association of Colleges of Nursing
AHRQ	Agency for Healthcare Research and Quality
AMIA	American Medical Informatics Association
ANA	American Nurses Association
AVG	active video game
CERT	community, emergency, response, teams
CHN	community health nurse
CHSE	Certified Healthcare Simulation Educator
CHSE-A	Certified Health Simulation Educator – Advanced
CHSOS	Certified Healthcare Simulation Operations Specialist
CNIO	chief nursing informatics officer
CPR	cardiopulmonary resuscitation
CVI	content validity index
EMR	electronic medical record
EMS	Education Management Solutions
ESL	English as second language
FAST SIM©	Faculty Administrators Students Technology Strategic Integration Model
FERPA	Family Educational Rights and Privacy Act
FNP	family nurse practitioner
GMO	genetically modified organism
H&P	history and physical
HCI	human–computer interaction
HEDEG	Heuristic Evaluation for Digital Educational Games
HIMSS	Heath Information Management Systems Society
HPS	human patient simulators
IM	instant message
INS	Informatics nurse specialist
IOM	Institute of Medicine
IPE	interprofessional education
IT	information technology
JIT	just-in-time
KSAs	knowledge, skills, and attributes
MOU	memorandum of understanding
NLN SIRC	National League for Nursing's Simulation Innovation Resource Center
OSCE	Objective Structures Clinical Examination
PBL	problem-based learning

PHEG	Playability Heuristic Evaluation for Educational Computer Games
PICO	population, intervention, comparison group, outcome
QSEN	Quality and Safety Education for Nurses Initiative
RCT	randomized controlled trial
ROI	return on investment
RWP	real-world practicum
SBLE	simulation-based learning experiences
SG	serious games
sim	simulator
SL	Second Life®
SLURL	Second Life uniform resource locator
SOAP	subjective data, objective data, assessment, plan
SOS	simulation operations specialist
SSH	Society for Simulation in Healthcare
START	simple triage and rapid treatment
SUN	simulation user network
TA	teaching assistant
TANIC	TIGER-based Assessment of Nursing Informatics Competencies
TeamSTEPPS	Team Strategies and Tools to Enhance Performance and Patient Safety
TIGER	Technology Informatics Guiding Education Reform
URL	uniform resource locator
USDoC	United States Department of Commerce
VGS	virtual gaming simulation
VLE	virtual learning environment
VP	virtual patient
VpNAM	virtual patient nursing activity model
VR	virtual reality
VWFTs	virtual world field trips
VWP	virtual world practicum
Wi-Fi	trademark of the *Wi-Fi* Alliance

GLOSSARY

Active learning is a process engaging students in learning activities that encourage inquiry, examination, analysis, synthesis, and assessment of the learning content.

Anytime–anywhere learning refers to the fact that learning can occur at different or various times and in different or diverse places.

Asynchronous is when something does not occur at the same time.

Authentic assessment is the measurement of scholarly achievements that are useful, important, and meaningful; the assessment strategies can be developed by the teacher or through teacher-learner dyad collaboration.

Authentic assignments are tasks or activities in which the learner is faced with real-world demands; they involve active learning in which students complete a project related to practicing professional roles.

Authenticity refers to instructional strategies and techniques that are designed to connect the dots for students to map their learning from the classroom to the real world; it helps students translate what they are learning to real-world issues, problems, applications, and skills such as reasoning, critical thinking, and skill development related to the real world or a specific profession such as nursing.

Avatar is a graphical representation of a human in a virtual space that interacts with other objects and avatars.

Burstiness refers to bursting data or data that are transmitted in uneven or irregular spurts or bursts rather than smoothly in a continuous, uninterrupted stream; it reflects intermittent or erratic increases and decreases in the frequency of an event and the time between contacts in a time-fluctuating system that can slow spreading processes over the network that can be used to study the spread of information or, in healthcare, diseases.

Certification provides an official or a formal recognition of certain characteristics that attest to the status or a level of achievement such as demonstrating, validating, or establishing a proficiency, ability, or talent within and comprehension or understanding of a specific body of knowledge provided by an external review, examination, assessment, meeting of certain standards, or education.

Certified refers to being officially recognized for a level of achievement such as demonstrating, validating, or establishing a proficiency, ability, or talent within and comprehension or understanding of a specific body of knowledge.

Click refers to pressing down and rapidly releasing a mouse button.

Click data refers to the systematic collection of the number of times a specific weblink is selected by a user to foster the study of the structure and dynamics of web traffic networks.

Cluster randomized trials uses group randomization as opposed to individual randomization.

Collaboration is working together to meet mutual goals or produce something; the collaboration could occur as for example, faculty to faculty, faculty to mentor, faculty to student, mentor to student, student to student, student to additional course faculty, and student to expert.

Collaboration-based refers to a focus on working together. In a virtual, immersive simulation, the interprofessional collaboration would require professionals and learners to share and explore profession-specific knowledge to build a relationship to complete a task or assignment.

Consequential validity is the positive or negative outcomes of a program or assessment such as the degree to which the program encourages good learning techniques.

Construct is a concept, idea, theory, paradigm, or hypothesis.

Construct validity is the degree to which a test measures what it claims to measure.

Content validity is the extent to which there is agreement about the content of the program to which an assessment logically measures all aspects of a defined construct.

Content validity index (CVI) refers to the extent to which a measure embodies or represents every aspect, factor, or component of a given construct.

Created space or **created environment** refers to environments or spaces existing within brick-and-mortar or digital spaces that have been specifically engineered to replicate real-world places, producing sufficient authenticity and environmental fidelity to allow for the suspension of disbelief.

Cross-sectional research obtains data from a specified point in time.

Cultural diversity refers to the reality of a mixture of ethnic or cultural groups; the inclusion or addition of different ethnicity and cultures in a group or organization; and differences in race, social status, gender, gender identity, disability status, or any other characteristic based on characteristics, values, roles, and traditions.

Cyber denotes an electronic medium or methods and a culture of computers, computing, or computer networks such as the Internet; it can extend to encompass information technology and virtual reality.

Cyber simulation is a simulation that can occur in cyberspace that replicates real-life situations.

Cybersickness is a collection of motion sickness–type symptoms experienced by people using virtual reality.

Cyberspace is a notional, virtual, or unreal space or environment within which interactions associated with the Internet occur; it is an area or space created by interconnected computers and computer networks on the Internet and can refer to anything associated with the Internet and its diverse culture of connectedness.

Cyberspace simulation is a simulation that can occur virtually on the Internet that replicates real-life situations.

Debrief or **debriefing** is an essential discussion that occurs after learners enact a simulation to help them reflect on and reframe the context and elucidate perspectives, assumptions, and outcomes. After the completion of each weekly interactive case study, students provide feedback to their faculty member on set questions to solicit ways to improve any aspect of the scenario or their experience for the week while connecting the knowledge, affect, and skills.

Deliberate practice is purposeful, engaged, and systematic, methodical repetition or practice, with focused attention conducted to improve performance by enhancing the quality of the practice, not relying on the quantity of practice or repetition.

Designed experience is created by subject matter experts to provide structured activities that facilitate interactions among learners and the environments to drive anticipated experiences. In other words, the designed experience embodies structured activity within an environment. Theme parks are often, in part, based on the theory of designed experience.

Development team or **game development team** is the group of people assembled to construct the game. Development teams are most successful when they include learning and evaluation scientists who have a firm grasp on educational pedagogy specific to digital media, game theory, and psychometrics or statistics. The team must also include subject matter experts to guide the content and context of the game. These team members, in addition to traditional development members, include, but are not limited to, producers, game designers, programmers, artists, and game testers.

Digital divide is the divide between those with access to new technologies and those without; it refers to the economic and social gulf between those who have ready access to information and communication technologies, computers, and the Internet and those who do not.

Ecology of Culturally Competent Design model is a framework for incorporating cultural diversity into a simulation, adding depth and breadth to the story it tells based on four factors: activities, context, characters, and narrative; this model can be applied to any type of diversity because "culture" does not apply to race alone and simulations can be developed to reflect characteristics such as gender, gender identity, or disability.

Educational design refers to the formulation of solutions that can include products, artifacts, processes, methods, programs, curricula or policies, strategies, and guidelines to address applied, real-world, practical, complex, multifaceted educational problems.

Educational game or **game** captures the act of interacting within the context of a learning environment structured by rules, a competition or contest, and educational goals or outcomes. The game mechanics (the rules or the way that the game operates), narrative, and designed experiences provide consequences for actions and inactions, motivating or pushing players toward discrete goals.

Elevator pitch is one way to conceptualize the pitch; you should be able to completely summarize the game concepts, educational outcomes, and return on investment in less than a minute, about the time you might spend on an elevator during a chance encounter with a stakeholder or decision maker, hence the term *elevator pitch*.

Emotional design is the development of things that people can connect with on a personal or emotional level when they interact with them to generate positive emotions; it refers to the emotions evoked by technologies or products' use, which can occur during use of a serious game.

Engagement refers to the amount of inquisitiveness, interest, consideration, attention, motivation, and passion that a student exhibits while learning.

Evidence-based education practice is a methodology to all facets of education ranging from processes and policies to teaching practice based on substantial and reliable evidence resulting from experiments.

Executive practicum refers to one of the final courses for students to complete their master's in nursing degree in the executive specialty track, in an online program.

Executive producer represents the funding agency or publisher of the game or product.

Experiential learning refers to the process of hands-on learning in which the learner develops knowledge, skills, and attitudes from authentic experiences outside of conventional academic settings; it is reflecting on doing.

External involvement refers to a professional assisting with the development of the virtual simulation but not playing a role in the enactment of the simulation.

External validity refers to the extent to which study results can be generalized or applied to other situations.

Face validity is a subjective judgement, often by a panel of experts, on the extent to which content is applicable or looks to be valid.

Face-to-face refers to real-world classrooms where the teachers and learners are present in the same space together.

Family Educational Rights and Privacy Act (FERPA) is a federal law designed to protect the privacy of students' education records. Any school receiving funds through the U. S. Department of Education must comply with this law.

Fealty represents the realism of the features of a simulation. In Second Life®, the realism comes from being present and immersed in a community of scholars within the virtual world.

Feasibility considers the practicality of the education program and is determined through theoretical risk management or is formally tested using a trial. Appraisal of feasibility requires consideration of technical, economical, operational, and scheduling aspects.

Feedback is when comments and information are communicated back to a learner; it should be focused on the learning objectives or outcomes and be relayed in a productive, constructive way that directly addresses explicit characteristics or aspects of the learner's performance.

Fidelity refers to the level of realism in a simulation or how well it mimics the real world; the higher the level of fidelity, the more authentic or life-like are the simulations, and they contain complex interfacing that includes people (teams), data, information, and advanced communication tools.

Fit or game fit refers to statements related to efficacy, efficiency, and appeal of the game.

Game or educational game captures the act of interacting within the context of a learning environment structured by rules, a competition or contest, and educational goals or outcomes. The game mechanics (the rules or the way that the game operates), narrative, and designed experiences provide consequences for actions and inactions, motivating or pushing players toward discrete goals.

Game design document provides the intention of the game for team members. The game design document needs to be highly detailed and provide a record of decisions made from game visioning, game-build processes, and game release. There are often different levels of documentation specific to different development team members, each team member having a different role; it is an evolving, living document.

Game designer refers to the *development team* member responsible for defining the gameplay process and vision; the game designer conceives and operationalizes the game mechanics or rules and structure of the game as communicated by the content and subject matter experts.

Game-development team or **development team** consists of writers, programmers, designers, artists, sound designers or composers, project managers, publishers, and quality assurance and testing personnel, all of whom collaborate to construct the game. Development teams are most successful when they include learning and evaluation scientists who have a firm grasp on educational pedagogy specific to digital media, game theory, and psychometrics or statistics. The team must also include subject matter experts to guide the content and context of the game.

Game dynamic refers to the evolving behavior that results from playing the game.

Game fit or **fit** describes statements related to efficacy, efficiency, and appeal of the game.

Game mechanics refers to the rules that determine and direct the types of entities (agents, objects, and elements), their relationship to the game, and the way that the user interacts with the game; it is the rules or the way that the game operates.

Game producers refers to the different types of *producers* related to video game production.

Game testers are key components of the quality-assurance process. (They are sometimes called *alpha* or *beta testers*, referring to the early and late stages of game development, respectively.) In the process of educational game development, it may be necessary to use paid game testers who are experts in gaming user interfaces, experiences, and mechanics, as well as subject matter experts who can evaluate best practices within the context of the situated discrete discipline portrayed during the game experience.

Gameability is the capacity for users to alter their answers or responses.

Games for learning refers to a computerized, virtual game in which the primary purpose is educational rather than entertainment. Sometimes, but not always, these games are simulation based; they are also known as *serious games*.

Gamification is when game theory is applied to endeavors or activities that are not game based; it is modifying a boring activity into a game.

Hardscape simulation center is a brick-and-mortar area that has patient simulators for learners.

Hit is defined as a single file request in the access log of a web server or a match of data in a search string against data that one is searching.

Heuristic refers to a standard or rule of thumb or a guide to follow when making decisions or judgements; it is allowing students or learners to discover, realize or learn something for themselves.

Human-computer interaction (HCI) is the discipline that studies how people interact with computers, analyzing the connection between design and computation from a humanistic and ergonomic perspective and considering the experience of use and user preferences.

Immersion refers to extensive or deep exposure to surroundings or conditions that are pertinent to the object of study, such as developing navigation skills and competencies using a computer to complete required activities; it is sometimes referred to as *presence*.

In situ is undisturbed in its natural or initial, original place or position, site, or location.

Informatics nurse specialist is a licensed nurse who has been formally prepared at the graduate level in informatics or a related field.

Information technology refers to the application of computers to capture, store, retrieve, examine, transmit, disseminate, and manipulate or process data or information.

Infrastructure refers to the foundation, framework. or structure that provides the scaffolding or support for the processing, storage, dissemination, and analysis of data and information for a system or an organization's computing, information technology, and technologies; it is composed of the physical and virtual resources that must be considered as technology tools are added to and eliminated from this framework.

Instructional environment is the teaching, learning, behavioral, social, and personal features of the learning experience whether it is within a classroom setting or online with a virtually simulated experience such as a virtual world, augmented reality, or virtual reality.

Intellectual property refers to an intangible asset or something that does not exist as a physical, touchable, or tangible object; it is the intangible rights that protect the products of the human intellect, such as such as music, poetry, art, software, inventions, or formulas used in commerce.

Interdisciplinary relates to more than one branch of knowledge or different professions.

Internal consistency reliability is the correlation or consistency between different items on the same test that measure the same construct.

Internal involvement refers to professionals participating within the virtual simulation; they assist with the enactment of the simulation.

Internal producer manages the day-to-day production process and *game-development team*.

Internal validity is the quality of a study and/or the extent to which direct cause and effect is demonstrated and confounding variables avoided.

Interprofessional means between two or more professions.

Interprofessionalism refers to effectively integrating professionals' separate knowledge and skill sets to provide a shared, collective knowledge base for problem solving, communication, and conflict resolution.

Inter-rater reliability is the degree to which raters/assessors of the same thing agree in assessment decisions.

Island is a land area or land mass surrounded by water; in Second Life®; they are as regions detached from the mainland that residents can use to mimic the real world for purposes of virtual simulation.

Journal club is a group of learners or people who meet regularly to analyze, evaluate, and synthesize an article retrieved from the literature published within the last 5 years.

Just-in-time (JIT) information refers to information that is accessible exactly when needed.

Just-in-time (JIT) learning refers to learning on demand or making learning available to the learner at the exact time the learner needs the data, information, knowledge, or skill.

Longitudinal research refers to the investigation of a sequence of exposures over time.

Memorandum of understanding (MOU) is a formal agreement between two or more parties. Companies and organizations can use MOUs to establish official partnerships. MOUs are not legally binding, but they carry a degree of seriousness and mutual respect; they are stronger than a unwritten agreement.

Mentee refers to a person who has a mentor to counsel, advise and help while preparing for a future role. It is a person who has a mentor to help establish goals, teach skills needed in Second Life®, promote a sense of community, design activities, and collaborate with each other. It can be a student or another person receiving coaching, leadership, role modeling, or instruction from a mentor in a formal, mutually beneficial mentor–mentee relationship.

Mentor refers to a person who counsels, advises, and helps to prepare students, recent graduates, or novices entering a profession for their future role; it is a person who helps mentees establish goals, teaches them skills needed in Second Life®, promotes a sense of community, designs activities, and collaborates with each other. It is a faculty member who provides coaching, leadership, role modeling, and instruction to students in a formal, mutually beneficial mentor–mentee relationship.

Mobile application pitch is defined under *pitch*.

Networking is the sharing of data, information, knowledge, or services among facilities or people; it is the design, building, and use of a network (two or more linked or connected computer systems).

NLN Jeffries Simulation Theory is a theory on elements of a nursing simulation necessary for meeting student learning outcomes; it was developed by Dr. Pamela Jeffries and the National League for Nursing.

Nontechnical skills refer to leadership, teamwork, situation awareness, and decision making.

Nursing education is the formal learning and practice of the science of nursing.

PICO is a mnemonic for population, intervention, comparison group, and outcome. Most well-operationalized research questions have all of these components. An example of a good research question follows: In a population of BSN students (P), do students who practice two hours a week to insert a peripherally inserted central catheter (PICC) line on a mobile application learning intervention (I) have a higher first-time passage rate when tested on a placement of a PICC line (O) compared with students practicing two hours a week inserting a PICC line in the simulation laboratory (C)? Note that the research question does not have to be phrased in the P-I-C-O order.

Pitch, video game pitch, or **mobile application pitch** refers to a short and discrete presentation that conveys how an educational game or application represents a measurable intervention and solves a problem within the context of a curriculum. It should attend to the concepts of *fit*. Think of the pitch as an executive summary of the game. It should address return on investment or a value proposition and include a discussion related to the complexity, cost, and time involved in game development or integration. In general, the pitch should be concise and not exceed one page. You should be able to completely summarize the game concepts, educational outcomes, and return on investment in less than a minute, about the time you might spend in an elevator during a chance encounter with a stakeholder or decision maker, hence the term *elevator pitch*.

Plus-Delta debriefing is a method in which the facilitator/mentor asks only a few questions such as "What went well?" and "What needs improvement."

Poseball is an object that is programmed or scripted to run an animation on an avatar that accesses it. In Second Life®, an avatar sitting on a poseball would behave as directed by the programming of the poseball. For example, a poseball could help one pose for a picture or snapshot.

Practicum is a course of study involving a mentored or supervised authentic experience in an actual setting, such as mentored nursing education students teaching students as part of their course of study.

Prebrief is the introduction to the learning activities that prepares the student to enact or perform the learning activity; it is critical to achieving the learning outcomes.

Predictive validity refers to the degree to which success in an educational program predicts an outcome such as good future performance.

Preintervention and postintervention are studies that examine subjects before and after an experience to determine whether there is any change based on the attributes of the intervention.

Presence refers to the feeling of being there with others (e.g., feeling as though you are present or in the same place as other students, a teacher, or a mentor); it is often thought of as immersion, or the subjective experience of being in one place, location, or environment.

Problem-based learning is a learner-centered methodology in which learners acquire the predetermined information, knowledge, and/or skills about the concept or topical area by interacting with trigger materials that permit them to actively experience the solving of an open-ended problem.

Problematization of a term, writing, opinion, ideology, identity, or person is consideration of the concrete or existential elements of those involved as challenges (problems) that invite the people involved to transform those situations. It is a method of defamiliarization of common sense.

Producer refers to the different types of producers or *game producers* related to video game production. The *executive producer* often represents the funding agency or publisher. The *internal producer* manages the day-to-day production process and *game-development team*.

Professional a person who is engages in one branch of knowledge or is qualified in a profession.

Professional nursing competencies refer to the ability to function in specific nursing roles and abilities, often based on the nursing process.

Professional nursing roles are specialties at the MSN level (e.g., nurse educator, nursing informatics, nursing professional development, nurse executive, clinical nurse specialist, nurse practitioner, nurse midwife, nurse anesthetist).

Project is a specific task that is conceptualized, planned, designed, and implemented.

Prototyping is the process of creating a basic version or model that can be constructed, tested, and reworked or reiterated until a suitable prototype or model is realized.

Psychological fidelity refers to how believable a simulated experience is and how well it approximates reality.

Psychometrics refers to the study of test measurements and test qualities.

Publisher refers to internal or external entities responsible for the distribution and, often, the technical support for a *game*. Very few academic institutions have the expertise or capacity to provide distribution or technical support for educational games.

Quasiexperimental is an empirical study that does not randomize its subjects and uses a control group to examine the causal impact of an intervention on the experimental group receiving the intervention.

Real world is the world we live in.

Real-world practicum (RWP) is a practicum in an actual setting, such as mentored nursing education students teaching students as part of their course of study.

Realism refers to the direct observation of the world and coping or dealing with the way things are by differentiating or distinguishing the actual or real from the abstract, theoretical, hypothetical, or speculative.

Reliability is the stability and consistency of virtual simulation program design and methods of assessment (i.e., does an assessment dependably pass and fail the right learners?).

Rigor is the scrupulous and meticulous conduct of virtual simulation through the structured and controlled planning of educational program design and methodological commitment to careful, consistent, and diligent assessment.

Scaffold or **scaffolding** refers to various instructional methods used by the teacher or mentor to move students incrementally toward a deeper comprehension and skill attainment, with the aim of developing a more independent learner; the teacher or mentor gradually and steadily transfers more responsibility over the learning process to the learner.

Scenario is a sequence of events and a course of action.

Scripted simulation is a situation or dilemma dramatized using a storyboard. Students act out the storyboard and then discuss the implications of the story and possible solutions to the problem while acknowledging how the story affected them emotionally and professionally; it is a simulation based on stories of characters, settings, individuals, and narratives designed to meet learning outcomes.

Second Life® (SL) is a virtual world where the residents are avatars (graphical representations of students) who navigate and interact with the environment, as well as with other avatars.

Second Life® Island is an area within Second Life purchased by individuals or organizations for development for a variety of purposes, including education.

Serious game (SG) refers to a computerized, virtual game in which the primary purpose is education rather than entertainment; sometimes, but not always, these games are simulation based; it is also known as *games for learning*.

Simulation is an attempt to digitally model a real-life or hypothetical situation on a computer that learners can experience in a safe environment. By mimicking real-life conditions, events, problems, or situations, simulation prepares learners for real-life events or for a the future role. In such simulations, nursing students can practice patient interactions in a safe environment in virtual or latex-based simulation. It refers to the imitation of something real or a representation of key design elements or variables of a system or process. From an educational perspective, simulation is a technique striving to leverage an artificial or created environment with situated narrative to drive a *designed experience.*

Simulation to Practice model refers to students being assigned study material for preparation prior to the simulation; as students work through the story, they begin to reflect on what is going on (reflection-in-action) and sometimes go off script as they react to the action. When the story ends, they begin debriefing; this phase is called *reflection-on-action*.

Simulation-based learning refers to learning that occurs in a simulation-based environment to develop the learner's knowledge, skills, attitudes, and behaviors in a safe environment that does not place patients at risk while providers learn how to care for them.

Simulation-based learning environment is an environment or setting for learning that is totally controlled by the developers and educators who designed and created it to mimic real-world conditions, situations, systems, and/or processes being examined, studied, or enacted by the learner.

Skill-based active learning focuses on practicing and performing tasks or skills. In a virtual, immersive simulation example, the skill-based interprofessional element is present if an assignment requires students to perform tasks typically associated with another profession.

Stakeholders refer to an individual, a group of individuals or an institution, business, organization, or association with an involvement, interest or concern in the institution's business', organization's, or association's actions, plans, goals, objectives, and policies.

Standardized feedback is feedback that is consistent across all simulations.

Storyboard is a sequence of drawings, pictures, or photographs that usually include instructions and dialogue depicting the scenes and shots planned for the video or production; for example, it consists of a series of images of the avatars in the three-dimensional (3D) virtual learning environment hospital, showing where the action would take place, where character avatars should be placed in each scene, and what they should say.

Teamwork refers to the process of the combined collaborative and cooperative action of groups of individuals to work together to achieve a mutual or common goal.

Tech-rover is a person hired to offer support to faculty integrating technology and support to students engaging in technology; it is a work-study student who is hired to assist faculty with the development of their virtual simulations and who can support students as they engage in the simulation.

Technological resistance is the opposition or resistance to the adoption of new educational technologies.

Technological solutionism is the belief that every problem has a technology-based solution and that technological advancement will save society.

Technology-enhanced healthcare simulation refers to a simulation in which the learner engages and interacts to mimic or simulate a facet of healthcare, such as patient care, for the intention of teaching, learning, and/or performance assessment.

Technology knowledge deficit is the lack or insufficiency of cognitive information related to a specific topic.

Technostress is an adaptation problem in which individuals struggle to cope with the adjustments to the use of technology; it is the pressure, anxiety, or psychosomatic illness caused by repeatedly working with computer technologies.

Test–retest reliability is the similarity of results when learners are tested and retested (without additional learning) to determine the stability of the assessment.

Three dimensional (3D) refers to objects that have three dimensions: height, width, and depth. The human body is 3D.

Unscripted simulation is one in which students must make decisions; they are given basic information about their task and need to figure out what they would do if they are the professional solving the problem at hand. Students clarify the issues, read about the topic, and derive a solution or a product that meets the goals of the simulation. It is a simulation in which students are presented with a problem or a case and must decide on the best course of action.

Validity is the accuracy and credibility of a virtual simulation program's design and methods of assessment (i.e., does an assessment truly represent what you are trying to measure?).

Video game refers to an electronic game in which the players control images on a monitor or a television screen by using a specialized gaming device.

Video game pitch is defined under *pitch*.

Virtual gaming simulation (VGS) is the blending of virtual simulation and serious gaming so that the user is immersed in an interactive simulated activity that resembles real life.

Virtual is anything simulated using a computer.

Virtual learning environment (VLE) is the integration of computer and Internet technologies into teaching and learning to improve learning.

Virtual patient Nursing Activity Model (vpNAM) is a model that allows for the adaptation of virtual patients to the nursing paradigm for student development of clinical reasoning skills; it provides a basic template for systematically developing different types of virtual patients from a common model, allowing for shared pedagogical designs across technical solutions.

Virtual patients (VP) are digital or simulated patients generated by a computer.

Virtual reality (VR) is the use of computerized applications to create interactive and immersive three-dimensional environments in which the user is given the impression of being physically present.

Virtual simulation is a simulation that can occur in a virtual learning or a virtual reality environment that replicates real-life situations. The user plays a central role by participating and interacting in the virtual environment via motor-control, communication, and decision-making skills. It refers to the use of a virtual learning environment such as Second Life®, where the learner can enact learning activities or real-life experiences in a virtual setting.

Virtual simulation–mediated learning is active learning facilitated by a human mentor who helps learners in the simulation gain insights, reflect on the intent of the learning, and connect the dots to translate the learning to their practice.

Virtual world is a digital or computer-based online world or environment designed for interaction in which customized simulations. Users can interact with each other as avatars, as well as interact with objects in the environment based on the customized programming.

Virtual world field trips (VWFTs) are field trips or excursions that take students to virtual settings or displays of places or experiences they would never be able to go to or do in the real world.

Virtual world practicum (VWP) is a practicum in a virtual world that emulates a practicum in the real world. Students can practice or learn techniques and skills and hone their critical-thinking and reasoning skills. One advantage is that students could engage in activities that they could not experience in real-world practicums, such as a mentored nursing executive student dealing with an impaired employee who is in a patient's room; due to legal and ethical issues, students would not be able to experience this process prior to graduation.

Wi-Fi is networks that do not have physical or wired connections between the sender and the receiver but instead use radiofrequency technology.

INDEX

accessibility, 5
active engagement, 39
active learning, 145
active video games (AVGs), 145
administrative stakeholders, 98
administrator preparation, 100
    financial issues, 100–101
    legal issues, 101–102
administrators
    buy-in, 254–255
    champions, identifying, 254–255
    and FAST SIM©, 248, 263–264
    influence, 37–39
    nursing curriculums, 252–253
    organizational impact, 256
    orientation and socialization, 256
    professional development, 255
    role of, 213–214, 249–251, 261–267
    simulation-based education, 248–249
    supports and barriers, 253–254
    virtual technology and mediated learning, 251–252
    virtual technology integration, 72–73
advocates, administrator, 264
Agency for Healthcare Research and Quality (AHRQ), 66
AHRQ. *See* Agency for Healthcare Research and Quality
American Association of Colleges of Nursing (AACN), 233
American Medical Informatics Association (AMIA), 233
American Nurses Association (ANA), 233, 234
AMIA. *See* American Medical Informatics Association
ANA. *See* American Nurses Association
Angoff technique, FIRST2ACT, 183, 184
anytime–anywhere learning, 117
AR. *See* augmented reality
artificial intelligence, 6
assessment, 11, 149–151, 273
assimilate technology, 33
asynchronicity, 183
asynchronous, 8
asynchronous learning activity, 35–36
augmented reality (AR), 7
authentic assignments, 214, 216–218
avatar manipulation, 203
avatars, 47, 160

AVGs. *See* active video games

back-end developers, 99
badges, 5
Bauman's Layered Learning Theory, 116, 120
BC Provincial Simulation Coordination Committee (BCPSCC), 248
Benner's experiential learning model, 119–120
blended learning, 116
budget, 262
budgeter, administrator, 265
budget plan and university support, 276
Burn Center, serious game, 9
burstiness, 122

Canadian Association of Schools of Nursing (CASN), 137
capstone courses
    concepts of, 44–45
    SL into, 45–47
    standard deliverables, 45
CASN. *See* Canadian Association of Schools of Nursing
CBE. *See* competency-based education
C-CEI. *See* Creighton Competency Evaluation Instrument
CDC. *See* Centers for Disease Control and Prevention, collaboration
Centers for Disease Control and Prevention (CDC), collaboration, 228–229
CERT. *See* community emergency response team
certifications, 99
Certified Healthcare Simulation Educator (CHSE), 103
Certified Healthcare Simulation Operations Specialist (CHSOS), 99
challenges, 276
champions, identifying, 254–255
CHN course. *See* community health nursing course
CHSE. *See* Certified Healthcare Simulation Educator
CHSOS. *See* Certified Healthcare Simulation Operations Specialist
clickers and smartphones, tool, 35
cloud-based technology, 7
Code Orange, serious game, 9
Code Studio, serious game, 10

collaboration, 224
collaboration-based, 225, 227–231
collaborative culture, administrator, 264
collaborative partnerships, 276
CoLoBot: Colonize with Bots, serious game, 10
community assessment, learning experience, 170–173
community emergency response team (CERT), 166
community health nursing (CHN) course, 109–111
competency-based education (CBE), 5
consequential validity, 178
constructivism, 11–12
construct validity, 186
content validity, 178
content validity index (CVI), 180
costs
   game development, 119
   VGS, 130
created spaces, 114
credentials, 5
Creighton Competency Evaluation Instrument (C-CEI), 38
cultural diversity, 218–220
CVI. *See* content validity index
cybersickness, 76
cyberspace simulation or cyber simulation, 44

data, 13
data analytics and machine learning, 5
data, information, knowledge, wisdom (DIKW) pathway, 13–14
debrief/debriefing, 89, 91–92, 148, 204
deliberate practice, 64
designed experiences, 114
DigesTower, SGs, 154–155
digital divide, 74
digital games, 115–116
DIKW pathway. *See* data, information, knowledge, wisdom pathway
direct costs, administrator, 263
director, administrator, 265
disaster-triage experience, learning, 166–170

e-Baby, SGs, 152–154
Ecology of Culturally Competent Design model, 120, 219
education, 6
educational design, 113
educational game(s), 114
   activities based on, 116
   development, 118–119
educational technology, 26, 27
Education Management Solutions (EMS), 65
edutainment, 8

e-learning, 8
electronic medical record (EMR), 82–84
elevator pitch, 267, 275
emerging technologies, 40
emotional design, 148
employers, 99–100
EMR. *See* simulated electronic medical record
EMS. *See* Education Management Solutions
enactment, 10, 91, 273
end-of-program competency testing, 252–253
engage, 6
engagement, 152
English as second language (ESL), 220
environments, 114
e-RAPIDS (Rescuing a Patient in Deteriorating Situations), 177
e-simulation, 176–177
ESL. *See* English as second language
ethical dilemmas, 14
ETHICAL Model for Ethical Decision Making, 14–18
   ethical dilemma, 18–22
evidence-based education practice, 121–122
executive specialty practicum, 88
experiential learning, 216
external involvement, 225–226
external validity, 185

face-to-face interaction, 53
face validity, 178
faculty
   influence, 33–37
   issues, instructional environment, 102–103
   learning communities, 254
   preparation, 104
   professional development, 254, 276
   stakeholders, 98
   in virtual simulations, 89–90
      debriefing, 91–92
      FAST SIM©, 88
      practicum project, 94–96
      SL, 88–89
      virtual journal club, 93–94
      VWP, 88
   virtual technology integration, 72
Faculty Administrators Students Technology Strategic Integration Model© (FAST SIM), 1–2, 25–26
   administrators and, 37–39, 248, 263–264
   application, 31–32
   description, 26–29
   faculty influence, 33–37
   game development and, 114–115
   instructional environment and, 97–98
   interprofessional simulation and, 223–224
   NI and, 234

nursing student simulation and, 161–165
rigor of virtual simulation and, 178
SGs and, 143–144
student influence, 39–40
synchronous and asynchronous tools, 35–36
VGS and, 128
virtual technology integration and, 60, 71–72
VLE and, 36–37, 196
VWP and, 88
Family Educational Rights and Privacy Act (FERPA), 102
family nurse practitioner (FNP), 78–82
FAST SIM. *See* Faculty Administrators Students Technology Strategic Integration Model©
fealty, 216
feasibility, 178
feedback, 63
Feedback Incorporating Review and Simulation Techniques to Act on Clinical Trends (FIRST2ACTWeb™), 176
FERPA. *See* Family Educational Rights and Privacy Act
fidelity, 101
financial issues
   administrator preparation, 100–101
   instructional environment, 100–101
FIRST2ACTWeb™. *See* Feedback Incorporating Review and Simulation Techniques to Act on Clinical Trends
FIRST2ACTWeb™ program, 176–177, 187
   development
      aims and objectives, 179–180
      designing materials, 180
      "real life" testing, 180–181
      adapting materials, 181–183, 184
      trial, implementation, and evaluation, 183–186
fit, 115, 118, 119
flexible learning, 251
Florence, serious game, 9
FNP. *See* family nurse practitioner
Free Dive, serious game, 9
front-end developers, 99
front-line managers, 98

gameability, 145
game-based
   learning, 114
   teaching, 114
game designers, 121
game development
   anytime–anywhere, 117
   educational, 118–119
   evidence-based education practice, 121–122
   and FAST SIM©, 114–115
   just-in-time learning, 117–118
   learning models, 119–120
   reliability and validity, 120–121
   teaching, motivation and learning, 115–117
game dynamic, 147
GAME2LEARN, serious game, 9
game mechanics, 8, 121, 147
gameplay, 8
games, 114
games for learning, 144
gamification, 144
genetically modified organisms (GMOs), 44
GMOs. *See* genetically modified organisms

hardscape simulation center, 102–103
HCI. *See* human-computer interaction
health assessment, 106–109
HEDEG. *See* Heuristic Evaluation for Digital Educational Games
Heuristic Evaluation for Digital Educational Games (HEDEG), 147
heuristics, 147
home health assessment, learning experience, 170–173
HPS. *See* human patient simulators
human-computer interaction (HCI), 148
human patient simulators (HPS), 75, 250

i-Human, 78
IM. *See* instant message
immersed, 90
immersion process, 7, 236, 241
implementation, 38
INACSL. *See* International Nursing Association for Clinical Simulation and Learning
indirect costs, administrator, 263
informatics nurse specialist (INS), 237
information, 13
information technology (IT), 73, 105
infrastructure, 100, 105
in-kind resources, 262
innovative learning methodologies, 250
INS. *See* informatics nurse specialist
instant message (IM), 49
Institute of Medicine (IOM), 233
institutional review board (IRB), 107
instructional environment, 98
   administration, 98
   CHN course, 109–111
   faculty, 98
   faculty issues, 102–103
   faculty preparation, 104
   and FAST SIM©, 97–98
   financial issues, 100–101
   health assessment, 106–109
   information technology, 105

instructional environment, 98 (cont.)
   legal issues, 101–102
   student issues, 103–104
   student preparation, 104–105
   students, 98
   technology experts, 98–100
interactive technology, 39
interdisciplinary elements, 224
internal consistency reliability, 181
internal involvement, 225
internal validity, 185
International Nursing Association for Clinical Simulation and Learning (INACSL), 63, 104, 135, 149, 248
interprofessional education (IPE), 65–67
interprofessionalism, 59
interprofessional simulation, 224
   collaboration-based, 225, 227–231
   external involvement, 225–226
   and FAST SIM©, 223–224
   internal involvement, 225
   skill-based, 224–225, 227–231
   volunteers, searching for, 226
inter-rater reliability, 178
involvement, interprofessional, 225–226
IOM. See Institute of Medicine
IPE. See interprofessional education
IRB. See institutional review board
IT. See information technology
IT professionals, game development, 147

journal club, 93–94
just-in-time (JIT) information, 117
just-in-time (JIT) learning, 117

knowledge, 13
knowledge, skills, and attributes (KSAs), 104–105
Kolb's experiential learning theory, 119, 132
KSAs. See knowledge, skills, and attributes

latex-based simulation, 8
learner centered, 11
learning/course management tool, 35
learning experiences. See student learning experiences
lecture-capture tool, 35
legal issues, instructional environment, 101–102

makerspaces, 5
massive open online courses (MOOCs), 7
mediated learning, virtual technology and, 251–252
memorandum of understanding (MOU), 254, 276
mentees, 213
mentor, 89, 91–92

mentoring, 212
   in SL, 215
   virtual simulation-mediated learning, 212–215
micro-credentials, 5
middle-level administrators, 98
M-learning, 6
mobile devices, 40
mobile first, 6
money, administrator, 262
MOOCs. See massive open online courses
MOU. See memorandum of understanding
multiprofessional education, virtual simulation, 66
Multi-User Programming Pedagogy for Enhancing Traditional Study (M.U.P.P.E.T.S.), serious game, 10
M.U.P.P.E.T.S. See Multi-User Programming Pedagogy for Enhancing Traditional Study

nasogastric tube (NGT) placement, virtual reality for, 64
National Council of State Boards of Nursing (NCSBN), 60
National League for Nursing (NLN), 29, 39
NCSBN. See National Council of State Boards of Nursing
The Neighborhood, 129
neonatal care, SGs, 152–154
network, 196
NGT placement. See nasogastric tube placement
NI. See nursing informatics
NLN. See National League for Nursing
NLN Jeffries Simulation Theory, 216
NMC Horizons Report, 144
nontechnical skills, 290
NP. See nurse practitioner
nurse practitioner (NP), VGS, 136–139
nursing education, 60
   VGS in (see virtual gaming simulation)
   virtual gaming (see serious games)
   virtual learning, 7–11
nursing education practicum, 211–212
nursing informatics (NI), 4, 12–13, 234
   challenges, 241
   and FAST SIM©, 234
   fundamentals of, 235–237
   skill and knowledge development, 238
   VLE and SL, 235–237, 238–240
   evaluation process, 240–241
nursing student simulation, 159–160
   community and home health assessment, 170–173
   disaster-triage experience, 166–170
   and FAST SIM©
      development, 162–164

evaluation, 164–165
selection, 161–162

Objective Clinical Structured Evaluations (OSCE), 252–253
online collaboration tool, 35
opportunities, 276
organizational impact, 256
OSCE. *See* Objective Clinical Structured Evaluations

PBL. *See* problem-based learning
PEDA. *See* prebrief, enactment, debrief, assessment
pediatric care, SGs, 154–155
peripherally inserted central catheter (PICC) line, 122
personnel, administrator, 262
"Peter the Service Dog" simulation, 216–218
PHEG. *See* Playability Heuristic Evaluation for Educational Computer Games
"Philippe the New Nurse" simulation, 218–220
PICC line. *See* peripherally inserted central catheter line
PICO. *See* population, intervention, comparison group, outcome
pitch, 267
Playability Heuristic Evaluation for Educational Computer Games (PHEG), 147
PlayLogo3D, serious game, 10
Plus-Delta debriefing, 218
population, intervention, comparison group, outcome (PICO), 121–122
practicum project, 94–96
prebrief, 90
prebrief, enactment, debrief, assessment (PEDA), 10, 90, 273
prebriefing, 148
predictive validity, 178
presence, virtual environment, 214
presentation software, tool, 35
problem-based learning (PBL), 38, 215
professional development, 255, 276
Prog & Play, serious game, 10
prototyping, 147
psychometrics, 120–121
Pulse!!, serious game, 9

QSEN. *See* Quality and Safety Education for Nurses Initiative
Quality and Safety Education for Nurses Initiative (QSEN), 162, 234

randomized controlled trial (RCT), 144
RCT. *See* randomized controlled trial
realism, 101
real-world practicum (RWP), 87
  faculty and, 90
reflection-on-action, 220
regional conferences, professional development, 255
reliability, 178
  game development, 120–121
remote collaboration, 65
return on investment (ROI), 256
rigor, 178
rigor of virtual simulation, 178–179
  development
    aims and objectives, 179–180
    designing materials, 180
    "real life" testing, 180–181
    adapting materials, 181–183, 184
    trial, implementation, and evaluation, 183–186
  and FAST SIM©, 178
    FIRST2ACT and FAST2ACTweb, 176–177, 177f
ROI. *See* return on investment
RWP. *See* real-world practicum

SBLE. *See* simulation-based learning experiences
scaffolding, 213
scaffolds, 119
scenarios, 89, 160
schedule debriefing sessions, 150
scripted simulations, 214
Second Life® (SL), 5, 43, 88, 129
  into capstone course, 45–47
  disaster-triage experience in, 166–170
  as educational strategy, 62
  faculty and mentors, tips for, 91–92
  mentoring in, 215
  student instructions for, 46–47
  technology and environment, 50–53
  technology and ethics of surveillance, 48–50
  virtual simulation-mediated learning in, 212–214
  VLE and, 235–237, 238–240
  in VWP, 88–89
Second Life® Islands, 212
serious games (SGs), 7, 8–10, 143. *See also* virtual gaming simulation
  assessment, 149–151
  development process, 146–148
  evaluation, 151–152
  and FAST SIM©, 143–144
  instruments, 147
  neonatal and pediatric nursing learning, 152–155
  prebriefing and debriefing, 148–149

serious games (SGs), 7, 8–10, 143. *See also* virtual gaming simulation (*cont.*)
   teaching–learning process, 144–146
   virtual simulations and, 128
setting, administrator, 263
SGs. *See* serious games
Shadow Health, 78
simple triage and rapid treatment (START), 163, 166
simulated electronic medical record (EMR), 82–84
simulation, 159. *See also* nursing student simulation
simulation-based-education, 248–249
simulation-based learning, 98
simulation-based learning environments, 97, 119
simulation-based learning experiences (SBLE), 63
simulation coordinators, 99
Simulation Innovation Resource Center (SIRC), 104
SIMULATIONiQ™ IPE, 65, 67
Simulation Operations Specialist (SOS), 99
simulations, 8, 27, 60, 97–98, 118
simulation scenario, 8
simulation team developer, administrator, 265
Simulation to Practice model, 219
Simulation User Networks (SUNs), professional development, 255
SIRC. *See* Simulation Innovation Resource Center
skill-based simulation, 224–225, 227–231
SL. *See* Second Life®
smart boards, 7
SOAP. *See* subjective data, objective data, assessment, plan
social media, 7, 40
Society for Simulation in Healthcare (SSH), 99, 103
SOS. *See* Simulation Operations Specialist
SSH. *See* Society for Simulation in Healthcare
staff, role of, 213–214
stakeholders, 98, 178, 264, 265
standard deliverables, capstone courses, 45
standardized feedback, 63
START. *See* simple triage and rapid treatment
storyboard, 215
strategic partnership, 263
strategic planning, administrators, 253–254
   champions, identifying, 254–255
   organizational impact, 256
   orientation and socialization, 256
   professional development, 255
   student learning experiences
      development, 162–164
      evaluation, 164–165
      selection, 161–162
students. *See also* nursing student simulation

influence, 39–40
instructions for SL, 46–47
issues, instructional environment, 103–104
orientation and socialization, 256
preparation, 104–105
role of, 214
stakeholders, 98
technology integration, 32, 33
virtual technology integration, 73–74
subjective data, objective data, assessment, plan (SOAP), 80
SUNs. *See* Simulation User Networks
synchronous, 8
synchronous learning activity, 35–36

tablets and laptops, 6
tablets tool, 35
TANIC. *See* TIGER-based Assessment of Nursing Informatics Competencies
target users, 146
TAs. *See* teaching assistants
teaching assistants (TAs), 255
teaching-learning process, SGs, 144–146
TeamSTEPPS. *See* Team Strategies and Tools to Enhance Performance and Patient Safety
Team Strategies and Tools to Enhance Performance and Patient Safety (TeamSTEPPS), 65, 66
technical support specialists, 99
technological resistance, 74
technological solutionism, 74
technology, 26
   administrators, 261
   and simulation, 27
   tools and learning advantages, 35
   virtual technology integration, 74–75
technology-challenged student, VLE, 198–202
technology-enhanced healthcare simulation, 59
technology experts, 98–100
Technology Informatics Guiding Education Reform (TIGER), 233
technology integration, 4, 27, 31, 273–274. *See also* virtual technology integration
   administrator, role of, 264–265
technology knowledge deficit, 196
technology trends, 4–7
technology user, administrator, 265
technostress, 75
tele-sitter project, VLE, 206–208
test–retest reliability, 181
3D VLEs, 212, 214
3DiTeams, serious game, 9
three-dimensional (3D) model, 47, 209
TIGER. *See* Technology Informatics Guiding Education Reform

TIGER-based Assessment of Nursing Informatics Competencies (TANIC), 235, 239, 240
time, administrator, 262
Time After Time, serious game, 9
2D model. *See* two-dimensional model
two-dimensional (2D) model, 209

USDoC. *See* United States Department of Commerce
United States Department of Commerce (USDoC), 74
unscripted simulation, 215

VA Critical Thinking, serious game, 8
validity, 178
  game development, 120–121
VGS. *See* virtual gaming simulation
video, 6, 7
video games, 115
Virtual ECG, serious game, 9
virtual education, 248–249
virtual environment, 44
virtual gaming simulation (VGS), 61, 127, 270. *See also* serious games
  and FAST SIM©, 128
  learning modules and, 132–136
  in nurse practitioner, 136–139
  requirements and costs, 130
  virtual learning environments and tools, 128–130
  virtual simulations and serious gaming, 128
virtual health assessment, 106–109
virtual journal club, 93–94
virtual learning environment (VLE), 27, 36–37, 61, 88, 159–160
  avatar manipulation, 203
  effectiveness, 205
  family nurse practitioner (FNP), 78–82
  and FAST SIM©, 196
  interprofessional in (*see* interprofessional simulation)
  NI (*see* nursing informatics)
  nursing student (*see* nursing student simulation)
  simulated EMR, 82–84
  and SL, 197, 235–237, 238–240
  technology-challenged student, 198–202
  tele-sitter project, 206–208
  and tools, 128–130
Virtual Learning Laboratory (VLL), 277–278
virtual learning landscape
  constructivism, 11–12
  DIKW pathway, 13–14
  ETHICAL Model for Ethical Decision Making, 14–18
  ethical dilemma, 18–22
  NI, 12–13
  in nursing education, 7–11
  serious game, 8–10
  technology trends, 4–7
Virtual Pain Manager, serious game, 8
virtual patient (VP), 11, 59, 252, 253
  assessment of, 63–64
virtual patient nursing activity model (vpNAM), 253
virtual reality (VR), 5, 6
  advantage to, 160
virtual simulation, 8, 60, 88, 101
  administrators, 248, 252, 253, 256, 263
  faculty in, 89–90 (*see also* faculty)
  for multiprofessional education, 66
  rigor of (*see* rigor of virtual simulation)
  and serious games, 128
  virtual technology integration, 75–76
  and VWP, 88
virtual simulation–mediated learning
  authentic assignments, 216–218
  cultural diversity, 218–220
  and FAST SIM©, 212
  mentoring, 212–215
  nursing education practicum, 211–212
  in SL, 212–214
  3D VLEs, 212, 214
virtual technology and mediated learning, 251–252
virtual technology integration
  accessibility and VPs, 63–64
  administrators, 72–73
  clinical experiences, 61–62
  clinical practicum hours, 60–61
  faculty, 72
  and FAST SIM©, 60, 71–72
  proficiency, 64
  remote collaboration and IPE, 65–67
  standardized feedback, 63
  students, 73–74
  technology, 74–75
  virtual simulation, 75–76
virtual world field trips (VWFTs), 214
virtual world practicum (VWP), 87
  and FAST SIM©, 88
  SL in, 88–89
  virtual simulation and, 88
virtual world practicum project development, 94–96
virtual worlds, 8, 45, 47
VLE. *See* virtual learning environment
VLL. *See* Virtual Learning Laboratory
volunteer, interprofessional, 226
vpNAM. *See* virtual patient nursing activity model

VP. *See* virtual patient
VR. *See* virtual reality
VWFTs. *See* virtual world field trips
VWP. *See* virtual world practicum

Ware Aurora toolset, serious game, 9
wearables, 6

web-based synchronous instruction, 35
web-based training courses, 36
Wi-Fi, 84
wireless infrastructure, 6
wisdom, 13

Zero Hour: America's Medic, serious game, 9

Made in the USA
Monee, IL
03 May 2026